Principles of Radiological Physics

For Churchill Livingstone

Editorial Director (Nursing and Allied Health): Mary Law
Project Manager: Valerie Burgess
Project Editor: Dinah Thom
Copy Editor: Sue Beasley
Sales Promotion Executive: Maria O'Connor

Principles of Radiological Physics

Donald T. Graham MEd TDCR

Director, Department of Radiography Education,
School of Health Sciences, Robert Gordon University, Aberdeen

THIRD EDITION

CHURCHILL
LIVINGSTONE

NEW YORK EDINBURGH LONDON MADRID MELBOURNE SAN FRANCISCO AND TOKYO 1996

CHURCHILL LIVINGSTONE
An imprint of Harcourt Publishers Limited

 is a registered trademark of Harcourt Publishers Limited

First Edition 1981
Second Edition 1987
Third Edition 1996
  Reprinted 1999

ISBN 0 443 04816 9

British Library of Cataloguing in Publication Data
A catalogue record for this book is available from the British Library.

Library of Congress Cataloging in Publication Data
A catalogue record for this book is available from the Library of Congress.

The
publisher's
policy is to use
**paper manufactured
from sustainable forests**

Printed in China
NPCC/02

Contents

Preface

In his preface to the first edition, Robin Wilks stated that *Principles of Radiological Physics* had been intended primarily for the student, although he hoped that teachers and others involved in the education of students might find it useful.

Within the last few years the education of student radiographers in Britain has altered significantly. Since the last edition of the book was published in 1987, radiography has changed from a profession with a national diploma qualification—the Diploma of the College of Radiographers (DCR)—to an all graduate entry to the profession. As well as changes in education, there have been equally significant advances in the use of technology in diagnostic imaging departments, resulting in the inclusion of new topics in radiography courses and the exclusion of other topics which have become less important. The new edition of *Principles of Radiological Physics* attempts to encompass both the changes in student education and the changes in technology.

In this edition the text has been extensively rewritten while the main structure of previous editions has been maintained. At the start of each chapter there is a contents list and the 'aim' of the chapter is delineated. This provides the student with a brief introduction to the chapter and enables easier access of information. At the end of each chapter, there is a summary, a self-test and a list of suggested further reading. As in previous editions 'insights' are used either to deal with topics at greater depth or to consider the relevance of the topics to radiographic practice. Throughout the textbook there is an emphasis on enabling readers to *understand* the basic principles which govern the operation of diagnostic imaging equipment so that they can optimise their ability to use it.

The chapters dealing with radiation protection have been updated to cover new legislation, and appendices have been added which include the basic principles of nuclear medicines CAT scanning, magnetic resonance imaging, digital imaging and ultrasound imaging. All of the above now play an increasingly important role in diagnostic imaging.

In editing a major textbook on radiological physics I have been dependent on the help and encouragement of many friends and colleagues. Firstly, I would like to thank Mary Law and Dinah Thom at Churchill

Livingstone for their encouragement throughout the project, and Sue Beasley for reading the script and making many useful comments and suggestions. Amongst my friends and colleagues I would especially like to thank Christine Gunn for reading the script of each chapter and suggesting a number of changes. The final form of the book has been much improved as a result of her helpful suggestions. Finally, I would like to thank my wife, Winifred, for her help and support throughout the project—without this support, re-editing this book would not have been such an enjoyable experience.

The study of physics is essential in helping us to understand how machines operate and thus enabling us to produce high quality images at minimum radiation dose to our patients and ourselves. If this textbook furthers this understanding, then I have succeeded in my task.

Aberdeen 1996   D.T.G.

Author and publisher's disclaimer

Please note that whilst every effort has been made to be accurate, the author and publisher disclaim any responsibility for any inaccuracies which remain or for any newer information which supersedes any part of this book, particularly in relation to the impact of legislation on radiation protection procedures and safety levels.

PART 1

Radiography and mathematics

PART CONTENTS

Principles of radiography

1.1 AIM

The aim of this chapter is to consider the basic principles of diagnostic radiography, therapy radiography and radiation protection. This should allow the reader to appreciate how the individual chapters within the text form part of a whole study.

1.2 DIAGNOSTIC AND THERAPY RADIOGRAPHY

X-rays (and other forms of radiation) can have two main uses in medicine. They can be used to investigate the patient's illness or physical state—this forms *diagnostic radiography*; or they can be used to produce cell changes in certain body tissues—this is the basis of *therapy radiography*.

1.2.1 Diagnostic radiography

In diagnostic radiography an image of a structure within the patient's body is produced on a film or a television monitor. Normally, of course, we cannot see inside each other's bodies because light photons, to which our eyes are sensitive, are absorbed and reflected very close to the surface of body tissues.

Insight
To examine internal body structures using light, an instrument called an endoscope must be inserted into the body. This consists of fibre-optic bundles which transmit the light to and from the region of interest and so allow the operator to view the organ. Such techniques are used in 'keyhole surgery'. This type of imaging does carry some risk, or it may be uncomfortable for the patient, and so radiography will often be considered as an alternative.

Light is a form of *electromagnetic radiation* (see Ch. 25) and it seems logical to suggest that, if we can take photons of electromagnetic radiation which have higher energies than light photons, then these may have sufficient energy to penetrate body tissues and allow us to visualise internal organs. *X-rays* are in this part of the electromagnetic spectrum and so will penetrate body tissues and allow us to image internal organs. The retina of the eye, unfortunately, cannot detect X-rays and so we cannot see an image of an organ just by shining an X-ray beam on it. This means that the X-rays which have passed through the body must be made to strike an imaging device which will produce a visible image, e.g. a piece of film.

Figure 1.1 shows the basic requirements for the formation of a radiographic image. The X-rays are produced in the X-ray tube by accelerating

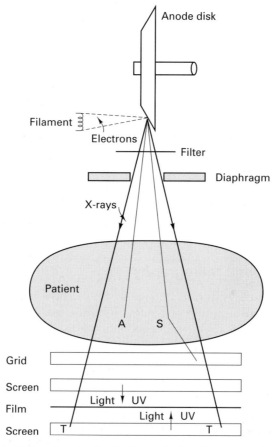

Figure 1.1   Principal interactions involved in the production of a radiographic image. A represents absorbed photons, S represents scattered photons and T represents transmitted photons.

electrons and causing these to collide with an anode. To understand how this works we need to know about *energy* (see Ch. 6) and *electricity* (see Chs 10 and 14) as well as the construction of the *X-ray generator* (see Chs 17 and 20) and the *X-ray tube* (see Ch. 22). The X-rays so produced are over a wide band of energies. Most of the photons which have insufficient energy to be of diagnostic value are removed from the beam using *filtration* (see Ch. 29) and the area of the patient irradiated is restricted using a *diaphragm* (see Ch. 22).

The beam now interacts with the patient and a number of things may happen to the X-ray photons. These may be:

- *transmitted* (*T* in Fig. 1.1). These photons pass through the patient without interacting with the patient's tissues. They are thus unaffected by their passage through the patient.
- *absorbed* (see *A* in Fig. 1.1). These photons interact with the patient's tissues and as a result lose all of their energy. As the photon consists only of energy, then these photons disappear from the spectrum of radiation transmitted through the patient.
- *scattered* (*S* in Fig. 1.1). These photons interact with the patient's tissues and are then deflected from their original path. Such a deflection may or may not result in a loss of some of the photons' energy.

Different materials absorb different amounts of radiation (see Ch. 30) and so a differentiated radiation pattern leaves the patient. The scattered radiation is not helpful to the image, so when the scatter production is significant, as much as possible of this is removed using a *secondary radiation grid* (see Ch. 32). Finally, the radiation strikes screens which are made of a material which will *fluoresce* (see Ch. 31), and the light from this is made to strike a film to create a *radiographic image* (see Ch. 32).

1.2.2 Therapy radiography

In therapy radiography, we are not trying to produce images but are using the *biological effects* of radiation to kill tumour cells. At the same time, we try to cause as little damage as possible to the healthy cells in the body.

Insight

There are four main methods of cancer treatment: surgery, chemotherapy, alteration of the hormone balance and radiotherapy. They may be used in isolation or together to give the optimum treatment regime for a given cancer in a given patient. The treatment may be *radical* or *palliative*. The former is an all out effort to achieve a cure and the latter is used to relieve pain and other distressing symptoms when no cure for the disease is possible. This is normally in the terminal stages of the disease.

The relative success of radiotherapy in the management of cancer lies in the fact that malignant cells are more sensitive to radiation than healthy cells in the same organ. The reasons for this will be discussed in Chapter 34. In spite of this, a number of healthy cells are affected by radiation and so must be given time to recover. Thus the radiation dose is delivered as a number of treatments rather than as a single dose. This technique is known as *fractionation* and may mean that a patient has 15–30 treatments over a period of 3–6 weeks.

Methods of radiation treatment

A detailed description of the different methods of radiation treatment is beyond the scope of this introductory chapter and the reader is directed to some of the more specialised texts on the subject. In considering the overview of radiation treatment methods we can, however, identify some distinct types which we will further discuss. These are:

- teletherapy
- brachytherapy
- radionuclide therapy.

Teletherapy. Here an external source of radiation (normally X-rays or gamma-rays) is directed at the tumour. The aim is to give the maximum dose to the tumour and the minimum dose to the healthy tissue. This is often achieved by treating the tumour from a number of fields (see Fig. 1.2). The areas in the patient which receive doses of equal value are joined by lines called *isodose lines*. The shape and the position of these lines may be altered by the use of absorbing wedges and compensators and also by altering the energy of the beam (where this is possible). When the treatment plan has been produced, the positions of the treatment fields on the patient are checked in a *simulator* where the treatment angles can be set up and the fields marked. In areas of the patient around the head and the neck, accurate positioning and immobilisation is achieved by placing this part in a specially prepared clear plastic shell.

Brachytherapy. When we use external radiation beams, the radiation must travel through healthy tissue to reach the tumour. There are some situations where tumours are relatively accessible from the body surface or are in body cavities where sealed *radioactive sources* (see Ch. 27) may be inserted. This technique is known as brachytherapy. The technique can often mean that a large dose can be delivered to the tumour while a much smaller dose strikes the surrounding tissues because of the effects of the Inverse Square Law (see Ch. 3). If the sources were implanted directly by the radiotherapist, the dose to the hands of the operator could be quite large. This is overcome by inserting a number of guides into the correct position and mechanically inserting the sources over the guides for the required treatment. This technique is called *afterloading* and is often used in the treatment of pelvic cancers.

Radionuclide therapy. A third possibility is that the radiation can be delivered to the tissue by allowing the tissue to absorb a certain *radionuclide*

Figure 1.2   Examples of radiotherapy treatment plans.

(see Ch. 27). This is probably best illustrated by considering the treatment of an overactive thyroid gland. The activity of the gland can be reduced by removing part of the gland surgically, or some of its tissue may be destroyed using radiation. To allow the thyroid to produce the required hormones it must absorb iodine. The patient may be given an oral solution of sodium iodide where the iodine is in the form of [131]I. Some of this *isotope* (see Ch. 27) is taken up by the gland and the rest is secreted in the urine.

^{131}I is a *beta particle* emitter (see Ch. 27) and this results in a radiation dose to the thyroid tissue which reduces its metabolic rate to normal. Because of the limited range of the beta particles produced, there is less radiation dose to structures around the thyroid than there would be if we used an external radiation beam. ^{131}I also has a relatively short *half-life* (8 days; see Ch. 27) and so the radiation hazard posed by the patient to others can be minimised.

1.3 RADIATION PROTECTION

All radiation to the cells which make up our bodies carries a risk of damage to those cells. It is also true that some tissues are more sensitive to radiation than others (see Ch. 33). The use of radiation in medicine is of great value to man, but it is the largest single factor which contributes to the *artificial radiation dose* received by the human race. A chart showing the contribution of the various radiation sources is shown in Figure 1.3.

Because of this we have a duty to minimise the dose to our patients and colleagues and so minimise the risk of radiation damage. The radiation dose is composed of *primary radiation* and *secondary radiation*, and so we need to look at the ways in which these are produced and absorbed. This will be considered in Chapters 28 and 30. Because of the known hazards of

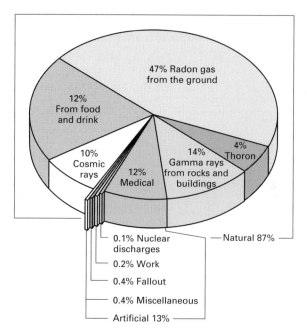

Figure 1.3 Sources of radiation exposure to man. (Data kindly supplied by The National Radiological Protection Board, Oxon.)

radiation, there are certain statutory requirements for *radiation protection* and *monitoring* in diagnostic and therapy departments (see Ch. 33). In terms of assessing the risk it is important to know the dose received both by patients and radiation workers and this will be discussed in Chapter 33 which deals with the topic of *radiation dosimetry*.

Summary

This brief overview should enable the reader to understand certain physical principles which underpin diagnostic radiography and therapy radiography. Patients and staff should be exposed to the minimum risk from the radiation and the principles governing this have been outlined.

FURTHER READING

This overview covers a very large subject area and so only the principal texts are identified. Further reading in specialised topics will be covered in the chapter bibliographies.

Diagnostic radiography
Stockley S M 1986 A manual of radiographic equipment. Churchill Livingstone, Edinburgh
Moores B M, Wall B F et al 1989 Optimisation of image quality and patient exposure in diagnostic imaging. British Institute of Radiology Report 18, London

Therapy radiography
Bomford C K 1993 Walter's and Miller's Textbook of radiotherapy. Churchill Livingstone, Edinburgh
Souhami R, Tobias J 1987 Cancer and its management. Blackwell Scientific Publications, Oxford

Radiation protection
National Radiological Protection Board (NRPB) 1985 Ionising radiation regulations 1985. HMSO, London
National Radiological Protection Board (NRPB) 1988 Guidance notes for the protection of persons against ionising radiations arising from medical or dental use. HMSO, London

2

Geometric radiography

2.1 AIM

The aim of this chapter is to explore the geometry involved in the production of certain radiographic images.

2.2 INTRODUCTION

The very nature of this chapter involves a basic knowledge of mathematics and especially geometry. If this fills you with foreboding, please read Appendix A before proceeding with the rest of the chapter.

Many of the concepts and calculations encountered in radiography are based on the application of geometry and trigonometry to the production of the image. These will be discussed in this chapter. To allow us to apply these to radiography there are some commonly used terms which we require to define:

Definitions

Field Size: This defines the size and the shape of the X-ray beam. As we will see later in this chapter (Sect. 2.4), the field size varies with the distance from the source of the radiation or *focus* of the X-ray tube.
FFD: Focus to Film Distance
FSD: Focus to Skin Distance
FOD: Focus to Object Distance
OFD: Object to Film Distance
FDD: Focus to Diaphragm Distance

The influence of these quantities on the image production will be described in the rest of this chapter.

2.3 EFFECTIVE (APPARENT) AND REAL FOCAL SPOT SIZES

As described in Chapter 22, X-rays are produced when a beam of electrons is accelerated from the cathode to the anode of the X-ray tube. At the anode the electrons are decelerated and their kinetic energy is converted to heat (99.5%) and X-rays (0.5%). The small area of the anode bombarded by the electrons is known as the *focus*. Because of the large amount of heat produced, the focus should occupy as large an area as possible, thus limiting the temperature rise. The size of the focus also affects the image sharpness (see Sect. 2.6) and so, from an imaging point of view, the focus should be as small as possible. These seemingly contradictory requirements are accommodated using the *line focus principle*. This is shown in Figure 2.1. The electron beam from the cathode is represented by AB and this strikes the anode at XZ. The distance XZ is one dimension of the *real focal spot*. The central ray of the X-ray beam is represented by CD. By viewing the focus along this line the *effective focal area* is seen. One dimension of this is represented by the line YZ. The angle between the central ray and the anode, θ, is referred to as the anode angle or target angle.

Consider the triangle XYZ in Figure 2.1. Since the lines XY and CD are parallel, the angle YXZ is also θ.

Also

$$\sin \theta = \frac{YZ}{XZ}$$

By cross-multiplying this can be arranged as:

$$XZ = \frac{YZ}{\sin \theta}$$

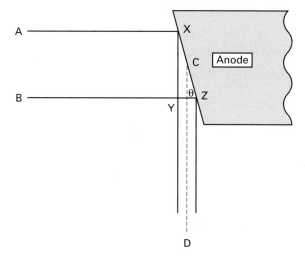

Figure 2.1 Relationships between the real and the effective focal spot sizes. The length AB represents the electron beam, the length XZ the real focal spot and the length YZ the effective focal spot.

$$\text{real focus} = \frac{\text{apparent focus}}{\sin \theta} \qquad \text{Equation 2.1}$$

This means that if the apparent focal spot and the target angle are known for an X-ray tube, the real focal spot can be calculated using the above formula.

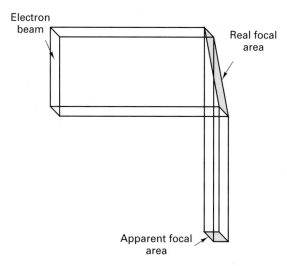

Figure 2.2 Three-dimensional nature of real and apparent (effective) focal spots.

It is important to remember that the focal spot has two dimensions (it has breadth as well as length) as can be seen from Figure 2.2. Because the breadth of the focal spot is at right angles to the electron beam and the central ray, it is not affected by the target angle.

Example

An X-ray tube has an apparent focal spot of 0.6 mm by 0.6 mm and the target angle of this tube is 17°. Calculate the size of the real focal spot.

Using Equation 2.1 we can say that:

$$\text{real focus} = \frac{\text{apparent focus}}{\sin \theta}$$
$$= \frac{0.6}{0.292}$$
$$= 2.05 \text{ mm}$$

As the breadth of the focus is unaffected by the target angle, the dimensions of the real focal spot will be 2.05 mm by 0.6 mm.

As the sine of an angle increases with the angle, it can be seen that the dimensions of the real focal spot (and hence the loading which can be applied to the X-ray tube) increases with smaller target angles. (Try the above calculation using a target angle of 10°.) The significance of this will be discussed in Chapters 22 and 23.

2.4 FIELD SIZE AND FFD

Figure 2.3 shows the divergence (in two dimensions) of the X-ray beam with increasing distance form the focus of the X-ray tube. Using the principles of similar triangles a number of deductions can be made.

Consider the triangles FCD and FAB.

It can be seen that

$$\frac{CD}{FG} = \frac{AB}{FJ}$$

or

$$\frac{S_1}{FFD_1} = \frac{d}{FDD}$$

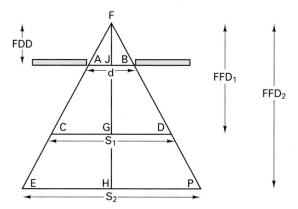

Figure 2.3 Variations of field size with focus to film distance (FFD).

Thus by cross-multiplication:

$$S_1 = \frac{d \times \text{FFD}}{\text{FDD}}$$

Equation 2.2

From this it can be seen that the size of the field for a given X-ray tube with a given focus to diaphragm distance, is related to the size of the diaphragm aperture and the focus to film distance.

Now consider the triangles FCD and FEP.

It can be seen that

$$\frac{CD}{FG} = \frac{EP}{FH}$$

or

$$\frac{S_1}{\text{FFD}_1} = \frac{S_2}{\text{FFD}_2}$$

Equation 2.3

From the above it can be seen that, if the diaphragm aperture is left unaltered, the field size is proportional to the focus to film distance.

Many *light beam diaphragms* used in radiography have a scale indicating the size of the field which will be covered at various focus to film distances. Similar techniques are applied in radiotherapy where the treatment field is altered by altering the *applicator size* or the position of the *jaws* on the unit.

Example

An X-ray beam has a field size of 20 cm by 20 cm at an FFD of 100 cm. At what FFD will the field size be 30 cm by 30 cm?

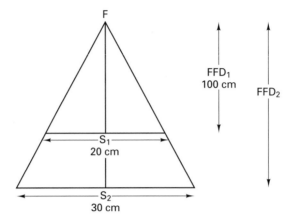

Figure 2.4 Field sizes at given FFDs.

It may be helpful to draw the triangles so that you can visualise the situation (see Fig. 2.4).
Using Equation 2.3:

$$\frac{S_1}{FFD_1} = \frac{S_2}{FFD_2}$$

By cross-multiplication:

$$FFD_2 = \frac{S_2 \times FFD_1}{S_1}$$
$$FFD_2 = \frac{30 \times 100}{20} \text{ cm}$$
$$= 150 \text{ cm}$$

(*Useful check:* The field size has increased by 50% (i.e. from 20 cm to 30 cm) so the FFD, which is directly proportional, must also have increased by 50% (i.e. from 100 cm to 150 cm).)

2.5 IMAGE MAGNIFICATION

Figure 2.5 represents the geometry of an imaging situation either in diagnostic radiography or on a radiotherapy simulator. AB is an object within the patient (e.g. a piece of bone) and CD is the radiographic image of that object. BD is the object to film distance (OFD) and FD is the focus to film distance (FFD).

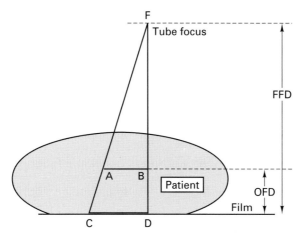

Figure 2.5   Magnification of the radiographic image. AB is an object within the patient and CD is the image of this object.

Obviously CD is greater than AB and so we can say that the image of the object will be magnified. There are occasions in radiography where it is necessary to measure the size of a structure and so the degree of magnification must be calculated.

Consider the triangles FAB and FCD:

$$\text{magnification} = \frac{\text{size of the image}}{\text{size of the object}}$$

$$= \frac{CD}{AB}$$

$$= \frac{FD}{FB}$$

$$= \frac{FFD}{(FFD - OFD)}$$

$$\text{magnification} = \frac{FFD}{(FFD - OFD)} \qquad \text{Equation 2.4}$$

Note that the magnification factor does not depend on the position of the object related to the central ray but only on the FFD and OFD. To limit the degree of magnification there are two possibilities:

● The patient should be positioned so that the object of interest is as close to the film as possible.
● If it is impossible to position the object close to the film (e.g. in the lateral view of the cervical spine) then the magnification can be limited by increasing the focus to film distance.

Example

Radiography of a child's femur is undertaken using the following exposure factors. The focus to film distance is 100 cm and the object to film distance is 6 cm. The length of the radiographic image of the femur is 25 cm. Calculate the true length of the femur.

Using Equation 2.4 the magnification can be stated as:

$$\text{magnification} = \frac{\text{FFD}}{(\text{FFD} - \text{OFD})}$$
$$= \frac{100}{(100 - 6)}$$
$$= 1.064$$

(Note that magnification has no units.)

$$\text{size of the object} = \frac{\text{size of the image}}{\text{magnification}}$$
$$= \frac{25}{1.064} \text{ cm}$$
$$= 23.49 \text{ cm}$$

2.6 GEOMETRIC UNSHARPNESS (PENUMBRA)

The focal spot in the X-ray tube is a finite size. Figure 2.6 represents the situation which exists because of this. (Note that the focal spot used for the calculation of image distortion is the apparent focal spot.)

AB represents the focus, CD the object and FG the image of the object. At either end of this image there is *penumbra* or *geometric unsharpness*

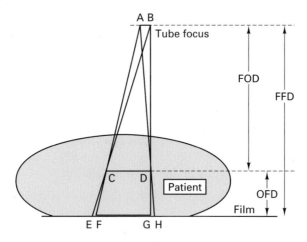

Figure 2.6 Geometry of penumbra or geometric unsharpness. AB is the effective focal spot, CD is the object, FG is the image and EF and GH represent the penumbra.

represented by EF and GH. (For simplicity it is assumed that the X-ray beam is centred to end D of the object.)

Using similar triangles the following can be seen:

$$\frac{GH}{AB} = \frac{GD}{BD}$$
$$= \frac{OFD}{FOD}$$

$$GH = \frac{AB \times OFD}{FOD}$$
$$= \frac{AB \times OFD}{(FFD - OFD)}$$

or

$$\text{penumbra} = \frac{\text{focus} \times OFD}{(FFD - OFD)} \qquad \text{Equation 2.5}$$

A similar situation exists for the value of the penumbra at EF.

In most radiographic imaging situations it is desirable to keep the penumbra as low as possible (or at least below 0.3 mm where it is below the resolution of the eye at normal viewing distances) and so we can deduce from Equation 2.5 that the following methods might accomplish this:

- The apparent focal spot should be as small as possible.
- The object to film distance should be as small as possible.
- The focus to film distance may be increased if the previously identified techniques are impossible.

Note: The unsharpness on a radiograph (Ut) is a combination of three types of unsharpness:

- *geometric unsharpness* (Ug)
- *movement unsharpness* (Um)—this is unsharpness of the image caused by movement of the patient or the imaging equipment
- *photographic unsharpness* (Up)—this type of unsharpness is caused by the film and intensifying screens used to produce the image.

These are linked by the equation:

$$Ut^2 = Ug^2 + Um^2 + Up^2 \qquad \text{Equation 2.6}$$

Care must be taken in considering ways of reducing geometric unsharpness if these have an effect on the other types of unsharpness which contribute to the total unsharpness.

Example

The following conditions exist for a lateral projection of the cervical spine:
FFD = 200 cm; OFD = 20 cm; focal spot size = 1.2 mm. Calculate the size of the
penumbra.

Using Equation 2.5:

$$\text{penumbra} = \frac{\text{focus} \times \text{OFD}}{(\text{FFD} - \text{OFD})}$$

$$= \frac{1.2 \times 200}{(2000 - 200)} \text{ mm}$$

$$= 0.13 \text{ mm}$$

2.7 PENUMBRA FROM DIAPHRAGMS

Figure 2.3 showed us how a movable diaphragm could be used to
delineate the field size of an X-ray beam. This diagram, however, assumes
that the radiation was produced at a point source. The situation for a focus
of finite size is shown in Figure 2.7. Here D_1 and D_2 represent one pair of
leaves of a diaphragm. As an alternative to a diaphragm, detachable cones
may be used but the principle is still the same.

The penumbra, *P*, is the 'shadow' of the edge of the diaphragm or cone
formed because of the finite size of the focal spot. The calculation shows

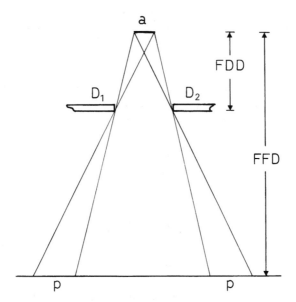

Figure 2.7 Penumbra, *P*, due to the diaphragms.

exactly the same progression as the calculation in the previous section. By substituting the appropriate values in Equation 2.5 then:

$$P = \frac{F \times (FFD - FDD)}{FFD}$$

Equation 2.7

This particular penumbra has very little significance in diagnostic radiography except that it explains why the edges of a long cone (e.g. the type used for imaging of the paranasal sinuses) are more clearly defined than the image of the leaves of a light beam diaphragm. The calculation of the diaphragm penumbra is important in *teletherapy radiation treatment* (see Ch. 1) where it is necessary to know the radiation dose to the whole treatment volume within the patient.

2.8 STRUCTURE LOCALISATION

In the past, a technique using similar triangles was used to locate foreign bodies in tissue to facilitate their surgical removal. This has been largely replaced by alternative techniques using either ultrasound imaging or computed tomography. There is, however, a similar technique that is utilised to accurately locate small impalpable lesions in the breast. These lesions may be found during breast screening but, because they are impalpable, they present practical difficulties in locating them for biopsy or surgical removal.

If the breast is considered as a three-dimensional structure, the position of the lesion, P, can be established in two dimensions using conventional radiography and a localising grid (see Fig. 2.8). This has located the position of the lesion relative to the medial and lateral aspects of the breast and the anterior and posterior aspects of the breast. The final dimension will allow us to locate the depth of the lesion within the breast. Because this is usually done to allow a biopsy guide to be inserted into the breast, the position of the lesion is usually established relative to the focus of the X-ray tube. One method of doing this is described in the following text.

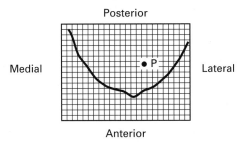

Figure 2.8 Example of breast outline superimposed on a localisation grid. The circular black area, P, represents the position of the lesion on this image.

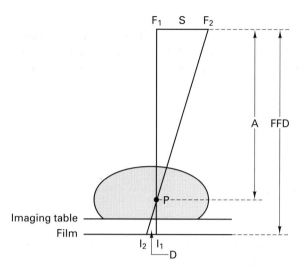

Figure 2.9 Breast lesion localisation. The tube is shifted a distance S from F_1 to F_2 and the image of the lesion P shifts from I_1 to I_2 through a distance D.

Consider the imaging situation shown in Figure 2.9. Two images of the lesion are produced on the film, the first with the tube in position F_1 and the second with the tube moved a known distance, S, to position F_2. These produce images I_1 and I_2 on the film. The distance, D, can also be measured on the film. Using similar triangles:

$$\frac{I_1 I_2}{F_1 F_2} = \frac{(FFD - A)}{A}$$

$$\frac{D}{S} = \frac{(FFD - A)}{A}$$

$$D \times A = S(FFD - A)$$
$$= S \times FFD - S \times A$$
$$D \times A + S \times A = S \times FFD$$
$$A(D + S) = S \times FFD$$

$$A = \frac{S \times FFD}{(D + S)}$$

Equation 2.8

This gives the distance between the focus of the tube and the lesion. Thus we now have the three coordinates necessary to define the position of the lesion relative to the tube focus and so a biopsy guide may be attached to the tube, the necessary coordinates set, and a needle inserted to localise or biopsy the lesion.

Example

The following exposure conditions are used to localise a small lesion in a breast: focus to film distance 75 cm; tube shift 20 cm. The images of the lesion showed an image distance shift of 1.2 cm. Calculate the depth of the lesion below the tube focus.

Using Equation 2.8:

$$A = \frac{S \times FFD}{(D + S)}$$
$$= \frac{20 \times 75}{1.2 + 20} \ cm$$
$$= 70.75 \ cm$$

Thus the distance of the lesion from the focus of the X-ray tube has been established as 70.75 cm.

2.9 TOMOGRAPHY

Tomography is a technique used to produce sharp images of a plane or section within the patient. This allows the clinician to identify the anatomy of this section of tissue without the distraction of superimposed shadows; for example, if the clinician is only interested in the renal areas, the shadows cast by the bowel in the abdominal radiograph may make these more difficult to visualise.

Tomography may be performed using a variety of techniques, many of which are outwith the scope of this text. For the purpose of this discussion about the geometry of image production, only linear tomography will be considered.

2.9.1 Principles of linear tomography

In linear tomography the X-ray tube and the film holder are linked by a rod mechanism. During the exposure the tube moves in one direction and the film holder moves in the opposite direction. This movement is around a fulcrum. The height of the fulcrum and the angle through which the tube moves during the exposure can be adjusted by the radiographer. We will now consider the effect of each of these adjustments.

2.9.2 Fulcrum height adjustment

Figure 2.10 shows the imaging situation in linear tomography. Points A, F and B are within the patient, with the point F being on the plane of the

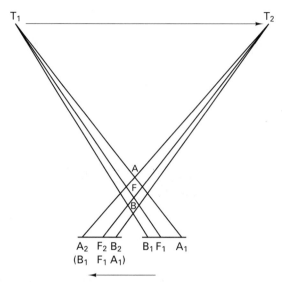

Figure 2.10 Images produced in linear tomography for a tube movement from position T_1 to position T_2. See text for further explanation of the diagram.

fulcrum. During the exposure the tube moves from position T_1 to T_2 and the film holder moves in the opposite direction from position 1 to position 2. The projection of the points A, F and B on the film produces images A_1, F_1 and B_1 when the tube is in position T_1 and A_2, F_2 and B_2 when the tube is in position T_2. From the diagram it can be seen that the projection of point F moves with the same velocity as the film and so F_1 and F_2 are super-imposed and will appear sharp on the radiograph. The projection of point A moves at a higher velocity than the film and so A_1 and A_2 are not superimposed and will appear unsharp. Similarly, the projection of point B moves at a lower velocity than the film and so will also appear unsharp. Thus we can conclude that:

The images of points on the plane of the fulcrum will be sharp on the radiograph, whereas the images of points above and below this plane will be unsharp.

By raising or lowering the fulcrum height, the radiographer can control the level of the layer within the patient which produces sharp images on each radiograph.

2.9.3 Tomographic angle adjustment

The eye is not a perfect optical instrument and so will tolerate a certain amount of movement unsharpness around a point. Consider the situation in Figure 2.11. If the eye will tolerate a movement unsharpness of X around the point F_1, then the projection of any point within the layer A and B will

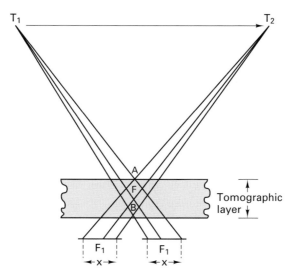

Figure 2.11 Tomographic layer thickness for a large tomographic angle. X represents the unsharpness tolerance of the eye when the image is viewed.

be accepted as sharp. Thus the tomographic layer has a finite depth, with the fulcrum being at the centre of this layer.

Now consider the situation where the tube moves through a smaller tomographic angle during the exposure. This situation is shown in Figure 2.12. If we accept that the tolerance of the eye is still a distance X around the point F_1, then we can see that the thickness of the tomographic layer is increased. Thus we can establish the relationship between layer thickness and tomographic angle namely:

The thickness of the tomographic layer can be increased by reducing the tomographic angle and can be reduced by increasing the tomographic angle.

Calculation of the exact thickness of the tomographic layer is a somewhat complex exercise as this also varies with the height of the fulcrum (the higher the fulcrum the thinner the layer) and the focal spot selected (the broader the focus the thinner the layer). This is beyond the scope of this introductory chapter. Students should refer to the manufacturers' literature for various tomographic units to note the layer thickness produced at different tomographic angles.

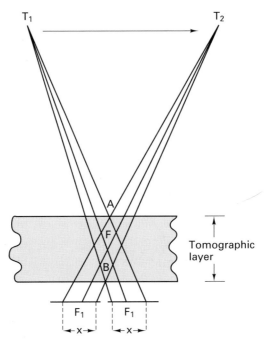

Figure 2.12 Tomographic layer thickness for a small tomographic angle. X represents the unsharpness tolerance of the eye when the image is viewed.

Example

Draw an imaging situation similar to the one shown in Figure 2.12. Now, allowing the same tolerance for movement unsharpness and the same tomographic angle, repeat the drawing with the fulcrum set at twice the height in the original drawing. Verify that the tomographic layer within the patient is thinner.

Summary

In this chapter you should have learnt:

- The relationship between the apparent and real focal spot sizes (see Sect. 2.3)
- The relationship between the field size and the focus to film distance (see Sect. 2.4)
- The factors which affect image magnification (see Sect. 2.5)
- The factors which affect geometric unsharpness and how to minimise this form of unsharpness in the radiographic image (see Sect. 2.6)
- How to localise a structure using similar triangles (see Sect. 2.7)
- The factors which affect the height and thickness of the tomographic layer (see Sect. 2.8).

SELF-TEST

$$RF = \frac{AF}{Sin\theta}$$

a. An X-ray tube used in a skull unit has a target angle of 10°. The apparent focal spots available on this tube are 0.6 × 0.6 mm (fine focus) and 1.2 × 1.2 mm (broad focus). Calculate the size of the real focal spots.

b. What are the dimensions of a diaphragm placed at a distance of 10 cm from the focal spot which will allow a field of 25 × 30 cm to be covered at a focus to film distance of 1 metre?

$$S_1 = \frac{FFD \times d}{FDD} \qquad \frac{si}{FFD} = \frac{S_2}{FFD}$$

c. A lateral radiograph of a patient's spine was taken at a focus to film distance of 1 metre. The distance between the spine and the film was 15 cm. On the resultant radiograph the height of a particular intervertebral disc was measured as 1.2 cm. Calculate the true height of the disc.

$$M = \frac{FFD}{FFD - OFD} \qquad M = \frac{O}{I}$$

d. If the effective focal spot size is 0.5 mm and an object is 8 cm from the film, what would be the size of the penumbra if the focus to film distance was:
(i) 1 metre
(ii) 2 metres?

$$P = \frac{focus \times OFD}{FFD - OFD} \qquad \frac{focus \times (FFD - FDD)}{FFD}$$

e. The following exposure conditions were used to localise the depth of a small breast lesion: focus to film distance = 75 cm; tube shift = 30 cm.
   The images of the lesion showed a shift of 1.6 cm between the two images. Calculate the depth of the lesion below the tube focus.

$$A = \frac{S \times FFD}{D + S}$$

f. With respect to linear tomography:
(i) Why are the images of points on the plane of the fulcrum sharp on the radiograph whereas images of points above and below this plane are unsharp?
(ii) What is the relationship, at a given fulcrum height, between the tomographic angle and the tomographic layer thickness?

FURTHER READING

Effective and real focal spots
Further information on this topic is available in Chapter 22 of this text. The following may also prove useful:

Foster E 1985 Equipment for diagnostic radiography. MTP Press, Lancaster, ch 5
Hendee W, Ritenour R 1992 Medical imaging physics, 3rd edn. Mosby Year Book, London, ch 5
Hill D R (ed) 1975 Principles of diagnostic X-ray apparatus. Macmillan Press, London, ch 8
Stockley S M 1986 A manual of radiographic equipment. Churchill Livingstone, Edinburgh, ch 6
Webb S (ed) 1988 The physics of medical imaging. Institute of Physics Publishing, Bristol, ch 2, sect. 2.5
Van Der Plats G J 1980 Medical X-ray techniques in diagnostic radiology. Macmillan Press, London, ch 1

Field size and FFD
Stockley S M 1986 A manual of radiographic equipment. Churchill Livingstone, Edinburgh, ch 8

Image magnification
Hendee W, Ritenour R 1992 Medical imaging physics, 3rd edn. Mosby Year Book, London, ch 15
Van Der Plats G J 1980 Medical X-ray techniques in diagnostic radiology. Macmillan Press, London, ch 5

Object localisation
Detailed description of this technique can be found in the manufacturer's literature for a mammography unit which has a localisation or biopsy attachment.

Tomography
Foster E 1985 Equipment for diagnostic radiography. MTP Press, Lancaster, ch 10
Hendee W, Ritenour R 1992 Medical imaging physics, 3rd edn. Mosby Year Book, London, ch 16, sect. 16.8
Hill D R (ed) 1975 Principles of diagnostic X-ray apparatus. Macmillan Press, London, ch 17
Stockley S M 1986 A manual of radiographic equipment. Churchill Livingstone, Edinburgh, ch 16
Van Der Plats G J 1980 Medical X-ray techniques in diagnostic radiology. Macmillan Press, London, ch 16

3

The Inverse Square Law

3.1 AIM

The aim of this chapter is to introduce the reader to the Inverse Square Law and to explore its applications in radiography and radiation protection.

3.2 INTENSITY OF RADIATION

To understand the Inverse Square Law we must first understand what is meant by the term *intensity*.

As we will see in Chapter 25, electromagnetic radiation is composed of quanta, each of which has an energy. If we draw a square of unit area at right angles to the path of a uniform beam of electromagnetic radiation (such as X-rays), then the total energy per second from all the quanta passing through the square is defined as the *intensity* of the beam, so that:

> **Definition**
>
> The *intensity* of a beam of electromagnetic radiation at a point is the total energy per second flowing past that point when normalised to a unit area.

It is not necessary at this stage to understand the units of energy or exposure to allow us to apply the Inverse Square Law; these will be dealt with in later chapters.

3.3 STATEMENT OF THE INVERSE SQUARE LAW

The intensity of the radiation emitted from a small isotropic source is inversely proportional to the square of the distance from the source, provided there is negligible absorption or scattering of the radiation by the medium through which it passes.

Note that this statement of the Inverse Square Law also gives the conditions under which the law may be directly applied:

- *small source*—in practice this means small compared to the distance from the source to the point of measurement.
- *isotropic source*—this means that it emits radiation in all directions. This is necessary in order that the intensity of the radiation is independent of the *direction* from the source.
- *no absorption or scattering of radiation*—this ensures that the radiation passing through an area is not affected by the medium through which the radiation passes. It is important to remember that back-scattering of the beam from objects beyond the point of measurement must also be eliminated as this would produce an increase in the intensity.

As we will see, it is not possible to meet all of these conditions in many situations in radiography. In such cases the law must be applied with caution or even with appropriate correction factors (e.g. absorption due to air may be important when we consider low-energy beams of X-rays).

Insight
A situation where the Inverse Square Law does not apply is in the case of a laser beam. This is because the light is essentially parallel, so the intensity is constant and does not depend on distance from the source.

3.4 MATHEMATICAL PROOFS OF THE INVERSE SQUARE LAW

3.4.1 Concentric spheres proof

Consider a small isotropic source (S) at the centre of two concentric spheres A and B of radii X and Y (Fig. 3.1). The total energy per second passing through the surface of sphere B is the same as that passing through the surface of sphere A (in the absence of absorption or scatter). Let this be E units.

As we identified in Section 3.2 the intensity is the total energy passing through unit area per second.

Let the intensity at the surface of sphere A be I_x and the intensity at the surface of sphere B be I_y.

Then

$$I_x = \frac{E}{4\pi X^2}$$

and

$$I_y = \frac{E}{4\pi Y^2}$$

(remember that the surface area of a sphere is $4\pi r^2$)

Thus

$$\frac{I_x}{I_y} = \frac{E \times 4\pi Y^2}{E \times 4\pi X^2}$$

or

$$\frac{I_x}{I_y} = \frac{Y^2}{X^2} \qquad\qquad \text{Equation 3.1}$$

This is the mathematical statement of the Inverse Square Law.

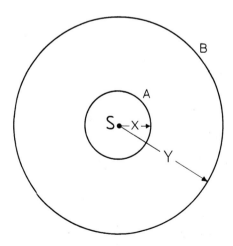

Figure 3.1   Concentric spheres with centre S and radii X and Y.

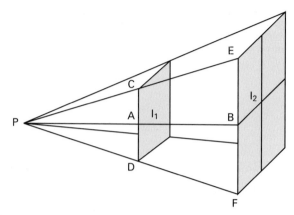

Figure 3.2 Similar triangles proof of the Inverse Square Law. Note that the radiation at I_2 is spread over four times the area of I_1 and so the intensity at I_2 is one-quarter of the intensity at I_1.

3.4.2 Similar triangles proof

It is sometimes easier for radiographers to use the similar triangles proof of the Inverse Square Law as this relates more closely to the geometry considered for image production.

Consider the situation shown in Figure 3.2. The radiation is produced at a point P and is allowed to fall on the square of side CD and the square of side EF.

PB is twice the length of PA.

From our consideration of similar triangles in the previous chapter, we can say that EF must therefore be twice the length of CD.

Thus the area of the square of side EF is four times the area of the square of side CD.

Remembering that the intensity is the total energy per unit time divided by the area we can calculate that I_1 must be four times the value of I_2.

Thus by doubling the distance between the point and the source of radiation we can see that the intensity of the radiation is reduced to one-quarter.

Stated mathematically this is:

$$\frac{I_1}{I_2} = \frac{d_2^{\,2}}{d_1^{\,2}} \qquad\qquad \text{Equation 3.2}$$

Using the relationship established above we can produce a table of intensities at given distances (see Table 3.1).

Table 3.1 Relationships between *distance* and *intensity*

Distance	Area	Intensity	1/(distance)^2
X	1	I_x	$1/X^2$
$2X$	4	$I_x/4$	$1/4X^2$
$3X$	9	$I_x/9$	$1/9X^2$
$4X$	16	$I_x/16$	$1/16X^2$
$5X$	25	$I_x/25$	$1/25X^2$
$10X$	100	$I_x/100$	$1/100X^2$

3.5 THE INVERSE SQUARE LAW AND THE X-RAY BEAM

If we consider the three conditions listed earlier for the Inverse Square Law to be applied we can see that, strictly speaking, the X-ray beam does not satisfy these conditions because:

- X-rays are not emitted from a true point source (see Sect. 2.3) as the focal spot has a finite size
- they are not emitted equally in all directions as the anode heel effect (see Ch. 22) causes the intensity to vary across the beam
- absorption and scattering of the X-ray beam (see Ch. 30) occur as it passes through air.

These effects are, however, small for X-ray beams generated above 50 kV$_p$, so the Inverse Square Law may be applied to such beams.

Examples

a. The absorbed dose rate in air at a distance of 60 cm from the focal spot of an X-ray tube is 0.5 mGy·s^{-1} (do not worry about the unit as this does not affect the calculation!). What is the absorbed dose rate at 75 cm from the focus?

Using Equation 3.2 we can say that:

$$\frac{I_1}{I_2} = \frac{d_2{}^2}{d_1{}^2}$$

where $I_1 = 0.5$ mGy·s^{-1}, $d_1 = 60$ cm and $d_2 = 75$ cm. I_2 is what we need to calculate.

The equation can be rearranged thus:

$$I_2 = \frac{I_1 \times d_1{}^2}{d_2{}^2}$$

(If you are unable to follow this, look at the section on cross-multiplication in Appendix A.)

$$= \frac{0.5 \times (60)^2}{(75)^2} \text{ mGy·s}^{-1}$$
$$= 0.32 \text{ mGy·s}^{-1}$$

Thus the absorbed dose rate at 75 cm will be 0.32 mGy·s^{-1}.

b. In the above example, at what distance would the exposure rate be 2.0 mGy·s^{-1}?

Again we start with Equation 3.2:

$$\frac{I_1}{I_2} = \frac{d_2{}^2}{d_1{}^2}$$

where I_1 = 0.5 mGy·s^{-1}, d_1 = 60 cm and I_2 = 2.0 mGy·s^{-1}. This time d_2 is unknown. We can arrange the equation in terms of d_2 thus:

$$d_2{}^2 = \frac{I_1 \times d_1{}^2}{I_2}$$
$$= \frac{0.5 \times (60)^2}{2.0}$$
$$= \frac{(60)^2}{4}$$
$$d_2 = \sqrt{\frac{(60)^2}{4}} \text{ cm}$$
$$= 30 \text{ cm}$$

Thus the absorbed dose rate will be 2.0 mGy·s^{-1} at a distance of 30 cm from the tube focus. (*Note:* By the Inverse Square Law, if we halve the distance the intensity will increase by a factor of four, so the calculation is correct.)

3.6 mAs AND THE INVERSE SQUARE LAW

In radiography, if the kV$_\text{p}$ is unaltered, the radiation output from the tube is altered by altering the mAs (defined in Table 6.3)—if the mAs is doubled, then the output will be doubled. We can see how this is affected by the Inverse Square Law from the discussion below.

Suppose a given setting of mAs produces a satisfactory radiograph at a given FFD; how will this setting of mAs have to be altered for a different value of FFD?

Consider the situation shown in Figure 3.3. If a radiograph was taken using an FFD of PA and the image produced was satisfactory, then this means that the film received the correct amount of radiation. If the film was repositioned for an FFD of PB and the exposure factors remained

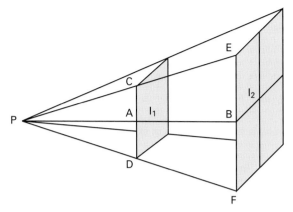

Figure 3.3   Radiographs taken at different FFDs. If we wish to get the same intensity of radiation on both radiographs then the mAs for PB must be four times the mAs required for PA.

unaltered, then the amount of radiation received by the film would be one-quarter of the correct exposure (the distance has been doubled and so the intensity is quartered). This second radiograph would be too light or *underexposed*. In order that the film at B receives the same exposure as the original film at A, the amount of radiation leaving the tube must be increased by a factor of four. This means that both these radiographs would have the same *optical density* or blackening.

From the above we can see that:

The mAs required to produce radiographs of the same density at different FFDs is proportional to the FFD squared.

This can be expressed mathematically as:

$$\frac{mAs_1}{mAs_2} = \frac{FFD_1{}^2}{FFD_2{}^2}$$

Equation 3.3

It is important to form a mental picture of the difference between the straightforward measurement of the intensity of the radiation at a point where the amount of radiation leaving the source is constant (this involves applying the Inverse Square Law) and this second case where the amount of radiation at a point is kept constant by altering the output from the X-ray tube (this involves using Equation 3.3).

Example

A chest radiograph was produced at an FFD of 2 metres and required the following exposure factors: 65 kV_p and 16 mAs. If this radiograph is to be repeated at an FFD of 1 metre at the same kV_p, what mAs will be required?

Using Equation 3.3 we can say that:

$$\frac{mAs_1}{mAs_2} = \frac{FFD_1^2}{FFD_2^2}$$

where $mAs_1 = 16$ mAs, $FFD_1 = 2$ metres and $FFD_2 = 1$ metre. mAs_2 is unknown.

The equation can be arranged in terms of mAs_2 thus:

$$
\begin{aligned}
mAs_2 &= \frac{mAs_1 \times FFD_2^2}{FFD_1^2} \\
&= \frac{16 \times (1)^2}{(2)^2} \, mAs \\
&= 4 \, mAs
\end{aligned}
$$

Note: By the Inverse Square Law, if we halve the distance then we will have four times the intensity. If we want to have the same intensity to the film then we need one-quarter of the original mAs. So the answer is correct.

The influence of the FFD on the mAs required can be seen by comparing the radiographs of a wrist phantom in Figure 3.4. Radiograph (a) was exposed at an FFD of 100 cm and was given an exposure of 16 mAs. Radiograph (b) was exposed at an FFD of 200 cm and was given an exposure of 16 mAs. Radiograph (c) was exposed at an FFD of 200 cm and was given an exposure of 32 mAs. Radiograph (d) was exposed at 200 cm and was given an exposure of 64 mAs. Note that radiographs (a) and (d) have the same optical densities.

Summary

In this chapter you should have learnt:

- The definition of radiation intensity (see Sect. 3.2)
- The Inverse Square Law and its use in calculating the intensity of radiation at a given distance form a source (see Sects 3.3, 3.4 and 3.5)
- How the mAs given for a radiograph is influenced by the FFD used because of the Inverse Square Law (see Sect. 3.6).

(a)

(b)

Figure 3.4a,b The effect of mAs and Inverse Square Law on the radiographic image: (a) FFD 100 cm and exposure of 16 mAs; (b) FFD 200 cm and exposure of 16 mAs.

(c)

(d)

Figure 3.4c,d The effect of mAs and Inverse Square Law on the radiographic image: (c) FFD 200 cm and exposure of 32 mAs; (d) FFD 200 cm and exposure of 64 mAs. Note the fact that images (a) and (d) have the same optical density.

SELF-TEST

a. What is meant by the *intensity* of electromagnetic radiation?

b. State the Inverse Square Law as applied to a beam of electromagnetic radiation.

c. The absorbed dose rate in air at a distance of 100 cm from the target of an X-ray tube is 1.8 mGy·s^{-1}.
   (i) What will be the absorbed dose rate in air at a distance of 150 cm?
   (ii) At what distance from the focus will the absorbed dose rate in air be 0.2 mGy·s^{-1}?

d. A radiograph of a lateral cervical spine required an exposure of 65 kV$_p$ and 24 mAs at an FFD of 200 cm. A repeat radiograph was later required but this time the distance was restricted to 100 cm. If all other factors remained unchanged, calculate the new mAs required to produce the same density on the radiograph.

FURTHER READING

Intensity of radiation
Ball J L, Moore A D 1986 Essential physics for radiographers, 2nd edn. Blackwell Scientific Publications, London, ch 15
Hay G A, Hughes D 1983 First year physics for radiographers. Baillière Tindall, London, ch 10

Inverse Square Law
Ball J L, Moore A D 1986 Essential physics for radiographers, 2nd edn. Blackwell Scientific Publications, London, ch 14
Hay G A, Hughes D 1983 First year physics for radiographers. Baillière Tindall, London, ch 9
Van Der Plats G J 1980 Medical X-ray techniques in diagnostic radiology. Macmillan Press, London, ch 4

mAs and the Inverse Square Law
Ball J, Price T 1989 Chesneys' Radiographic imaging. Blackwell Scientific Publications, London, ch 12
Jenkins D 1980 Radiographic photography and imaging processes. MTP Press, Lancaster, ch 7

4

The Exponential Law

4.1 AIM

The aim of this chapter is to introduce the Exponential Law and consider its applications to radiographic science. The law is fundamental to an understanding of radioactive decay and the attenuation of certain electromagnetic radiations (e.g. X-rays and gamma-rays).

4.2 DESCRIPTION OF THE EXPONENTIAL LAW

Perhaps the best everyday example of the Exponential Law concerns money. If £100 is invested with a financial institution which gives a fixed interest rate of 5% per annum then the growth of that money over a 25-year period is shown in Table 4.1.

Table 4.1 Growth of £100 at 5% per annum

Year	Interest rate	Money at end of year	Net increase for year
1	5%	£105.00	£5.00
2	5%	£110.25	£5.25
3	5%	£115.76	£5.51
4	5%	£121.55	£5.79
5	5%	£127.63	£6.08
6	5%	£134.01	£6.38
7	5%	£140.71	£6.70
8	5%	£147.74	£7.03
9	5%	£155.13	£7.39
10	5%	£162.90	£7.77
11	5%	£171.03	£8.13
12	5%	£179.59	£8.56
13	5%	£188.56	£8.97
14	5%	£197.99	£9.43
15	5%	£207.89	£9.90
16	5%	£218.29	£10.40
17	5%	£229.90	£10.91
18	5%	£240.66	£11.46
19	5%	£252.70	£12.04
20	5%	£265.33	£12.63
21	5%	£278.60	£13.27
22	5%	£292.53	£13.93
23	5%	£307.15	£14.62
24	5%	£322.51	£15.36
25	5%	£338.64	£16.13

Notice that the net increase per year is initially quite small (£5.00 in the first year) but the rise increases with time (£16.13 in the twenty-fifth year). This is an example of exponential growth in that as the time increases by *equal amounts* (1 year) the money increases by *equal fractions* (5%).

If we draw a graph of the total money with the financial institution we get a smooth curve as shown in Figure 4.1. This is the typical shape of an increasing exponential.

For a second example consider a situation where we possess an initial sum of £100. If we consider a tax system where 5% of this money is removed each year as a tax, then the fate of the original £100 is shown in Table 4.2.

Again we can note that the net decrease is greatest during the first year (£5.00) and is least during the twenty-fifth year (£1.46). The rate of decrease is, however, the same, at 5% per annum. This is an example of exponential decay in that as the time increases by *equal amounts* (1 year) the money decays by *equal fractions* (5%). Also note that the amount of money left will never reach zero (*i.e. there will always be some money left*).

If we draw a graph of the total money left, we get a smooth curve as shown in Figure 4.2. This is the typical shape of a decaying exponential.

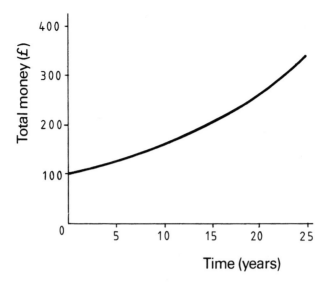

Figure 4.1 Growth of £100 at 5% per annum. Note that the rate of growth becomes greater with time. This is an example of *exponential growth*.

Table 4.2 Decrease of £100 at 5% per annum

Year	Tax rate	Money at end of year	Net increase for year
1	5%	£95.00	£5.00
2	5%	£90.25	£4.75
3	5%	£85.74	£4.51
4	5%	£81.45	£4.29
5	5%	£77.38	£4.07
6	5%	£73.51	£3.87
7	5%	£69.83	£3.68
8	5%	£66.34	£3.49
9	5%	£63.02	£3.32
10	5%	£59.87	£3.15
11	5%	£56.88	£2.99
12	5%	£54.04	£2.84
13	5%	£51.33	£2.71
14	5%	£48.77	£2.56
15	5%	£46.33	£2.44
16	5%	£44.01	£2.32
17	5%	£41.81	£2.20
18	5%	£39.72	£2.09
19	5%	£37.74	£1.98
20	5%	£35.85	£1.89
21	5%	£34.06	£1.79
22	5%	£32.35	£1.71
23	5%	£30.73	£1.62
24	5%	£29.20	£1.53
25	5%	£27.74	£1.46

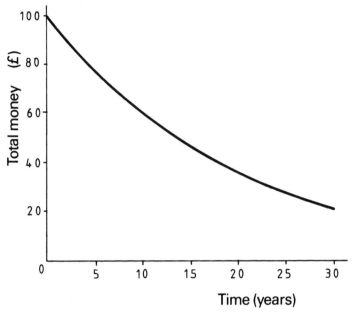

Figure 4.2 'Decay' of £100 at 5% tax per annum. Note that the rate of decay decreases with time and the amount of money left never reaches zero. This is an example of *exponential decay*.

The common factor in these two examples is that the change each year is 5%. This is characteristic of all exponential change and may be expressed as:

Definition

A quantity *y* is said to vary *exponentially* with *x* if equal changes in *x* produce equal *fractional* (or *percentage*) changes in *y*.

Insight

For students familiar with calculus, the mathematical equivalent of the above statement is:

$$\frac{dy}{y} = k \times dx$$

or

$$\frac{dy}{dx} = ky$$

If we integrate this equation then we get:

$y = y_0 \times e^{kx}$

Here the independent variable x forms part of the exponent of the number e and hence the term *exponential* law.

Note also that the equation $y = y_0 \times e^{kx}$ represents exponential growth. The equivalent for exponential decay would be expressed as $y = y_0 \times e^{-kx}$.

The two major examples of the Exponential Law in radiographic science are radioactive decay and the attenuation of electromagnetic radiation by matter. Both of these are described in the following sections.

4.3 RADIOACTIVE DECAY AND THE EXPONENTIAL LAW

Radionuclides are said to *decay* when they change from one nuclear configuration to another. This decay takes several forms including the ejection of alpha particles, beta particles (both positive and negative) and gamma-rays from the nucleus. These and other modes of decay are discussed more fully in Chapter 27. The particular mode of decay is, however, not important to our discussion in this section as the application of the Exponential Law is valid for all the modes. It can be stated as:

Definition

The *law of radioactive decay* states that the rate of decay of a particular nuclide (i.e. the number of nuclei decaying per second) is proportional to the number of such nuclei left in the sample (i.e. it is a fixed fraction of the number of nuclei left in the sample).

It can be seen that this is exactly analogous to the changes which occurred in the decaying exponential sum of money, in that a fixed fraction (or percentage) will decay each unit time (similar to the loss of money from the lump sum). Figure 4.3 shows a graph depicting the above situation. You will note that the initial fall in number of atoms is steep but slows down as less and less of the original nuclei are left. Also note that the number of original nuclei never reaches zero. This is exactly the same as happened in the case of the lump sum of money and you should note the similarities between Figure 4.3 and Figure 4.2.

4.4 MEASURES OF RADIOACTIVITY

In practice it would be extremely difficult to measure the number of nuclei remaining and so draw a graph as shown in Figure 4.3. What we can measure more easily is the *effects* of the nuclear disintegrations by counting the number of gamma-rays (for example) emitted, using a suitable counter. In this way we may make an estimate of the total number of disintegra-

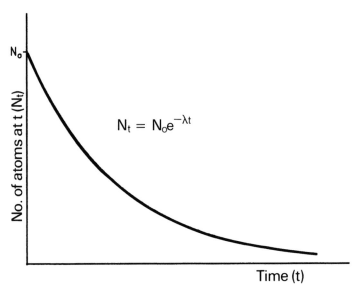

Figure 4.3 Exponential decay of the *number of atoms* of a particular radionuclide. Note the similarity to Figure 4.2.

tions per second occurring within the radioactive sample at any given time. This quantity is known as the *activity* of the sample and is measured in becquerels where 1 becquerel is 1 nuclear disintegration per second. We may now plot *activity* against *time* (see Fig. 4.4) and we obtain exactly the same curve as in Figure 4.3.

The equation for this curve is expressed as:

$$A_t = A_0 e^{-\lambda t} \qquad \text{Equation 4.1}$$

where A_t is the activity after a time t, A_0 is the initial activity, e is the exponential constant, λ is the decay constant and t is the time after the initial measurement.

Insight

In practice it is often easier to use Equation 4.1 in its logarithmic form. Consider the equation:

$$A_t = A_0 e^{-\lambda t}$$

If we take logarithms to the base e of both sides of the equation then we get:

$$\log_e A_t = \log_e A_0 - \lambda t$$

This equation and its use with logarithmic graph paper will be considered further at the end of this chapter.

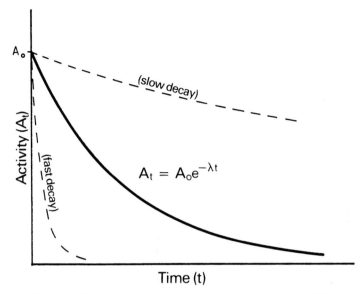

Figure 4.4 Exponential decay of the *radioactivity* of a particular radionuclide.

Figure 4.4 shows the decay curves for radionuclides which have different rates of decay. As we cannot consider the time it will take a nuclide to reach zero as a measure of its rate of decay, a quantity called the *half-life* is used to describe the rate of decay. This is further considered in the next section.

4.5 HALF-LIFE AND DECAY CONSTANT

Definition

The *half-life* of a radionuclide is the time required for the activity of the radioactive sample to decay to one-half of its original value.

An illustration of the half-life of a particular radionuclide is shown in Figure 4.5. The activity of the sample when $t = 0$ is A_0. When the activity is reduced to $A_0/2$ then the radionuclide has undergone one half-life. This is indicated by the time $t_{1/2}$. If another half-life passes, then the activity is reduced by a further factor of 2 and is now $A_0/4$, and so on for further half-lives. Notice that as in our monetary example (Fig. 4.2) the curve never reaches zero activity, so no radioactive source is ever completely *dead*.

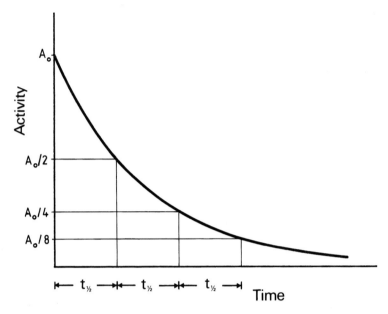

Figure 4.5 Half-life ($t_{1/2}$) and the radioactive decay. Note that each $t_{1/2}$ reduces the level of radioactivity by one-half.

If we now consider Equation 4.1 we can use this to establish a relationship between the decay constant and the half-life:

$$A_t = A_0 e^{-\lambda t}$$

Now, by definition, at the half-life, $A_{t_{1/2}} = A_0/2$. Thus the equation can be rewritten in the form:

$$\frac{A_0}{2} = A_0 e^{-\lambda t_{1/2}}$$
$$\frac{1}{2} = e^{-\lambda t_{1/2}}$$
$$2 = e^{\lambda t_{1/2}}$$
$$\log_e 2 = \lambda t_{1/2}$$
$$0.693 = \lambda t_{1/2}$$

$$\lambda = \frac{0.693}{t_{1/2}} \qquad\qquad \text{Equation 4.3}$$

The decay constant is thus measured in time^{-1} since it is inversely related to the half-life.

Example

The half-life of $^{99}Tc^m$ is 6 hours. What is its decay constant?

From Equation 4.3:

$$\lambda = \frac{0.693}{t_{\frac{1}{2}}}$$

$$= \frac{0.693}{6} \text{ hours}^{-1}$$

$$= 0.1155 \text{ hours}^{-1}$$

Because of this relationship between the half-life and the decay constant we may also write Equation 4.1 as follows:

$$A_t = A_0 e^{-(0.693t/t_{\frac{1}{2}})} \qquad\qquad \text{Equation 4.4}$$

Another important point is that it does not matter from which time, measurement of the half-life is begun. Figure 4.6 shows the decay of a radionuclide over a time of one half-life starting from an arbitrary time, T. Note that the value of $t_{\frac{1}{2}}$ shown in Figure 4.6 is exactly the same as the value shown in Figure 4.5. Thus, over an interval of $t_{\frac{1}{2}}$ the activity is reduced by a factor of 2 independent of the starting time, T.

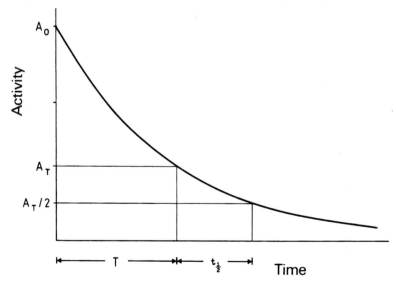

Figure 4.6 The half-life ($t_{\frac{1}{2}}$) is measured from an arbitrary time, T, in the above figure. It is found that the value of $t_{\frac{1}{2}}$ so obtained does not depend on the value of T, so the half-life may be measured from any starting time.

Example

A radioisotope of iodine, ^{131}I, has a half-life of 8 days. Its activity was measured as 14.4 MBq at 09:00 on 3 February. What will be its activity at 09:00 on 27 February?

The time interval over which we are considering the decay of the nuclide is 24 days. With a half-life of 8 days, this represents decay through three half-lives.

After one half-life the activity will be reduced by a factor of 2
After two half-lives the activity will be reduced by a factor of $(2 \times 2) = 4$
After three half-lives the activity will be reduced by a factor of $(4 \times 2) = 8$

i.e. each successive half-life reduces the activity by a factor of 2.

Thus the activity after three half-lives = 14.4/8 = 1.18 MBq.

The activity at 09:00 on 27 February will therefore be 1.18 MBq.

This example gives some clue as to the general method of solving such problems, for assuming n half-lives of decay, the decayed activity A_n can be calculated from the formula:

$$A_n = \frac{A_0}{2^n}$$ Equation 4.5

where A_0 is the original activity.

Similarly we can use this equation to *look back* to consider how much original activity would be required on a certain date to give us the required activity at the time of use of the isotope. Here the unknown is A_0 and the equation can be rearranged as follows:

$$A_0 = 2^n \times A_n$$ Equation 4.6

Example

An activity of 36.5 MBq of ^{99}Tc^m is required at 17:00 on 22 March. The radionuclide has a half-life of 6 hours. What activity of the isotope must be dispensed at 05:00 on 22 March to give the required activity?

Using Equation 4.6:

$$
\begin{aligned}
A_0 &= 2^n \times A_n \\
&= 2^2 \times 36.5 \text{ MBq} \\
&= 146 \text{ MBq}
\end{aligned}
$$

4.6 PHYSICAL HALF-LIFE, BIOLOGICAL HALF-LIFE AND EFFECTIVE HALF-LIFE

In all the considerations of radioactive decay so far we have considered the *physical half-life* of an isotope—the half-life as it would be measured using a quantity of isotope in the laboratory. In *nuclear medicine* there are two other types of half-life we need to consider:

• The *biological half-life* is the time taken for the concentration of a certain chemical in an organ to be reduced to half its original concentration. In this case, the concentration of the chemical is the important part and its activity is not important. This value is affected by the body's ability to excrete the chemical.

• The *effective half-life* is the time taken for the activity of a certain radionuclide in a certain organ to be reduced to half of its original activity. This will be affected by the physical half-life and the biological half-life.

The three types of half-life are connected by the equation:

$$\frac{1}{t_{\frac{1}{2}(\text{eff})}} = \frac{1}{t_{\frac{1}{2}(\text{phys})}} + \frac{1}{t_{\frac{1}{2}(\text{biol})}}$$

Equation 4.7

4.7 ATTENUATION OF ELECTROMAGNETIC RADIATION BY MATTER

The attenuation of electromagnetic radiation by matter constitutes the other major application of the Exponential Law in radiography.

The types of interactions which electromagnetic radiation undergoes when it passes through matter are explained in Chapter 30. A detailed knowledge of these mechanisms is not required at this stage. If we consider a slab of material which has 100 units of radiation incident on it and the transmitted radiation measures 90 units then we can say that the material *attenuates* 10 units of radiation (the differences between absorption and attenuation will be explained in Ch. 30).

For the Exponential Law to be applied, certain conditions must be satisfied:

• The radiation beam must be parallel. This means that it is not affected by the Inverse Square Law.
• The radiation beam must be homogeneous (i.e. the photons must all have the same energy). This means that the beam is not 'hardened' by the removal of low-energy photons by the attenuating material.
• The attenuator must be homogeneous. This means that the attenuating properties must be the same in different parts of the attenuator.

Consider the situation in Figure 4.7. Here, a parallel beam of radiation

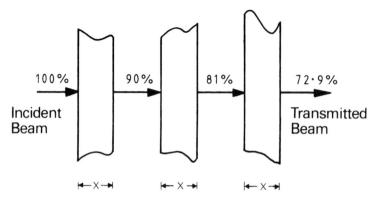

Figure 4.7 Exponential attenuation of a parallel beam of electromagnetic radiation by matter. Equal thickness (*x*) of the attenuator will transmit equal fractions (in this case 9/10) of the incident radiation.

(e.g. gamma-rays) is incident on a slab of uniform attenuating material of thickness *x*. Suppose there is 10% attenuation in the first slab, then 90% of the original beam is transmitted. If we put a further identical attenuator in the path of the beam, then it is found that it also attenuates 10% of the radiation incident upon it and 81% ($0.9 \times 90\%$) will be transmitted. A third identical attenuator transmits 90% of this amount (72.9%) and so on for further attenuators. Thus we can say that *equal changes in x produce equal fractional (or percentage) changes in the transmitted radiation intensity.* This is again an exponential relationship so we can say that:

The attenuation of a mono-energetic parallel beam of electromagnetic radiation by a uniform attenuator will vary exponentially with the attenuator thickness.

A graph of the transmitted intensity I_x through the attenuator of thickness *x* is shown in Figure 4.8. The incident radiation I_0 is the value of I_x when there is no attenuator ($x = 0$). Note the similarities between this curve and the other exponential curves shown in this chapter. The mathematical relationships between the quantities can be given using the equation:

$$I_x = I_0 e^{-\mu x} \hspace{3cm} \text{Equation 4.8}$$

where μ (mu) is the *total linear attenuation coefficient* and so takes into account all the processes of attenuation. The equation therefore refers to the variations of transmittance with *linear distance, x.*

Definition

The *total linear attenuation coefficient* is the fractional change in the intensity of a parallel beam of mono-energetic radiation per unit thickness of homogeneous attenuator.

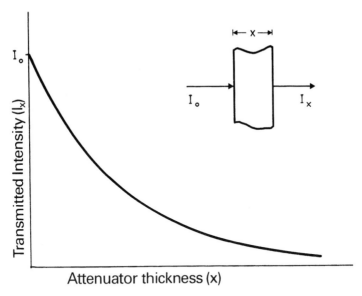

Figure 4.8   Graph showing changes in transmitted intensity due to exponential attenuation of radiation by a uniform attenuator. Note the similarity to Figure 4.3.

Note the similarities between the exponential relationships for radioactive decay (Equation 4.1) and exponential attenuation (Equation 4.8). This would suggest that there is a term similar to '*half-life*' which can be used to describe the penetrating properties of a beam of radiation. This term is the '*half-value thickness*' (often abbreviated to HVT).

4.8 HALF-VALUE THICKNESS (HVT)

If we consider Figure 4.9 we can see that successive HVTs reduce the intensity by factors of 2. We are therefore in a position to define HVT more precisely.

> **Definition**
>
> The *half-value thickness* (HVT) is that thickness of a substance which will transmit exactly one-half of the intensity of radiation incident upon it.

The HVT therefore depends on the attenuating properties of the substance itself and the penetrating power of the beam of electromagnetic radiation incident upon it. Thus in diagnostic radiography we might compare the penetrating properties of two beams using aluminium to measure the HVTs, whereas in therapy radiography we would do this using copper as our attenuator.

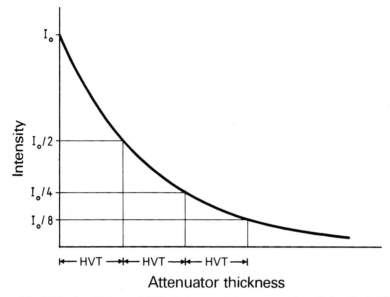

Figure 4.9 Half-value thickness (HVT) of a beam of electromagnetic radiation. Each HVT of the attenuator reduces the intensity by one-half. Note the similarities to Figure 4.5.

To complete the analogy with radioactive decay, Equation 4.3 is paralleled by:

$$\mu = \frac{0.693}{HVT}$$

Equation 4.9

Example

a. The HVT for a beam of radiation is found to be 2.8 mm of aluminium. What is the total linear attenuation coefficient of this beam in aluminium?

From Equation 4.9:

$$\mu = \frac{0.693}{HVT}$$

$$= \frac{0.693}{2.8}\, mm^{-1}$$

$$= 0.2475\ mm^{-1}$$

b. The HVT for a particular beam of gamma-rays is 3 mm of lead. What thickness of lead must be placed in the beam such that only 0.1% of it is transmitted?

There are several ways of tackling this and similar problems. Below is one method.

100% of the beam is incident on the lead and 0.1% is transmitted. This gives a reduction factor of 100/0.1 = 1000.

Now each HVT gives a reduction factor of 2 between the incident and the transmitted radiation as shown in the table below:

Number of HVTs	Intensity reduction factor
1	2
2	4 (i.e. 2×2)
3	8
4	16
5	32
6	64
7	128
8	256
9	512
10	1024

This sort of table is very easy to check so there should be little chance of arithmetic errors.

After 10 HVTs the intensity reduction factor is 1024, which is very close to the required factor of 1000.

Thus 30 mm of lead (10 HVTs) must be used to reduce the transmitted intensity to 0.1% of the incident intensity.

As was the case with radioactive decay (see Equation 4.5), we can use a formula to calculate the intensity (I_n) after n HVTs:

$$I_n = \frac{I_0}{2^n}$$

Equation 4.10

4.9 TENTH-VALUE THICKNESS (TVT)

It should be clear at this stage that values of absorber thickness other than the HVT will produce equal fractional changes in transmission and so it is possible to define a 'fifth-value thickness' or a 'tenth-value thickness', etc. Although the HVT is a very common method of measuring the attenuation of electromagnetic radiation through matter, the tenth-value thickness (TVT) is also used when considering large amounts of attenuation. An example of this would be when designing the walls of a radiotherapy treatment room when a very high intensity of radiation from the treatment machine must not be allowed to penetrate through the wall in significant quantities. One TVT would reduce the intensity by a factor of 10, two would reduce the intensity by a factor of 100 and so on.

4.10 THE USE OF THE LOGARITHMIC FORM OF THE EXPONENTIAL LAW

Consider Equation 4.2 which is the logarithmic form of the Exponential Law:

$$\log_e A_t = \log_e A_0 - \lambda t \qquad \text{Equation 4.11}$$

If we look at this equation, we see that it is in the form of $y = c - mx$ and so we would expect its graph to be in the form of a straight line. If we plot $\log_e$ of the activity on the Y-axis and time on the X-axis, we get the graph shown in Figure 4.10.

The requirement to calculate the logarithm for each result and the antilogarithm for each reading from the graph is overcome by the use of logarithmic graph paper (for a fuller description see Appendix A). Suitable graph paper in this case is log/linear graph paper, i.e. the Y-axis is logarithmic and the X-axis is linear.

An example of such a graph for the attenuation of a beam of electromagnetic radiation is shown in Figure 4.11. Note that equal spaces on the log scale represent changes by factors of 10, and so the logarithmic scale

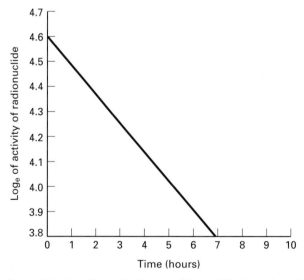

Figure 4.10 Graph of the logarithm to the base e of the activity of a radionuclide plotted against time. Note that the previous *exponential curve* (see Fig. 4.4) is now a *straight line*.

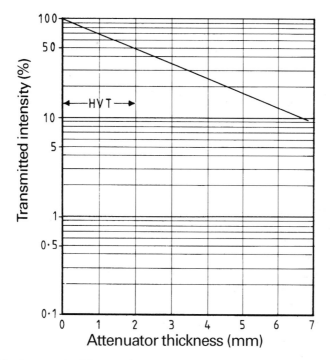

Figure 4.11 An example of the use of logarithmic graph paper to plot an exponential relationship. Note that the previous *exponential curve* (see Fig. 4.8) has become a *straight line*. The HVT for the beam of radiation is 2 mm, as read from the graph. Haif-lives may also be determined in this manner.

never reaches zero. This type of paper allows us to plot the points directly on the paper and then draw the best straight line through them. Such a linear graph makes it easier to interpolate and to extrapolate (see Appendix A) information from the graph.

Summary

In this chapter we have considered the following factors pertinent to the Exponential Law:

- The description of the Exponential Law (see Sect. 4.2)
- Radioactive decay and the Exponential Law (see Sect. 4.3)
- Measures which can be made of the activity of a radionuclide (see Sect. 4.4)
- The relationship between the half-life and the decay constant for a radionuclide (see Sect. 4.5)
- The relationships between the physical half-life, the biological half-life and the effective half-life (see Sect. 4.6)
- How the attenuation of electromagnetic radiation by matter obeys the Exponential Law (see Sect. 4.7)
- The half-value thickness for a beam of radiation and a given attenuator (see Sect. 4.8)
- The use of the tenth-value thickness (see Sect. 4.9)
- The use of the logarithmic form of the Exponential Law (see Sect. 4.10).

SELF-TEST

a. Some swabs have been contaminated with $^{99}Tc^m$ at 09:00 on 16 February. The half-life of the isotope is 6 hours. The level of activity from the swabs was measured at 64 MBq. If the activity of the swabs must be 1 MBq or less before they can be disposed of, what is the earliest time the swabs can be sent for disposal?

b. The decay constant for ^{75}Se is 0.0057 d^{-1}. What is its half-life?

c. An isotope of iodine, ^{131}I, has a half-life of 8 days. 16.8 MBq is required for a study starting at 10:00 on 19 March. If this isotope is to be dispensed at 10:00 on 3 March, what activity should be dispensed?

d. What is the equation which links the *biological half-life*, the *effective half-life* and the *physical half-life*?

e. The HVT for a particular beam of gamma radiation is 1.8 mm of lead. The absorbed dose in air at the front of a barrier is 15 mGy.h^{-1}. We wish the dose at the far side of the barrier to be 7.5 µGy.h^{-1} or less. What is the minimum thickness of lead required in the barrier?

f. (*For this final item it is desirable to have access to 3 cycle log/linear graph paper. If this is not available, it is possible (but less convenient) to plot the line using $\log_e$ of the activity against time on linear graph paper.*) Below are a set of readings of the activity of a certain isotope at the stated time intervals:

Time (hours)	Activity (MBq)
0	78.2
5	43.9
10	24.6
15	13.8
20	7.8
25	4.4
30	2.4
35	1.4
40	0.8

(i) Draw a graph of the activity against time (preferably on logarithmic graph paper).
(ii) Using the graph, estimate the half-life of the isotope.
(iii) What is the decay constant for this isotope?
(iv) Using the graph, estimate the activity of this isotope after 50 hours.

FURTHER READING

Radioactivity and the Exponential Law
Chapter 27 of the current text contains more information on this topic.

Ball J L, Moore A D 1986 Essential physics for radiographers, 2nd edn. Blackwell Scientific
  Publications, London, ch 19
Hay G A, Hughes D 1983 First year physics for radiographers. Baillière Tindall, London,
  chs 16, 18
Webb S (ed) 1988 The physics of medical imaging. Institute of Physics Publishing, Bristol,
  ch 6

Exponential attenuation of radiation
Ball J L, Moore A D 1986 Essential physics for radiographers, 2nd edn. Blackwell Scientific
  Publications, London, ch 16
Hay G A, Hughes D 1983 First year physics for radiographers. Baillière Tindall, London,
  ch 14

PART 2

General physics

5

Laws of physics (classical)

5.1 AIM

The aim of this chapter is to introduce the reader to some of the laws of classical physics. An understanding of these laws will aid an understanding of some of the physics discussed in later chapters of the book. (Some of the physics in the later chapters of this book (e.g. pair production as an absorption mechanism) cannot be explained in terms of the laws of classical physics. Before these concepts are considered (Ch. 25 onwards) the laws of modern physics will be considered in Ch. 24.)

5.2 LAW OF CONSERVATION OF MATTER (MASS)

Statement of the law

Matter is neither created nor destroyed, but it may change its chemical form as the result of a chemical reaction.

This law tells us that the total mass of the ingredients after a chemical reaction is equal to their mass before the reaction.

Insight

If we consider the reaction below:

$$AgNO_3 + KBr = AgBr + KNO_3$$

Here silver nitrate is mixed with potassium bromide to form silver bromide (used as the light-sensitive salt in the photographic emulsion) and potassium nitrate. The total mass of silver nitrate plus potassium bromide is equal to the total mass of silver bromide plus potassium nitrate. Matter has neither been created nor destroyed by the reaction.

5.3 LAW OF CONSERVATION OF ENERGY

Statement of the law

Energy can neither be created nor destroyed but can be changed from one form to another. The amount of energy in a system is thus constant.

This law tells us that energy is never used up but changes from one form to another.

Insight

When an electron is released from the filament of an X-ray tube it has potential energy. As it is accelerated across the tube, this potential energy is converted to kinetic energy. When it makes contact with the target of the tube, this kinetic energy is converted to heat and X-ray energy. At any time the sum of all the energies remains constant.

Some of the common forms of energy are listed below:

Chemical	Kinetic
Gravitational	Sound
Electrical	Radiation
Potential	Heat.

These two laws of conservation of mass and energy are combined into one law by modern physics (Ch. 24).

5.4 THE LAW OF CONSERVATION OF MOMENTUM

Statement of the law

The total linear or rotational momentum in a given system is constant.

This law is important when we consider collisions between two bodies.

Insight

There are two types of collision which occur, elastic and inelastic. An *elastic* collision is one where all kinetic energy is conserved, as in the case of a 'perfect' billiard ball colliding with a similar but stationary billiard ball; the moving ball stops while the ball which was previously stationary moves with the same velocity as the first ball had before collision. In an *inelastic* collision the total kinetic energy is not conserved, as in the case of two billiard balls colliding with a glancing blow, so that both continue to move after the collision. In both cases the *momentum* is conserved although the velocities of the bodies in each case will be different.

In radiographic science, conservation of momentum is mainly concerned with the interactions of X-rays with matter and these will be dealt with in Chapter 30.

5.5 NEWTON'S LAWS OF MOTION

Newton's Laws of Motion can be derived from the above laws, but they are so useful as to merit a separate section. They are defined as follows:

Law 1

A body will remain at rest or will travel with a constant velocity unless acted upon by a net external force.

Law 2

The rate of change of momentum of a body is proportional to the applied force.

Law 3

The action of one body on a second body is always accompanied by an equal and opposite action of the second body on the first.

Note: The terms 'velocity' and 'momentum' in the first two laws imply *direction,* as both are vector quantities (see Ch. 6).

A body of mass m and velocity u has a force F applied to it. After a time t its velocity has changed to v. Then the second law of motion can be stated thus:

$$\frac{(mv - mu)}{t} \propto F$$

$$\frac{m(v - u)}{t} \propto F$$

Now $(v - u)/t$ is the rate of change of velocity or the *acceleration*, *a*, of the body (see Ch. 6).

Hence we can say that:

$ma \propto F$ or $F = kma$, where k is the constant of proportionality (see Appendix A).

If we choose suitable units it can be arranged that k is equal to 1 and we finally have:

$F = ma$ Equation 5.1

In SI units (see Ch. 6) F is measured in Newtons, m is measured in kg and a is measured in $m \cdot s^{-2}$. This makes Equation 5.1 the familiar mathematical statement of Newton's Second Law and can also be used as the basis for the definition of the Newton (1 Newton = $1 \text{ kg} \times 1 \text{ m} \cdot s^{-2}$).

Insight

As an illustration of the use of this law, we are now in a position to calculate the kinetic energy of a body of mass m travelling with a velocity v. If we apply a steady force F in the opposite direction to that of v, the body will slow down and eventually come to rest. The work done in bringing the body to rest must be equal to its kinetic energy. This we can state mathematically as:

$E = -F \times s$ Equation 5.2

where s is the distance taken for the body to come to rest. (The force, F, and its associated acceleration, a, are regarded as negative as they are applied in the opposite direction to v.)

From Equation 5.1 we can now change Equation 5.2 as follows:

$E = -m \times a \times s$ Equation 5.3

The acceleration, a, is the change in velocity per unit time. Stated mathematically this is:

$$-a = \frac{(v - 0)}{t}$$

$$a = \frac{-v}{t}$$

As the action of the force is consistent throughout the deceleration, the time take for the body to stop can be calculated by dividing the distance travelled by the average velocity ($v/2$). So:

$$t = \frac{s}{\frac{1}{2}v}$$

$$= \frac{2s}{v}$$

Thus we get:

$$a = \frac{-v}{t}$$

$$= \frac{-v}{(2s/v)}$$

$$= \frac{-v^2}{2s}$$

$$as = -\tfrac{1}{2}v^2$$

If we now consider Equation 5.3, this can be rewritten:

$$E = -m(as)$$
$$= -m(-\tfrac{1}{2}v^2)$$

$$E = \tfrac{1}{2}mv^2 \hspace{4cm} \text{Equation 5.4}$$

Newton's Third Law is usually paraphrased as: 'To every action there is an equal and opposite reaction'. There are many examples of this in everyday life, such as a hammer hitting a nail, but it is important to realise that there need not necessarily be physical contact between the two bodies for one to act on the other. If we take two charged bodies and bring these close together (but not actually touching), the forces between the two bodies will be equal and opposite. The significance of this in the design of the cathode of the X-ray tube will be considered in Chapter 21.

5.6 AVOGADRO'S HYPOTHESIS, THE MOLE AND AVOGADRO'S NUMBER

As we will see in Chapter 26, all substances consist of atoms or molecules. These may react chemically with the atoms or molecules of other substances. These reactions occur with fixed proportions in order to produce a given chemical compound and it is possible to predict the number of molecules of the compound from a knowledge of the number of molecules of the original elements or compounds, for example:

$$2H_2 + O_2 = 2H_2O$$

In the case of gasses, Avogadro's hypothesis postulated that *'equal volumes of gasses at the same temperature and pressure contain equal numbers of molecules'*. This hypothesis was first postulated in the early nineteenth century and has been verified by a number of experiments since then.

This is taken one stage further within the SI system in the more general statement that *'the number of molecules per mole is the same for any substance'*. The mole is the SI unit of the amount of substance and is defined as:

Definition

The *mole* is the amount of substance which contains as many elementary particles as there are atoms in 0.012 kg of carbon-12.

Here, carbon-12 is used as the standard for technical experimental reasons. From this we can predict the number of atoms or molecules in a substance by knowing its atomic mass number and comparing this with carbon-12. For example, if we consider cobalt-60, then there will be the same number of atoms in 0.060 kg of cobalt-60 as there will be in 0.012 kg of carbon-12 as each consists of one mole of substance.

The number of molecules in a mole is given by *Avogadro's number* (or constant) and is 6×10^{23} molecules.

Insight

If we consider X-ray photons being attenuated by matter, this is a reaction between the photons and the electrons of atoms of the material through which they pass. If we know the number of atoms per mole of the material we can calculate the number of atoms per unit mass. By knowing the atomic number of the material it is then possible to establish the electron density and so predict the likelihood of an X-ray photon interacting with an electron. This will be further discussed in Chapter 30.

Summary

In this chapter you should have learnt:

- The Law of Conservation of Matter (see Sect. 5.2)
- The Law of Conservation of Energy (see Sect. 5.3)
- The Law of Conservation of Momentum (see Sect. 5.4)
- Newton's Laws of Motion (see Sect. 5.5)
- Avogadro's hypothesis, the mole and Avogadro's number (see Sect. 5.6).

SELF-TEST

a. State the Law of Conservation of Matter.

b. State the Law of Conservation of Energy.

c. State the Law of Conservation of Momentum.

d. State Newton's Laws of Motion.

e. The rest mass of an electron is 9.11×10^{-31} kg. Such an electron is accelerated across the X-ray tube and at the point of contact with the target its kinetic energy is 1.6×10^{-14} J. Calculate its velocity at the point of contact.

f. Iodine-131 is a common isotope of iodine which is used in thyroid studies (its mass number is 131). Calculate the mass of the substance required to give 12×10^{23} atoms.

FURTHER READING

Further reading on the laws of classical physics can be found in most textbooks which are used in schools for the study of A-level or Higher grade physics. In addition the following may prove useful:

Allan E, Harris J 1991 Higher grade chemistry. Hodder & Stoughton, London, ch 3
Ball J L, Moore A D 1986 Essential physics for radiographers, 2nd edn. Blackwell Scientific Publications, London, ch 1
Hay G A, Hughes D 1983 First year physics for radiographers. Baillière Tindall, London, ch 1
Macgregor J 1992 Higher chemistry. Oliver & Boyd, London, ch 4

Units of measurement

6.1 AIM

The aim of this chapter is to introduce the reader to the main units which are used in measurement in radiographic science.

6.2 UNITS OF MEASUREMENT

Science has three fundamental tools which are used in its attempts to understand the external world:

- experimental measurements
- logic
- theory.

These will be discussed in this chapter and in Chapter 7.

Problems arise when making experimental measurements as to what quantities to measure and how to measure them. In particular, the *units* in which these quantities are expressed must be defined so that, when two people make the same measurement, they get the same results. Also there are obvious advantages if one set of units is universally adopted as the basis for all measurements.

Each of the *base* units discussed in the next section relies on the appropriate *standard* to which each measurement is compared. Thus there are units of standard length, standard mass, standard time interval and so on. Without such standards no really accurate measurements can be made. This in turn retards the development of adequate theories, or models, of the world.

6.3 SI BASE UNITS

There are a plethora of units of measurement used throughout the world. The international system of units (SI) attempts to replace this with seven standard units. These standards are termed *base units* (Table 6.1) and represent the fundamental measurements which we might wish to make of a body:

- what is its size? (unit of *length—metre*)
- how massive is it? (unit of *mass—kilogram*)
- how bright is it? (unit of *luminous intensity—candela*)
- how much electrical current flows through it? (unit of *electrical current—ampere*)
- how many elementary particles does it contain? (unit of *amount of substance—mole*)
- how hot is it? (unit of *temperature—kelvin*)
- how do all the quantities vary with time? (unit of *time—second*).

Table 6.1 SI base units

Quantity	Unit of measurement	Symbol
Length	metre	m
Mass	kilogram	kg
Luminous intensity	candela	cd
Electric current	ampere	A
Amount of substance	mole	mol
Temperature	kelvin	K
Time	second	s

The very precise definitions of the units are not required for the rest of this text but if you wish to see them they are given in Appendix G.

The base units of mass, length and time are termed *fundamental units* since one or more of them is always involved in the measurement of any other quantity.

These seven SI base units may be combined to give *derived units* as described in the next section.

6.3.1 Derived SI units

A number of derived SI units can be formed by the combination of the seven base units. Some of these are sufficiently important to be given their

Table 6.2   Derived SI units and their definitions

Quantity	Definition	SI unit	Scalar/vector
Speed	Distance travelled in unit time	metre/second ($m \cdot s^{-1}$)	Scalar
Velocity	Distance travelled in unit time in a given direction	metre/second ($m \cdot s^{-1}$)	Vector
Acceleration	Change of velocity in unit time	(metre/second)/ second ($m \cdot s^{-2}$)	Vector
Force	The application of unit force to unit mass produces unit acceleration	newton (N) ($kg \cdot m \cdot s^{-2}$)	Vector
Pressure	Force applied per unit area	pascal (P) ($N \cdot m^{-2}$)	Vector
Weight	Force acting on a body due to gravity	newton (N) ($kg \cdot m \cdot s^{-2}$)	Vector
Work	This is the product of the force acting on a body times the distance the body moves	joule (J) ($N \cdot m$)	Scalar
Energy	Kinetic energy: work which can be done by a system because of its velocity	joule (J)	Scalar
	Potential energy: work which can be performed because of the position or state of a system	joule (J)	Scalar
Power	Rate of doing work	watt (W) ($J \cdot s^{-1}$)	Scalar
Momentum	The product of the mass and the velocity of the body	($kg \cdot m \cdot s^{-1}$)	Vector

own names and are listed in Table 6.2 and discussed in the rest of this chapter. Further derived units are of a more specialised nature (e.g. absorbed radiation dose) and will be discussed in the specific chapters which require such measurement.

Insight

For some quantities we can consider a body moving between two points. For certain measurement it is important to know how far the body has travelled between the two points. In other cases we wish to know how far it has travelled and also the direction it has travelled. Measurements where the direction is important are termed *vector* quantities whereas those where the direction is not important are known as *scalar* quantities.

6.3.2 Speed and velocity

The speedometer on a car is calibrated in terms of kilometres per hour (kph) or miles per hour (mph). Either of these shows that *speed* means distance travelled in unit time.

In SI units, speed (*S*), distance (*d*) and time (*t*) are related by the equation:

$$S = \frac{d}{t}$$

Equation 6.1

where d is in metres, t is in seconds and S, therefore, is in metres/second ($m \cdot s^{-1}$). The speedometer on a car gives no indication of the *direction* in which the car is moving so we can see that speed is a scalar quantity. *Velocity* is measured in the same units as speed ($m \cdot s^{-1}$) but this time the *direction* of movement is also measured. Thus a car travelling at a constant speed around a roundabout is continuously changing its velocity.

6.3.3 Acceleration

Acceleration implies a change in velocity and is defined as the *change in velocity per unit time*. For example, the acceleration due to gravity is approximately 9.8 metres per second per second (9.8 $m \cdot s^{-2}$). This means that for a free-falling body the velocity increases by 9.8 $m \cdot s^{-1}$ after each second. Thus, if a body is dropped, its downward velocity is 9.8 $m \cdot s^{-1}$ after the first second, 19.6 $m \cdot s^{-1}$ after the next second and so on.

The acceleration due to gravity causes a free-falling body to increase its velocity, but if the accelerating force is in the opposite direction to the direction of movement of the body, then it will cause it to lose velocity. This force causes a negative acceleration or a *deceleration*.

Also notice that acceleration is a vector quantity as the acceleration has direction.

6.3.4 Force

Newton's Second Law of Motion (see Sect. 5.5) shows that the net force acting on a body is proportional to the mass of the body multiplied by the acceleration produced on the body. The units of force are therefore $kg \cdot m \cdot s^{-2}$ in SI units. However, this quantity is sufficiently important to be given its own special name and is known as the *newton*. This can be defined as follows:

Definition

A net force of 1 *newton* acting on a body of mass 1 kg causes it to have an acceleration of 1 $m \cdot s^{-2}$.

Force is a vector quantity as it has direction. The acceleration produced by the action of the force (also a vector quantity) is in the same direction as the force.

6.3.5 Pressure

Pressure is defined as the *force exerted per unit area*. The units of pressure would therefore be $N \cdot m^{-2}$. Again it is sufficiently important to merit its own unit known as the *pascal* and is defined as follows:

> **Definition**
>
> The pressure acting on a body is 1 *pascal* if 1 newton of force is applied per square metre of body surface.

The difference between force and pressure can be readily appreciated if one considers crossing some snow wearing either shoes or skis. In both cases the force is the same but this force is applied to a smaller area in the case of shoes (the pressure on the snow is greater) so they tend to sink into the snow.

6.3.6 Weight and mass

As we have already seen **mass** is a base SI unit and is defined as *the amount of matter in a body* and is defined against the standard kilogram. This is sometimes confused with the mole (the amount of substance in a body) and so it is possibly easier to understand the concept of mass if we consider it in terms of inertia. We know that a force acting on a body will produce an acceleration and that the force, the mass and the acceleration are linked by the equation $F = m \times a$ (see Equation 5.1) so that inertia can be defined as the body's resistance to acceleration. From the equation it can be seen that as the mass of the body increases so the force required to produce a given acceleration also increases, i.e. *the inertia of the body increases with mass.*

The **weight** of a body is the downward *force* on the body due to the gravitational attraction of earth. Hence, the weight of a body is expressed in newtons not in kilograms. An equation similar to Equation 5.1 links weight, mass and gravity:

$$w = m \times g \hspace{4cm} \text{Equation 6.2}$$

From the above discussion and equation we can see that a body always has mass but it only has weight in the presence of a gravitational field. Hence a body in deep space has no weight (because of the zero gravitational field) but it has mass as it still requires a force to cause it to change its velocity (i.e. it has inertia).

6.3.7 Work and energy

Both *work* and *energy* are measured using the same units. A force is said to do work if it moves its point of application in the same direction as the applied force. This can be expressed as:

$$W = F \times d \hspace{4cm} \text{Equation 6.3}$$

Thus the units of work are newtons and metres (N·m). Again the concept of work is sufficiently important to merit its own unit which is the *joule*.

Definition

---

1 *joule* of work is performed when a force of 1 newton moves its point of application through a distance of 1 metre.

Energy can be considered as the capacity of a body to do work. There are two types of energy which we need to consider separately:

a. kinetic energy
b. potential energy.

a. Kinetic energy

Kinetic energy is energy which a body possesses by virtue of its motion. This motion may be *translational* (movement along a path) or *rotational* or a combination of both types. The kinetic energy is simply the work which must be done in the process of bringing the body to rest. We have already looked at this when we considered Newton's Laws of Motion and established an equation (Equation 5.4) for the kinetic energy of a body of mass m having a velocity of v.

$$E = \tfrac{1}{2}mv^2$$

Insight

Consider an electron which has been accelerated across the X-ray tube and is travelling with a velocity v at the point when it starts to collide with the atoms of the target. It has a kinetic energy ($= \tfrac{1}{2}mv^2$) and then starts to liberate some of that energy in the form of X-ray photons.

b. Potential energy

Potential energy is energy possessed by a body (or a system) by virtue of its condition or state. Thus a stationary body has potential energy if it is in a condition which allows it to release its stored energy. The potential energy of the system can be thought of as the work which the system will perform in bringing its potential energy to zero. If we consider a body of mass m which is at a height h above the ground, then we can apply Equation 6.3 to this situation:

$$W = F \times d$$

The force at work here is the weight of the body (mg) and the distance it can move is its height above the ground, so we now have the equation for the potential energy (PE):

$$PE = mgh$$ Equation 6.4

> **Insight**
>
> Consider the case of a hospital lift sitting at the ground floor. Attached to this lift, over a pulley system, is a counterweight. This counterweight has potential energy because of its position. If the brakes on the lift are released, it will assist in moving the lift up to the top floor (i.e. the counterweight performs work).
> Work and energy are both scalar quantities as they do not have direction.

6.3.8 Power

A particular car may reach a speed of 60 mph in 6 seconds while another car of the same mass does the same in 20 seconds. The first car is said to be more *powerful* than the second. If we assume that the cars are both travelling in the same direction, then their velocity is the same and so their kinetic energy ($= \frac{1}{2}mv^2$) is the same, but the first car reached that energy more quickly. Hence *power* can be expressed as the *rate at which energy is expended* and, since energy and work are basically the same thing, we can say that:

> **Definition**
>
> *Power* is the rate at which work is done.

Thus, power is measured in joules per second ($J \cdot s^{-1}$) but is again an important enough concept to merit its own unit, the *watt*. Thus:

$$watts = \frac{joules}{seconds}$$

or 1 *watt* is 1 joule of work per second.

6.3.9 Momentum

In everyday speech, *momentum* expresses the ability of a moving body to 'keep going'. This depends on the mass of the body and its velocity and so momentum is defined:

> **Definition**
>
> The *momentum* of a body is the product of its mass and its velocity.

We have already, briefly, come across the concept of momentum in the Law of Conservation of Momentum (Sect. 5.4).

Insight

Consider the situation where a projectile (e.g. a bullet) strikes a barrier. The depth to which it penetrates the barrier is dependent on the *mass* of the projectile and its *velocity* at the point of impact. This fits in with our concept of *momentum* as the ability of a body to keep going.

6.4 UNITS USED IN RADIOGRAPHY

Many derived SI units (such as the joule, coulomb, etc.) are used in radiographic science. However, other units outside the strict adherence to the SI system are especially useful to radiography and are unlikely to be discontinued, because of their practical convenience. These are shown and defined in Table 6.3.

6.4.1 kV$_p$

The potential difference (see Ch. 9) existing between the cathode and anode of an X-ray tube is measured in kilovolts, where $1 \, kV = 10^3 \, V$. In many X-ray generators, however, this potential difference is not constant but varies, with a given frequency, during the exposure time. Hence, it is conventional practice to quote the *peak* (i.e. maximum) value of the potential difference across the X-ray tube. Thus, when a radiographer selects $50 \, kV_p$ he/she is selecting a maximum voltage of $50 \, kV$ to be applied to the tube during the exposure. The effects of this voltage on the beam will be discussed in later chapters (Chs 28 and 29) of this text and also later in this chapter when we consider keV.

Table 6.3   Units used in radiography

Unit	Definition
kV$_p$	The maximum kilovoltage applied across an X-ray tube in a forward direction during an exposure
mA	The average electrical current passing through an X-ray tube during an exposure (measured in milliampere)
mAs	The average current passing through the tube during an exposure multiplied by the exposure time in seconds (1 mAs = 1 millicoulomb)
keV	The energy imparted to an electron when passing through a potential difference of 1 kV in a vacuum
HU	This is a measure of the heat energy deposited in the anode by an exposure and is the product of the kV$_p$ and the mAs

6.4.2 mA and mAs

X-rays are produced in an X-ray tube when electrons from the cathode, with high kinetic energy, strike the anode (see Chs 28 and 29). If we assume that each electron has a chance of producing X-rays, then the intensity of X-ray production is proportional to the number of electrons striking the anode per second. The number of electrons flowing per second is related to the *current* flowing through the tube (see Ch. 10). The SI unit of current is the ampere (A), as we saw earlier in this chapter, and it is equivalent to a current of 6×10^{18} electrons per second. This unit of current is too large a unit for radiography so current is measured in milliamperes ($1 \text{ mA} = 10^{-3} \text{ A}$).

We only wish the tube to produce X-rays in sufficient quantity to produce the image on the recording medium (e.g. film) and so an exposure time is set by the radiographer. It can be seen that, all other factors remaining constant, the amount of blackening (or optical density) of the film will be determined by the number of X-rays leaving the tube. From the above arguments this is determined by the total number of electrons striking the anode of the tube.

The total number of electrons striking the target (and hence the X-ray output) is determined by the number of electrons flowing in unit time (related to the mA) and the length of time for which the current flows (the exposure time in seconds, *s*). Thus the X-ray output from a tube (if all other factors remain unaltered) is determined by the mAs.

Any combination of mA and time which produces a given mAs will result in the same quantity of X-rays being emitted by the tube. If 60 mAs was required to produce an acceptable image, this could be delivered in the ways listed in Table 6.4.

The reasons why we might wish to use the different combinations of mA and time will be discussed in Chapters 29 and 32.

As we shall see in Chapter 10, the mAs is equivalent to the *millicoulomb* (10^{-3} C) which is the unit of electrical charge. The mAs is, however, used in preference to the millicoulomb as it makes it more obvious that this can be altered by altering the tube current (mA) or the exposure time (s).

Table 6.4   Different combinations of mA and time to produce a given mAs

Current (mA)	Exposure time (s)	mAs
10	6.0	60
20	3.0	60
100	0.6	60
200	0.3	60
300	0.2	60
600	0.1	60

6.4.3 keV

Energy, as we have already seen in this chapter, is measured in joules. When we come to consider the energies involved in the atom or the energies of the photons of the X-ray beam, the coulomb is an extremely large unit. The electron-volt (eV) or the kiloelectron-volt (keV = 10^3 eV) are much more convenient units of measurement for such energies.

Definitions

If an electron is accelerated from rest across a potential difference of 1 volt in a vacuum, it gains a kinetic energy of 1 *electron-volt*.
  Similarly an electron accelerated from rest across a potential difference of 1 kilovolt in a vacuum gains a kinetic energy of 1 *kiloelectron-volt*.

The energy (E) in joules can be calculated from the equation:

$$E = e \times V \hspace{4cm} \text{Equation 6.5}$$

In this equation e is the charge on the electron (1.6×10^{-19} coulomb) and V is the potential difference measured in volts. Thus:

$1 \text{ eV} = 1.6 \times 10^{-19} \text{ joule}$
$1 \text{ keV} = 1.6 \times 10^{-16} \text{ joule}$

Insight

If 75 kV_p is selected by a radiographer for a specific exposure then some of the electrons travelling across the X-ray tube will have a kinetic energy of 75 keV when they strike the anode. If we assume that some of these electrons give up all their energy as a single X-ray photon, then the energy of this photon will be 75 keV and it will represent the maximum photon energy in this beam. Thus by altering the kV_p, the radiographer can alter the maximum photon energy of the X-ray beam.

6.4.4 Heat Units (HU)

When electrons strike the anode of the X-ray tube, their kinetic energy is given up in a small area of the anode known as the focus (see Chs 2 and 28). Some of this energy is converted into X-ray photons but most of it (about 99%) is converted into heat. It is important to know how much heat an exposure or series of exposures produces as too much heat could produce sufficient temperature rise to melt the focal spot. In the case of most modern X-ray tubes, this is quoted by the manufacturer in kilojoules and will be considered in Chapter 23. For some of the older X-ray tubes, rating is quoted in Heat Units (HU) which give a useful measure of the heat energy imparted to the anode. In Chapter 10 we will show that the total energy (joule) dissipated by a current I (amp) driven by a potential difference V (volt) for a time t (seconds) is given by the equation:

$$E = V \times I \times t$$

This equation is correct only if V and I remain constant for the time t, which is not necessarily the case for the X-ray tube. Thus to find an *absolute* value of the heat produced (in joules) we would need to know the effective values for the tube voltage (kV) and tube current (mA). As we have already seen, the kV selector allows us to select the kV_p and we will see that the value of the mA which we select is the *average* value. Thus we can adapt the above equation to give:

Heat Units $= kV_p \times mA \times t$ Equation 6.6

But we already know that the product of the *mA* and the *exposure time* is the *mAs* and so we can say that:

Heat Units $= kV_p \times mAs$ Equation 6.7

Provided the manufacturer quotes the maximum permissible heat loading in Heat Units, this allows us to check if an exposure or a series of exposures is within the permissible rating for a particular focal spot. The importance of the rating of a particular focal spot will be considered in more detail in Chapter 23.

Summary

In this chapter we considered the following factors related to units of measurement:

- The SI base units for length, mass, luminous intensity, electric current, amount of substance, temperature and time (see Sect. 6.3)
- The SI derived units for speed, velocity, acceleration, force, pressure, weight, work, energy, power and momentum (see Sect. 6.3.1)
- Units of measurement used in radiography in the form of kV_p, mA, mAs, keV and Heat Units (see Sect. 6.4).

SELF-TEST

a. Give the derived SI unit in which each of the following are measured: velocity; acceleration; force; pressure; weight; work; energy; power.

b. Calculate the heat generated (in Heat Units) by the following exposure 75 kV_p, 200 mA, 0.5 s. If the maximum heat storage capacity of the anode disk is 10 000 Heat Units, state why this exposure cannot be repeated immediately.

FURTHER READING

Further information on the precise definition of SI units is found in Appendix G of this text and information on the loading of X-ray tubes is found in Chapter 23. In addition the following may prove useful:

Ball J L, Moore A D 1986 Essential physics for radiographers, 2nd edn. Blackwell Scientific Publications, London, ch 1

Foster E 1985 Equipment for diagnostic radiography. MTP Press, Lancaster, ch 5

Gifford D 1984 A handbook of physics for radiologists and radiographers. John Wiley & Sons, Chichester, chs 4, 22

Hay G A, Hughes D 1983 First year physics for radiographers. Baillière Tindall, London, ch 1

Hendee W, Ritenour R 1992 Medical imaging physics, 3rd edn. Mosby Year Book, London, ch 5

Johns H E, Cunningham J R 1983 The physics of radiology, 4th edn. Charles C Thomas, Illinois, USA, ch 1

Ohanian H C 1994 Principles of physics. W W Norton, London, ch 1

Stockley S M 1986 A manual of radiographic equipment. Churchill Livingstone, Edinburgh, ch 10

Thompson M A 1994 Principles of imaging science and protection. W B Saunders, London, chs 2, 6

Experimentation and statistics

7.1 AIM

The aim of this chapter is to introduce the reader to techniques which allow the accuracy and precision of various experimental measurements to be calculated and also to consider basic statistical methods which allow us to manipulate experimental data.

7.2 INTRODUCTION

Much of our knowledge in radiographic science is based on experimentation. It is important in dealing with such experiments that we know the limitations of our measurements and that we have sufficient statistical skill to allow us to draw correct conclusions from the measurement which we take.

7.3 EXPERIMENTAL ERRORS

7.3.1 How exact is accurate?

As we saw in Chapter 6, physics attempts to be an exact science based on accurate measurements of defined quantities such as mass, length, temperature and time. However, no instrument is able to give a truly exact value of the quantity being measured, since errors of measurement or of observation will always be present. Used in this sense, an error of measurement is not the same thing as a mistake but just an uncertainty as to the correct value of a measured quantity. It is also possible that the act of undertaking a measurement may alter the quantity we are trying to measure.

For example, suppose that we are using a non-digital meter to measure an electrical current. Among many possible sources of error, the following may be present:

- an observational error due to the thickness of the pointer on the scale
- an observational error due to incorrect interpolation between scale markings
- an observational error due to poor technique (e.g. not looking at right angles to the scale)
- a measurement error due to an incorrect 'zero', i.e. the pointer is not on the scale zero mark when no current flows
- a measurement error due to the scale being incorrectly calibrated
- a measurement error due to the act of measuring the current changing the current being measured.

Finding and reducing the effects of possible sources of error in a measurement is essential if an accurate, even if not exact, reading is to be taken.

How accurate do we need to be? Well, this depends upon why a particular measurement is being performed. If we make an error of 2 mm in an FSD (Ch. 2) setting of 50 cm, then the effect will be negligible on a conventional radiograph. However, a fault in an X-ray tube which produced the same error of 2 mm in an effective focal spot size of 1 mm (Sect. 2.3) will have the observable effect of increasing the unsharpness (Sect. 2.6) quite markedly. The fractional (or percentage) error is important, therefore, and is discussed in more detail in this chapter (Sect. 7.3.3).

Basically, the errors of measurement are sufficiently small if they do not affect the conclusions drawn from a result of a measurement or affect a procedure being undertaken (e.g. radiograph or radiotherapy treatment). In radiography or radiotherapy practice, errors of 1 mm when setting a distance or 1 degree when setting an angle are usually considered to be sufficiently accurate.

7.3.2 Random and systematic errors

Random errors are those errors which, on repeated measurements of the same quantity, are variable in size and have no discernible pattern or sequence. This may be due to the quantity itself varying in a random manner (e.g. number of radioactive disintegrations per second; see Ch. 27) or due to slight differences in the measurement technique of the observer on each occasion. Alternatively, the ambient conditions of temperature, pressure or humidity, etc. may affect the instrument being used in an apparently random manner.

Systematic errors may arise either from the observer or from the instrument itself, and may be constant or vary in some regular (i.e. non-random) manner. For example, the measurement of a length using a ruler with the zero incorrectly positioned will give rise to results which are systematically in error by a constant amount, e.g. 10.3 cm and 4.6 cm when the correct values are 10.0 cm and 4.3 cm respectively, when the zero is displaced by 3 mm.

Many sources of error are either wholly random or wholly systematic, but most errors encountered in practical situations are the result of both types. You may like to inspect the list of meter errors in the previous section and decide where the random and systematic errors might lie.

The existence of random and systematic errors leads to the concept of *accuracy* versus *precision*. *Precision* is a measure of the repeatability of a series of measurements, while *accuracy* is a measure of the correspondence between the result obtained and its exact value. The precision of a series of readings may be quite high in that they all might lie close to each other, but the accuracy may be poor if there is a significant systematic error involved. A faulty scale on a meter or a ruler, for example, will give the 'wrong' answers even though the readings taken from the scale may be highly repeatable. Precision leads to accuracy, therefore, if the systematic errors have been eliminated or corrected. It is the usual practice in physics to record a result with the estimated error in the form:

true value = measured value ± estimated error

If we have the statement that FSD = 50.0 ± 0.2 cm, then it is implied that the true value of the FSD lies somewhere between the values 49.8 cm and 50.2 cm.

Mathematically, if the error is e, the measured value is m and the true value is t, then $e = m - t$, since the error is just the difference between the measured and true values. Rearranging this, we have:

$$m = t + e \hspace{4cm} \text{Equation 7.1}$$

where the error e may be positive or negative.

The magnitude of e may be reduced by careful measurement technique and, where possible, the recording of a large number of readings so that a mean value (Sect. 7.4.1) may be taken.

7.3.3 Fractional and percentage errors

In practice, it is often useful to express an error in relation to the magnitude of the quantity being measured. If it is possible to measure to within 1 mm when using a particular ruler, then this error will become progressively less important as lengths of 1 cm, 10 cm, 1 m, 1 km are taken. Expressing the error of 1 mm as a fraction of the measured value, we obtain 0.1, 0.01, 0.001, 0.000001 or 10%, 1%, 0.1%, 0.0001% respectively. This concept of a fractional or percentage error is important because it helps us to predict what accuracy we need for our individual measurements in order to achieve a given percentage error in the final result. If we wish to measure the area of a rectangle to within 1%, for example, then it may be shown (Sect. 7.3.4) that it is necessary to measure the sides to an accuracy of 0.5%. Hence, a 10% error would be much too high while a 0.001% error would be unnecessarily restrictive for our purpose. A knowledge of the accuracies required also has an effect on the experimental apparatus used, for a 0.5% error in a 1 mm length is 0.005 mm—well beyond the capabilities of a ruler, so that a travelling microscope would be more suitable—while a 0.5% error in a length of 10 cm is 0.5 mm, enabling an accurate ruler to be used.

If we give the fractional error in a quantity the symbol f, then f is just the size of the error (i.e. measured value, m, minus true value, t) divided by the true value, t, of the quantity, so that $f = (m - t)/t$. Rearranging this equation, we have:

$$m = t(1 + f) \hspace{4cm} \text{Equation 7.2}$$

7.3.4 Combining errors

This section illustrates how to combine errors in some simple examples to obtain an error in the final result.

Error in a product

To take the previous example of measuring the sides of a rectangle, then the measured area A is just the product of the measured lengths of the sides. Now, if the exact lengths are a and b, and the fractional errors are taken as f_a and f_b, then from Equation 7.2 the measured lengths are just $a(1 + f_a)$ and $b(1 + f_b)$ respectively. Hence:

$$
\begin{aligned}
A &= a(1 + f_a) \cdot b(1 + f_b) \\
&= ab(1 + f_a) \cdot (1 + f_b) \\
&= ab(1 + f_a + f_b + f_a \cdot f_b)
\end{aligned}
$$

Now, the product, $f_a \cdot f_b$, is very small compared with f_a and f_b (e.g. if f_a and $f_b = 0.01$, then $f_a \cdot f_b = 0.0001$) and may be neglected, so that we obtain:

$$A = ab(1 + f_a + f_b)$$

We now relate this to f_A which is the fractional error in the exact area, ab, due to the errors involved in measuring the sides a and b. Equation 7.2 gives us: $A = ab(1 + f_A)$. Thus, by comparison with the above formula we can say that $ab(1 + f_A) = ab(1 + f_a + f_b)$. This simplifies to $f_A = f_a + f_b$. Hence, the fractional error in the area, f_A, is just the sum of the fractional errors f_a and f_b produced when measuring the two sides.

Generally, if we have a product involving several terms then, in words:

The fractional (or percentage) error in a product is the sum of the individual fractional (or percentage) errors of each term in the product.

As another example, if the mA is in error by +5% and the exposure time is in error by –2%, then the percentage error in the mAs (Sect. 6.4.2) is +3%. Frequently, however, the signs of the errors are unknown, so they are both taken as either positive or negative to obtain an error band about the measured value. This constitutes the 'worst case' size of the error.

Error in a quotient

If we divide one measured value of an exact quantity, a, by another measured value of an exact quantity, b, then the result obtained, R, is given by:

$$R = \frac{a(1 + f_a)}{b(1 + f_b)}$$

where f_a and f_b are the fractional errors in a and b.

$$R = \frac{a}{b} \cdot (1 + f_a)(1 - f_b) \qquad \text{(approximately)}$$

Expanding the two brackets and ignoring $f_a \cdot f_b$ as described above, we have:

$$R = \frac{a}{b}(1 + f_a - f_b)$$

so that the fractional error in R is $f_a - f_b$.
  Hence:

The fractional error in a quotient is obtained by subtracting the fractional error of the denominator from that of the numerator.

If the signs of the errors are unknown, however, then the worst case is obtained by *adding* the fractional errors.

Error in a sum

If S is obtained by summing measured quantities a and b (whose exact values are $a0$ and $b0$, and whose errors are e_a and e_b) then:

$$S = (a0 + e_a) + (b0 + e_b)$$
$$= a0 + b0 + e_a + e_b$$

Hence, as may be expected:

The error in a sum is the sum of the individual errors.

As in the two previous cases, if the signs of the errors are unknown, then the worst case error is still obtained by adding the errors, i.e. assuming both are either positive or both negative. The fractional error in S, f_s, is given by the formula:

$$f_s = \frac{(a0 \cdot f_a + b0 \cdot f_b)}{a0 + b0}$$

so that the fractional error in a sum depends upon the relative magnitudes of the individual terms and their fractional errors.

Insight

Calculus may be used to obtain an expression for an error by differentiating and treating dx and dy as errors in x and y as shown in the examples in the table below:

Expression	Error	Notes
$y = a + b$	$dy = da + db$	See paragraph above
$y = a \cdot b$	$dy = a \cdot db = b \cdot da$	Fractional error in $a \cdot b$
	$dy/y = db/b = da/a$	
$y = a/b$	$dy = (b \cdot da - a \cdot db)/b \cdot b$	Fractional error in a/b
	$dy/y = da/a - db/b$	
$y = x^2$	$dy = 2x \cdot dx$	
	$dy/y = 2dx/x$	
$y = k/x^2$	$dy = -2k \cdot dx/x^3$	This shows that the relative error in the measurement of radiation from a source using the Inverse Square Law decreases as the distance from the source increases, i.e. dx/x decreases as x increases
	$dy/y = -2dx/x$	

7.3.5 Examples of errors in practical radiography and radiotherapy

Whenever a measurement is made or a procedure is undertaken, inexact quantities will be involved. These are present in even the best and most careful of techniques and do not necessarily invalidate the results of the measurements or procedures performed. It is important to be aware of the magnitude of the errors, however, in order to be confident of the validity of the procedure. This is particularly important in radiotherapy, where the radiation dose delivered to the patient over a course of treatment must be as accurate and as reproducible as can be realistically achieved. For example, an inherent 'chain of errors' exists in the calibration procedure of a therapy machine which involves errors in the following:

- errors of measurement from an ionisation chamber (see Ch. 33) placed in the beam
- errors in correcting the above reading for temperature and pressure
- errors in correcting for various calibration factors
- errors in the positioning of the chamber
- errors in the reproducibility of the therapy machine's output doserate 'switch-on' and 'switch-off' errors, i.e. the output doserate does not immediately assume its steady value on switch-on, nor immediately drop to zero on switch-off
- errors in relating the measured doserate to the '100%' value of an isodose distribution (see Ch. 1) since, in many cases, it is not practicable to measure the 100% value, but some known percentage depth-dose at, say, 5 cm in water.

If all of these errors act in the same direction, for example all tending to make the doserate larger than it really is, then an overall error of 5% or greater is possible. Hence, great attention to detail is required in order to reduce the percentage error to 1% or less.

Further examples of areas where significant errors may occur are shown in Table 7.1.

Table 7.1 Areas of significant potential error

Measurement/procedure	Method	Potential source of error	Comment
FSD/SSD setting (see Ch. 2)	Applicator	Incorrect length	Systematic
	Pointer	Reading error	Random and systematic
	Optical indicator	Incorrect alignment	Systematic
Radiation field size adjustment	Adjustable collimator	Calibration or mechanical error	Random and/or systematic
Image magnification	Measurement of image of an object of known size placed in the appropriate position	Incorrect positioning of the object	Affects magnification
		Incorrect angulation of object to the central ray	May cause elongation or foreshortening of the image
		Inaccurate measurement of image size	Results in an incorrect magnification formula

7.4 STATISTICS

In the preceding sections it was described how repeated measurements of the same quantity will reduce, but not eliminate, the errors of measurement associated with that quantity. This is the situation where a quantity (e.g. a length) has an exact value but where the measured values are clustered around the exact value.

There is another class of measurements which involves a cluster (or population) of values, and that is when measurements are made on different objects belonging to the same category. In this case, the errors of measurement on an individual object may be completely negligible when compared to the magnitude of the natural variation among the objects themselves. For example, the heights of all the radiographers within a given department will probably exhibit quite a large variation and certainly more than the errors involved in measuring the height of one radiographer.

The body of knowledge which concerns itself with the analysis of information (data) obtained from observations is known as *statistics*. There are two types of statistics: *descriptive* and *inferential*. *Descriptive statistics* is concerned solely with such things as the organisation of the data, its graphical display, numerical calculations of means, etc., while *inferential statistics* may be described as the science of making decisions in the face of uncertainty (i.e. on the basis of incomplete information). The latter is the situation frequently encountered in the field of medical statistics where complete information is rarely available.

A group of items belonging to the same category is known as a *population*. A population may be very large (e.g. the number of atoms in a radioactive sample) or small. Note that 'population' as used here does not necessarily imply that people are involved.

Where it is difficult or impossible to collect data on every member of a population, it is necessary only to select a representative sample of that population such that the smaller and more manageable sample has all the important characteristics of the population from which it was drawn, except that of size. This technique is known as 'random sampling', and is much used in public opinion polls, for example. If the sample were not 'random', then there would be a bias in the data collected which would not be present in the larger population, and false conclusions may be drawn. For example, we would not get a reasonable indication of the average weight of patients attending the X-ray department if we happened to select our 'random sample' from patients who were attending a clinic for unexplained weight loss—our sample is not representative of the typical patient population of the X-ray department.

7.4.1 Measures of location and deviation

The graphical representation of the data associated with a population is usually drawn with the measured values on the X-axis and the number of each measured value on the Y-axis. The position of the graph so obtained on the X-axis is known as the *location* of the population, and the width of the graph is its *deviation*. The statistical quantities (usually just called 'statistics') which are used to measure location are the *mean*, *mode* or *median*, while the statistic used to measure deviation is the *standard deviation*. These are described below, together with some other statistical measures.

Mean, mode and median of a population

The *mean* value of a population is the same as the average, and is obtained by dividing the sum of all the data by the number of items in the population. This is shown by the formula:

$$\bar{x} = \frac{\sum\limits_{i=1}^{n} x_i}{n}$$

Equation 7.3

Here, $\bar{x}$ is the mean value, x_i is the ith measured value of the population and n is the number of items. Hence i takes values between 1 and n. The term $\sum\limits_{i=1}^{n} x_i$ means the sum of all the values of x from $i = 1$ to $i = n$, i.e. the sum of the values of all the measurements. Dividing by n produces a value which is somewhere between the minimum and maximum values of the data which form the population. An alternative way of considering the mean is to subtract it from all the other values of x. When this is done, the positive values exactly cancel out the negative values.

The value which occurs most frequently in a given population is not necessarily the mean value, however. Figure 7.1(a–d) shows that there are two other measures, or statistics, of curve location: the *mode* and the *median*. The *mode* is defined as the value which occurs most frequently, and the *median* is the middle value of all the measurements (e.g. in a series of measurements: 1, 2, 4, 4, 5, 6, 6, 6, 7 the median is 5 and the mode is 6). The figures show how these three statistics vary with asymmetrical distributions of values, for 'positive skewness' in Figure 7.1(b) and 'negative skewness' in Figure 7.1(c).

The *standard deviation* is a measure of the variation in the values of a distribution, i.e. by how much the distribution deviates from the mean value. Two symmetrical distributions with the same mean but different standard deviations are shown in Figure 7.2. In a population of n samples and where the ith measured value (i varies from 1 to n) is x_i, either of the two formulae shown below may be used to calculate the standard deviation, σ, of the distribution:

(a)

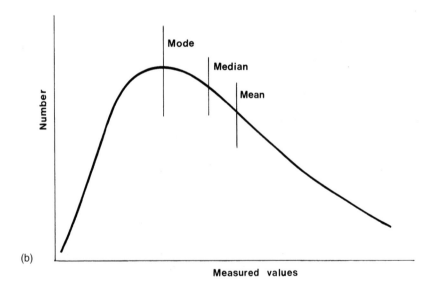

(b)

Figure 7.1a&b Measures of location of a population: (a) shows a symmetrical distribution; and (b) shows a positive skewness.

(c)

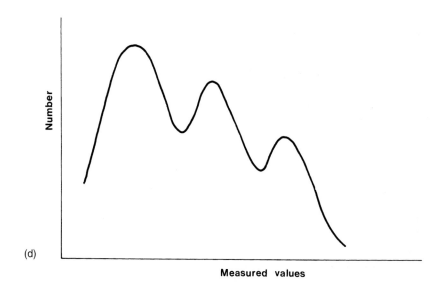

(d)

Figure 7.1c&d Measures of location of a population: (c) shows a negative skewness; and (d) shows a multimodal distribution.

$$\sigma = \sqrt{\frac{\sum_{i=1}^{n}(x_i - \bar{x})^2}{n-1}}$$

$$\sigma = \sqrt{\frac{\sum_{i=1}^{n}(x_i)^2 - \frac{\left(\sum_{i=1}^{n} x_i\right)^2}{n}}{n-1}} \qquad \text{Equation 7.4}$$

The second formula is particularly convenient when using a calculator or computer, since the mean need not be calculated first.

The *coefficient of variation* expresses the standard deviation as a percentage of the mean of a distribution and is equal to $100\sigma/\bar{x}\%$.

Standard error of the mean

There will inevitably be an uncertainty, even if small, in the practical measurement of a mean value, due to the errors inherent in the original observations (Sect. 7.3.2). This uncertainty may be expressed as the standard error of the mean, and is given by:

$$\text{S.E.} = \frac{\sigma}{\sqrt{n}} \qquad \text{Equation 7.5}$$

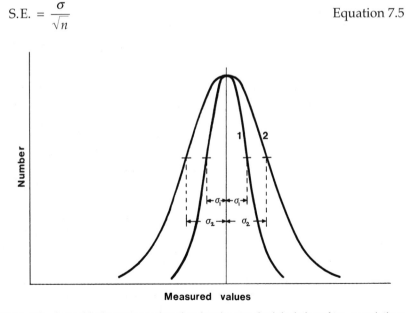

Measured values

Figure 7.2 A graphical representation showing the standard deviation of two populations, 1 and 2, where both distributions have the same mean.

It may be shown that it is 68% probable that the true value of the mean (ignoring systematic errors) lies within 1 standard error above or below the measured mean. Notice that both the standard deviation and standard error of the mean become smaller as the number of measurements, n, increases.

Statistics and diagnostic and therapy radiography

Statistical methods are used widely in all aspects of diagnostic imaging and radiotherapy, and this section touches upon a few examples.
   Quality control:

● The analysis of sizes and types of X-ray films used in different diagnostic investigations is a useful method for predicting future film requirements, and hence reducing waste.
   ● Similarly, the reasons for repeated investigations may be itemised and numbered in a reject analysis, so leading to a clearer understanding of the commonest causes of faulty radiographs. From this analysis, steps may be taken to reduce the number of repeated investigations leading to reduced film wastage, better financial management, and a lower radiation dose to the patient.

Neither of these two examples imposes a complex mathematical or statistical burden on a department, but there are real advantages to be gained in using them.
   Quantum noise. A rather more fundamental (and visible) example of statistics in X-ray imaging is the so-called 'quantum mottle' seen on a television monitor during a fluoroscopic examination of a patient using an image intensification system. This mottle, or quantum noise, is particularly noticeable at low mA or when short-persistence phosphors are used in the intensification system. It is due to the statistical variation of the video signal, which in turn is caused by the random variation in the production of electrons from the faceplate of the image intensifier. At the desired low dose rates for fluoroscopy, there is random variation in the mean values of the X-ray intensity transmitted through the patient, and hence in the production of electrons from the faceplate of the image intensifier and thus the light emitted from the intensifier output phosphor and reaching the television camera tube. This in turn causes variations in the generation of an electrical video signal from the target of the television camera tube. The standard deviation of an average of N electrons produced per second is just $\sqrt{N}$, so that increasing the mA by a factor of 4 increases the mottle by an absolute factor of 2 (i.e. $\sqrt{4}$). However, the *relative* quantum mottle has been reduced from $\sqrt{N}/N = 1/\sqrt{N}$ to $\sqrt{4N}/4N = \frac{1}{2}\sqrt{N}$, so that there has been a halving of the perceived 'noise' on the television monitor. Hence, the effect of quantum mottle on the image is reduced as the mA (or quantity of

radiation) is increased. Obviously a balance must be struck between using such a low doserate that the picture obtained is not adequate for diagnostic purposes or using such a high doserate that the patient receives an unnecessarily high radiation dose. A high-output X-ray tube is required on a CT scanner, for example, in order to reduce the quantum noise in the reconstructed sectional image which otherwise would hide structural detail.

Assessing fetal maturity. A measurement of the fetal biparietal diameter or the crown–rump distance may be used to estimate the age of the fetus. However, not all fetuses grow at the same rate, so a range of normal values for different fetal ages and ethnic groups is first determined by ultrasonic methods, and an unknown age may then be read from an appropriate graph. This is a simple technique, but how may we assess the accuracy of the age read from such a graph—is it within 1 day, 1 week or 1 month? Figure 7.3 shows a plot of the mean biparietal diameter (bpd) against age together with a pair of lines separated from the mean by 2 standard deviations. This means that at any given age, the bpd will be about 95% certain to lie somewhere between the –2σ line and the +2σ line. A measured bpd may be used to estimate an age by drawing a horizontal line on the graph and reading the intersections of the three lines on the Age axis. We may then say that a normal fetus' age is 95% probable to lie between these three lines, with the most likely age given by the mean value. Note that the lines separate more as the age increases, so that there is more uncertainty closer to 40 weeks than at 16 weeks. A typical age estimated by the graph will be accurate to within 1 to 2 weeks, and it is quite unrealistic to expect to be more accurate than this—not because the

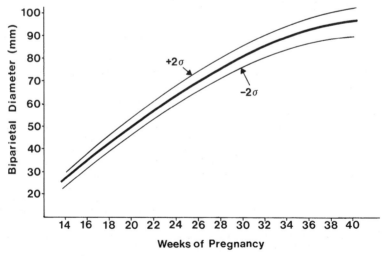

Figure 7.3 Typical appearance of a graph relating the age of a fetus to its mean biparietal diameter (bpd). Also shown are the 2 standard deviations limits within which 95% of the normal values lie.

measurement technique needs improvement, but because of the natural variation in the population of bpds.

Calculation of radiotherapy dose. In radiotherapy, the absorbed radiation dose to a tumour volume is specified by the radiotherapist. However, in a practical situation, it may be known that the absorbed dose is not constant over the whole of the volume to be treated. The radiotherapist may therefore specify a particular dose to a given point, a mean dose or a modal dose depending upon the clinical situation. The mean or modal dose to a volume may be calculated from a computer printout of the dose distribution.

Evaluation of procedures. Statistical methods may be used to select between two different diagnostic or treatment regimes in order to discover which one gives better diagnostic information or treatment results. It is important to select appropriate parameters to measure the relative performance of the two techniques. These may include the number of 'false positives' or 'false negatives' for a diagnostic test, or the '5-year survival rate' or suitably defined 'quality of life' for a therapeutic regime. In any event, a population of values will exist for each regime, and statistical tests of the differences between populations may be used to distinguish between the two techniques in question.

Epidemiology. Finally, statistical methods are employed to find correlations between disease and the environment. This branch of study is known as *epidemiology* and is valuable in suggesting causal links between our way of life, or the pollution in our environment, and the diseases we suffer. This may be performed on a local, national or international level. Obvious examples include smoking and lung cancer or diet and heart disease.

Summary

In this chapter we have considered the following factors which relate to experimentation and statistics:

- Experimental measurements are always subject to errors, both random and systematic (see Sect. 7.3.2).
- The precision of a set of measurements is a measure of their repeatability, while their accuracy is how close they are to the exact result (see Sect. 7.3.2).
- Accuracy is improved by taking a large number of measurements and correcting for the sources of systematic errors (see Sect. 7.3.2).
- The fractional error is the error divided by the mean value (see Sect. 7.3.3).
- The fractional error in a product is obtained by adding the individual fractional errors of each term in the product, and the fractional error in a quotient by subtracting them. If the signs of the errors are unknown, they are added to obtain the 'worst case' error (see Sect. 7.3.4).
- The location of a distribution of measurements (a 'population') may be defined either by the mean, the mode or the median (see Sect. 7.4).
- A measure of the spread of a population is given by the standard deviation, where 68% of all values lie between −1 and +1 standard deviation from the mean, and 95% of values lie within −2 and +2 standard deviations (see Sect. 7.4.1).

SELF-TEST

a. What are the fractional and percentage errors in an mA value which is set to 20, but which is really 22?

b. If a kV_p setting is in error by +5%, the mA by −1%, and the timer overestimates by 2%, what is the percentage error in the Heat Units delivered during an exposure? (For the calculation of Heat Units use Equation 6.7)

c. A particular exposure-timer is always in error by 0.01 s. What is the percentage error in the actual exposure time for the following set times:
   (i) 0.01 s
   (ii) 0.02 s
   (iii) 0.1 s
   (iv) 0.5 s
   (v) 1.0 s?

d. Which condition results in a greater effect on the intensity of an X-ray beam:
   (i) an error of 10% in the mA
   (ii) an error of 10% in the kV_p?
   (*Note:* Intensity is proportional to $mA \times kV_p^2$; see Ch. 28.)

e. Find the mean and the median of the following samples:
   (i) 37, 34, 40, 35, 33, 36, 37
   (ii) 10, 4, 6, 11, 13, 8, 11
   (iii) 52, 70, 37, 55, 42, 31, 47

f. The following readings are taken with a dose-measuring system for a series of 1 minute exposures on a therapy machine: 69.92, 70.20, 69.95, 70.14, 70.14, 69.97, 70.02, 70.24, 70.10, 70.00. Calculate the mean, standard deviation and standard error of the mean of this population. State the range within which 95% of all such readings would lie.

FURTHER READING

There are many specialised textbooks which deal with the topics of experimentation and statistics. Below is a list of titles which may be found in a radiography education library:

Anderson A J B 1991 Interpreting data—a first course in statistics. Chapman & Hall, London
Bland M 1987 An introduction to medical statistics. Oxford University Press, Oxford
Gollnick D A 1978 Experimental radiological health physics. Pergamon Press, New York
Polgarth S, Thomas S 1988 Introduction to Research in Health Sciences. Churchill Livingstone, Edinburgh
Rowntree D 1991 Statistics without tears—a primer for non-mathematicians. Penguin Books, London
White B 1991 Studying for science—a guide to information, communication and study techniques. E & F M Spon, London

Heat

8.1 AIM

The aim of this chapter is to consider heat as a transfer of energy. Links between heat and temperature are also established. The mechanisms of transferring heat are explored and their applications to the cooling of the stationary anode and rotating anode X-ray tube are considered.

8.2 INTRODUCTION

We are familiar with the feelings of *hot* and *cold*; indeed we are crucially dependent on our bodily temperature staying within a very limited range in order to survive. Compared to the vast ranges of temperature which exist across the universe our experience of 'hot' and 'cold' is very limited indeed.

> **Insight**
>
> We are, in fact, better at noticing 'hotter' or 'colder' than we are at determining an absolute value of 'hot' or 'cold'. This can readily be shown from a simple experiment for which you require a bowl of hot water, a bowl of cold water and two bowls of tepid water. Place the right hand in the bowl of hot water and the left hand in the bowl of cold water and leave them in position for about 2 minutes. Now transfer both hands to the bowls of tepid water. You will note that this water feels cold to the right hand and warm to the left hand. This shows that we are better in detecting changes in temperature than we are at detecting absolute values of temperature.

In order to investigate heat further, we must use objective measures of heat and cold as described in the following sections.

8.3 HEAT ENERGY AND TEMPERATURE

When heat is given to a body its atoms or molecules are given increased kinetic energy in the form of increased lattice vibration (this is the reason why substances expand when heated). Thus a body whose atoms have a higher kinetic energy than those of another body is said to be *hotter* or at a higher *temperature*. If two bodies are placed in contact, then heat will be transferred from the hotter body to the cooler body by collisions between the molecules at the point of contact. Thus the molecules of the cooler body receive a net increase in kinetic energy and so its temperature rises. The molecules of the hotter body have lost kinetic energy and so its temperature falls. This process continues until the two bodies are at the same temperature when no further exchange of energy takes place. The bodies are now in a state of *thermal equilibrium*. Notice that the thermal energy is always transferred from the body at the higher temperature to the body at the lower temperature irrespective of the size of the bodies. Also note that the temperature existing at thermal equilibrium will always lie somewhere between the initial temperatures of the two bodies.

> **Insight**
>
> If a body is made to give away thermal energy, then the lattice vibrations of its atoms or molecules will decrease. It is logical to assume that there must therefore be a temperature at which no lattice vibration exists. As all movement of molecules ceases to exist at this temperature, this is the lowest temperature which we can attain. This temperature is known as *absolute zero* and will be further discussed in the next section.

8.3.1 Temperature scales

There are two temperature scales used in modern physics: Celsius (also called centigrade) and Kelvin. The Celsius scale is defined as 0°C at the temperature of melting ice, and 100°C at the temperature of boiling water at an atmospheric pressure of 1.01×10^5 newtons per square metre (76 cm of mercury). On this scale the temperature of absolute zero (see previous Insight) is approximately –273.15°C. This temperature is zero on the Kelvin scale (0 K) while the temperature of melting ice is 273.15 K. From this we can see that the units of temperature are the same on both scales but the scales have different starting points, i.e. one unit on the Celsius scale is equivalent to one unit on the Kelvin scale. Note that temperature on the Kelvin scale does not have the degree symbol in front of the 'K'. It is a convenient approximation to assume that 0°C = 273 K so that the simple conversion formula may be used:

$$T°C = (T + 273) K$$ Equation 8.1

8.3.2 Units of heat energy, specific heat capacity and thermal capacity

As we have already discussed, if heat is given to a body, then its molecules will have a higher kinetic energy and its temperature will rise. Hence it is convenient to express a quantity of heat in terms of the temperature change it produces in a given body. Consider the situation where we wish to apply an amount of energy (Q) which will raise the temperature of a body by 1 kelvin unit (assume for simplicity that this does not change the state of the body, i.e. it does not change from a solid to a liquid). This will be affected by the mass and the type of material of the body. It also seems logical to assume that we would need twice the amount of heat to raise the temperature of the body by 2 kelvin units. If we take all these factors together we can write the equation:

$$Q = mc(T_2 - T_1)$$ Equation 8.2

where Q is the heat energy required to raise the temperature of a body of mass m from T_1 to a temperature T_2. The factor c is approximately constant for a particular material and is known as the *specific heat capacity* of the material. We can rearrange Equation 8.2 to get:

$$c = \frac{Q}{m(T_2 - T_1)}$$ Equation 8.3

so that c, the specific heat capacity, is in units of joules per kilogram per kelvin ($J \cdot kg^{-1} \cdot K^{-1}$). Specific heat capacity can be defined thus:

Definition

The *specific heat capacity* of a body is the energy in *joule* which is required to raise the temperature of *1 kg* of the body by *1 kelvin unit*.

The specific heat capacity is thus unique to a substance and it allows us to predict the behaviour of different masses of the same substance.

Example

The specific heat capacity of water is about 4.2 kJ·kg^{-1}·K^{-1}. How much heat energy is required to raise a mass of 10 g of water from 280 K to 285 K? (Remember that the unit of energy is the joule and the unit of mass is the kilogram.)

Using equation 8.2 we have:

$$Q = mc(T_2 - T_1)$$
$$= 10^{-2} \times 4.2 \times 10^3 \times (285 - 280)$$
$$= 210 \text{ joules}$$

In the situations considered so far we have considered the amount of heat required to raise the temperature of 1 kg of the material. Another unit of heat energy which is useful in practice is the *thermal capacity*.

Definition

The *thermal capacity* of a body is the heat energy in joule which is required to raise the temperature of the body by 1 *kelvin unit*.

Note that this definition differs from the previous one for *specific heat capacity* in that no mention is made of *unit mass*. Thus the thermal capacity refers to the whole of the body and not just 1 kg of it. It should also be noted that the *thermal capacity* of a body is the *specific heat capacity* of the body multiplied by the *mass* of the body. The units of thermal capacity are J·K^{-1}.

Example

The anode disks of two X-ray tubes are made of the same material but one has twice the mass of the other. If the same amount of heat is applied to each anode, which will have the higher temperature rise at the end of the exposure?

The thermal capacity is the product of the mass and the specific heat. Thus the larger anode will have twice the thermal capacity of the smaller one. If the same amount of heat is applied to each, the smaller one will experience twice the temperature rise of the larger one. The importance of this will be considered when we consider the rating of the X-ray tube (Ch. 23).

8.4 TRANSFER OF HEAT

As we mentioned at the beginning of this chapter, heat can be given to a body from some other structure with greater thermal energy than the body. Similarly, if a body can be isolated from its environment or is in a state of thermal equilibrium with its surroundings, there is no net gain or loss of heat from the body.

The mechanisms of heat transfer form an important part of the study of radiography because of the large amounts of heat energy produced at the target of the X-ray tube. The mechanical and thermal stress associated with this make it possible to damage the X-ray tube unless adequate precautions are taken. The anodes of all X-ray tubes must therefore be designed to transfer heat away from the focal spot as quickly as possible in order to minimise the temperature rise in this region. To understand how this is achieved, we must first understand the different mechanisms of heat transfer and then we will look at the practical application of this knowledge to the design of X-ray tubes. The three methods of heat transfer are *conduction*, *convection* and *radiation*.

8.4.1 Conduction

Conduction is the transfer of heat between bodies by physical contact of those bodies and therefore results in a transfer of kinetic energy by interatomic collision, thus forming the main process by which heat is transferred through a solid. If we apply heat to one end of a metal bar, the atoms at this end of the bar receive copious supplies of kinetic energy. These atoms, because of their increased vibrational energy, collide with neighbouring atoms and so kinetic energy is transferred gradually along the bar. This method of heat flow along the bar is known as *conduction* of heat.

We can find by experiment that the rate of flow of heat, q (joules per second or watt; see Sect. 6.3.7), by conduction is controlled by a number of things:

- $q \propto A$ (the cross-sectional area of the rod)
- $q \propto (T_1 - T_2)$ (the temperature difference between the ends of the rod; this is known as the temperature gradient)
- $q \propto (1/l)$ (where l is the length of the rod)
- q depends on the material of the rod.

Combining all these factors we have:

$$q \propto \frac{A(T_1 - T_2)}{l}$$

$$q = \frac{kA(T_1 - T_2)}{l}$$

Equation 8.4

Here k is the constant of proportionality and this is a constant for any given material. This is known as the *thermal conductivity* of the material. Materials are classed as 'good' or 'bad' conductors depending on the value of k. Typical values of k are shown in Table 8.1.

Table 8.1 Thermal conductivity of materials

Material	Thermal conductivity $(W \cdot m^{-1} \cdot K^{-1})$	Comments
Copper	386	Excellent conductor—used as the anode material in the stationary anode tube
Tungsten	202	Fairly good conductor—used as the target material in X-ray tubes
Molybdenum	147	Relatively poor conductor—used as the anode stem in the rotating anode tube
Glass	1.0	Poor conductor—is involved in the transfer of heat to the oil in the tube housing
Rubber	0.05	Very poor conductor
Air	0.02	Very poor conductor—removes heat from the housing of the X-ray tube by convection

Also note that the rate of flow of heat along a bar can be altered by altering the length, the cross-sectional area and the temperature gradient as well as by altering the material.

8.4.2 Convection

Convection is the main process by which heat is transferred in fluids (i.e. liquids and gases). If we consider heat being applied to a liquid in a beaker (see Fig. 8.1), then the liquid near the source of heat has thermal energy

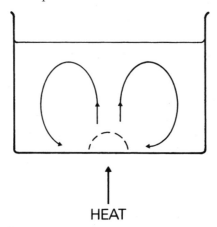

HEAT

Figure 8.1 Principles of convection. Applied heat causes the dotted region of fluid to expand, become less dense and rise, being replaced by cooler parts of the fluid. This sets up convection currents.

transferred to it by conduction. This increase in thermal energy causes the liquid to expand and consequently become less dense than the surrounding liquid. This causes the heated liquid to rise (as a result of hydrostatic pressure) and, as it rises, it transfers heat to the surrounding molecules by conduction. Thus the temperature of the small section of heated liquid returns to the same temperature as the surrounding liquid and so sinks back into the beaker to be heated a second time. Thus *convection currents* are established as shown in the diagram. The overall effect is that the whole volume of fluid is heated and not just the region where the heat is applied.

Some interesting points emerge from this:

- Convection can only occur where the molecules are free to move through the medium, i.e. in liquids and gases.
- It is not possible to have convection currents without some conduction.
- It is necessary to have a gravitational field in order for the convection currents to be initiated as the warm fluid moves in the opposite direction to the gravitational force, by hydrostatic pressure.

8.4.3 Radiation

In this process, heat is lost from a body with high thermal energy in the form of electromagnetic radiations. Radiation is the only heat transfer process which will take place through a *vacuum*. The most obvious and striking example is the heat we can feel from our sun where the radiation must pass through a near perfect vacuum for 93 million miles. Light and heat also reach us from other stars but we are able to discern only the light as we are not sufficiently sensitive to small amounts of heat (although the latter can be detected with infra-red sensors).

We are able to feel heat by radiation because it imparts kinetic energy to molecules of our tissues, which we discern as an increase in temperature. Heat radiations occur in a band of energies just beyond the red part of the visible spectrum (see Ch. 25 for further detail of the electromagnetic spectrum). This band of energies is known as *infra-red radiations*. All bodies radiate electromagnetic energies if their temperature is above absolute zero. This does not necessarily mean that we can discern the radiations as we perceive only a narrow band of energies extending from violet light to infra-red. Bodies of different colours and different surface compositions radiate somewhat differently and so it is conventional to consider *black body radiation*. This we will do next.

8.4.4 Black body radiation

A body looks black because very little of the light incident upon it is *reflected* or *transmitted*. A *black body* is defined as one which will absorb

100% of all radiations at all frequencies incident upon it. If such a black body is in a state of thermal equilibrium with its surroundings, then equal amounts of radiation must be absorbed and emitted per second. Hence it can be deduced that the black body must radiate more energy than any other type of body since no other body absorbs 100% of the energy incident upon it. The foregoing statements can be summarised thus:

- All bodies are capable of emitting radiation.
- A black body absorbs 100% of all radiations incident upon it.
- A black body is the most efficient emitter of radiation of any body.

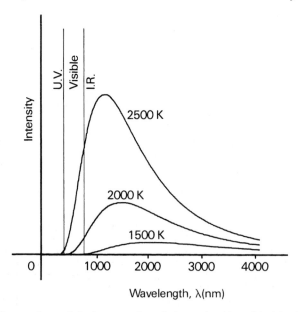

Figure 8.2 The spectrum of electromagnetic radiation emitted by a 'black body' at different temperatures. The total intensity is a function of the kelvin temperature ($I \propto T^4$).

We now need to know in more detail the spectrum of radiations emitted by a black body. Figure 8.2 shows such a spectrum for a black body at different temperatures. The following should be noted from the graph:

- The wavelength corresponding to the peak radiation progressively decreases as the temperature of the body increases.
- The height of the graph (intensity of radiation) is very sensitive to changes in temperature.
- The spectrum of the radiation is a smooth curve of which we perceive only a small part (violet to infra-red).
- The total intensity of the radiation emitted by a body at a given temperature is the sum of the intensities at each wavelength. This is therefore related to the area under the curve in each case. *Stefan's Law*

states that the total intensity of the emitted radiation is proportional to the *fourth* power of the *kelvin temperature*. Thus:

$$I \propto T^4$$

or $I = \sigma T^4$ Equation 8.5

where σ is Stefan's Constant.

Thus a doubling of the kelvin temperature results in the amount of heat radiation emitted being increased by a factor of $2^4 = 16$ times. As we can see from this, the intensity of the radiation emitted varies greatly with the body temperature. This has important consequences in the design of the rotating anode X-ray tube disk as we shall see later in this chapter.

A curve of emitted radiation at about 1000 K is equivalent to a metal rod which has been heated until it is glowing cherry red. As the temperature increases, the colour changes through light red to white since an increasing amount of the violet end of the spectrum is emitted along with the red (see 2000 K and 2500 K graphs in Fig. 8.2). At higher temperatures, objects emit white light—this is true of the filament of an electric light bulb or the anode disk of the rotating anode tube after a large exposure.

Insight

The mechanism which causes the emission of radiation is the acceleration and deceleration of the charged particles which make up the atoms or molecules of the body involved. An example particularly relevant to radiography is the sudden deceleration of electrons when they strike the anode of the X-ray tube—the *Bremsstrahlung* or *braking radiation*. Here some (or all) of the kinetic energy of the electron is transformed into an X-ray photon (see Ch. 28). Another example is the production of radio waves, where electrons are forced to oscillate at high frequencies in a radio transmitting aerial.

Thus the interactions of energetic atoms produce a broad band of emitted quanta wavelengths because of the range of interactions which are possible. All of these radiations form part of the electromagnetic spectrum. A narrow range of frequencies (in the infra-red part) are capable of being absorbed by the whole atom (as opposed to the electron shells or the nucleus) and so these atoms gain kinetic energy. This increase in the kinetic energy of the atoms is in the form of heat. Higher frequencies of radiation interact with the electrons in the orbitals and even higher frequencies will interact with the atomic nuclei.

8.5 THERMAL EXPANSION

Most substances expand when heated owing to the increased kinetic energy of the atoms. The *linear expansivity* is a measure of this thermal expansion and is defined as *the fractional change in unit length per unit change in kelvin temperature*. The thermal expansion of different parts of the X-ray tube is an important design consideration as the tube is subject to large temperature variations during its working life. If materials of very different thermal expansivity are used, this can cause mechanical stress which could result in fracture of one of the components. A particularly weak point in this respect is the seal between the glass and the copper anode in a stationary anode tube. A special type of glass with a thermal expansivity very similar to copper is chosen. This reduces the mechanical stress and thus the chances of fracture of the glass envelope and loss of vacuum in the tube.

8.6 EVAPORATION AND VAPORISATION

We are all familiar with the evaporation of liquids which occurs when heat is applied to them, e.g. boiling kettles. Evaporation is caused by the loss of *whole atoms* from the surface of the liquid. Some of the atoms are given sufficient kinetic energy to escape from the forces of attraction of their neighbours near the surface of the liquid and produce a vapour in the free space above this surface.

Whole atoms may also be liberated from the surfaces of *solid* materials under the action of heat. There is a stronger force of attraction between the atoms in a solid compared to a liquid and so liberation of the atoms is more difficult to accomplish. This means that in a solid the atoms require higher kinetic energy for liberation, i.e. solids need to be subjected to a higher temperature. The tungsten at the target and in the filament of the X-ray tube is subjected to such high temperatures that a certain amount of *vaporisation* takes place. The tungsten vapour can condense to form a thin layer of tungsten on the inside of the glass of the envelope (see Fig. 8.3). The major effect of this is to reduce the electrical insulation provided by the glass as tungsten is a reasonable conductor of electricity. This can produce an effect called a 'gassy tube', which renders the X-ray tube inoperable. Fortunately this does not occur too readily as tungsten has a low *vapour pressure* so does not readily vaporise at its normal working temperatures.

8.7 HEAT LOSS FROM AN X-RAY TUBE

The mechanisms of heat loss discussed earlier in this chapter will now be discussed in relation to the heat loss from the anode of both a stationary anode and a rotating anode X-ray tube. In the case of all X-ray tubes, a large amount of heat is generated during the X-ray exposure and so efficient heat loss is necessary to protect the tube against thermal damage and to allow short exposures of high intensity.

8.7.1 The stationary anode tube

Figure 8.3 shows the construction of a typical stationary anode tube in its housing. Superimposed on the figure are arrows originating from the focal spot which represent the paths taken by the heat energy to remove the heat from this small area of high temperature. The arrows marked (R) represent heat loss by radiation, while those marked (C) represent heat loss by conduction and those marked (CV) represent convection. The sequence of events is as follows:

- An exposure is made resulting in a considerable amount of heat energy being deposited at the focal spot of the tungsten target. This energy must be quickly dispersed otherwise the temperature rise at the target will cause thermal damage.
- Some of the heat is lost from the focal spot by radiation through the vacuum to be absorbed by the glass envelope and the oil.
- The main heat loss is by conduction through the tungsten target into the copper anode block and along the anode stem.
- The end of the stem is in contact with the oil and so sets up convection currents which warm up the whole of the oil. The oil expands as its temperature increases and, at a certain temperature, it will cause the ex-pansion bellows to trip the microswitch, preventing further exposures.
- Heat from the oil passes through the metal casing by conduction.
- The warm casing sets up convection currents in the air of the room.

Thus all three processes of conduction, convection and radiation are involved in the removal of heat from the focal spot. However, the stationary anode tube is designed to remove the majority of the heat from

Figure 8.3 Stationary anode X-ray tube and housing. Heat is lost from the target mainly by conduction (C) but convection (CV) and radiation (R) also play a part in the dissipation of heat from the target to the atmosphere of the room. *Key:* H—housing; L—lead lining; M—microswitch; B—expansion bellows; E—envelope; V—vacuum in envelope; K—cathode; F—filament; T—tungsten target; A—copper anode.

the target by *conduction*. From Equation 8.3 we can see that conduction depends on the type of material, the cross-sectional area, the temperature gradient and the length of the conductor. To maximise heat transfer by conduction:

- a material of high thermal conductivity (copper) is chosen
- a large cross-sectional area of anode block is used
- one end of the anode stem is surrounded by oil to achieve a temperature gradient
- the anode length is as short as possible.

The tungsten insert itself is not as good a thermal conductor as copper so is kept as thin as possible. The melting point of copper is 1083°C and this imposes a practical limit on the amount of heat which can be applied to the anode. The anode is, however, constructed with a fairly large mass thus increasing its thermal capacity and limiting the temperature rise in the copper.

8.7.2 The rotating anode tube

All three processes are again involved in the heat loss from the focal spot of the rotating anode tube, but in this case the main mechanism of heat loss is *radiation*, not conduction.

Figure 8.4 shows the main parts in the construction of the insert of the rotating anode X-ray tube. The focal track is made of a mixture of tungsten and rhenium and the main structure of the disk is made of molybdenum. Molybdenum has approximately twice the specific heat capacity and half the density of tungsten and so the thermal capacity of the disk can be increased without increasing its mass. As we saw earlier (see Stefan's Law)

Figure 8.4 The rotating anode X-ray tube insert. *Key:* A—anode disk; F—focal track; S—anode stem; R—rotor sleeve; B—ball bearings; T—rotor spindle; E—envelope; K—cathode; W—stator windings.

the heat loss from a body by radiation is proportional to T^4 and so heat loss from the disk by radiation can be encouraged by allowing it to reach a high temperature—during large exposures it gets 'white hot'. Thermal equilibrium may be achieved during longer exposures where the rate of heat loss balances the rate at which heat is deposited.

The heat radiated from the anode disk is absorbed by the glass envelope and the oil, setting up convection currents in the oil. Heat is then conducted through the casing and convected in the air of the room as in the case of the stationary anode tube.

While we wish the disk to dissipate its heat by radiation, we wish to prevent heat from travelling along the anode stem by conduction in order to prevent overheating of the ball bearings. This is achieved in three ways:

- the stem is made of molybdenum which has fairly poor thermal conductivity
- it is made with as small a cross-sectional area as possible
- it is made as long as mechanically practicable.

The anode rotor is also blackened to encourage heat loss by black body radiation.

Overheating of the anode disk may result in mechanical damage to the disk (e.g. cracking or pitting) or it may cause softening of the stem which will result in instability of the anode.

Summary

In this chapter you should have learnt:

- That heat is a form of energy produced by the kinetic energy of atoms in a body (see Sect. 8.3)
- The greater the kinetic energy of the atoms the higher the *temperature* and vice versa (see Sect. 8.3)
- That bodies which are in *thermal equilibrium* with their surroundings lose heat as fast as they gain heat and so experience no change in temperature (see Sect. 8.3)
- *Absolute zero* temperature corresponds to zero atomic kinetic energy and has a temperature of 0 kelvin (see Sect. 8.3.1)
- On the Kelvin scale the temperature at which ice melts is approximately 273 K (see Sect. 8.3.1)
- The link between heat and temperature provided by *specific heat capacity* and *thermal capacity* (see Sect. 8.3.2)
- Heat may be transferred from one point to another by *conduction* (mainly in solids), *convection* (in fluids) and *radiation* (may travel through a vacuum) (see Sects 8.4.1, 8.4.2 and 8.4.3)
- Heat must be transferred quickly from the focal spot of an X-ray tube if thermal damage is to be avoided (see Sect. 8.7)
- For a stationary anode tube *conduction* is the main mechanism of heat loss— therefore a copper anode with a large cross-sectional area is used (see Sect. 8.7.1)
- For a rotating anode tube *radiation* is the main mechanism of heat loss. Higher anode temperatures are required to give efficient heat loss (Stefan's Law: intensity $\propto T^4$) (see Sect. 8.7.2).

SELF-TEST

a. Why does a metal bar expand if it is heated?

b. The boiling point of water is 100°C. What is this in kelvin units?

c. The specific heat capacity of water is 4.2 kJ·kg^{-1}·K^{-1}. Calculate the power required to raise the temperature of 10 litres of water from 20°C to 32°C in 10 minutes.

d. The specific heat capacity of molybdenum is approximately twice the specific heat capacity of tungsten. If the same amount of heat is applied to two disks, one made of tungsten and one made of molybdenum each having the same mass, what will be the relationship between the temperature change produced in each disk?

e. Describe the mechanism by which heat is transferred by conduction.

f. Describe the mechanism by which heat is transferred by convection.

g. Describe the mechanism by which heat is transferred by radiation.

h. Compare the methods of heat loss from the target of the stationary anode and the rotating anode X-ray tubes.

FURTHER READING

Further information on X-ray tube design and rating is available in Chapters 22 and 23 of this text. The following may also prove useful:

Heat and heat transfer processes
Ball J L, Moore A D 1986 Essential physics for radiographers, 2nd edn. Blackwell Scientific Publications, London, ch 2
Hay G A, Hughes D 1983 First year physics for radiographers. Baillière Tindall, London, ch 1

X-ray tube design and cooling pathways
Ball J L, Moore A D 1986 Essential physics for radiographers, 2nd edn. Blackwell Scientific Publications, London, ch 12
Hay G A, Hughes D 1983 First year physics for radiographers. Baillière Tindall, London, ch 11
Hendee W, Ritenour R 1992 Medical imaging physics, 3rd edn. Mosby Year Book, London, ch 5
Johns H E, Cunningham J R 1983 The physics of radiology, 4th edn. Charles C Thomas, Illinois, USA, ch 2

9

Electrostatics

9.1 AIM

The aim of this chapter is to introduce the reader to the concepts involved in understanding the electrostatics which is relevant to radiographic science. This involves the consideration of electrical charge, charge distribution and electrical potential and potential difference.

9.2 INTRODUCTION

Electrostatics, as the name implies, is the study of static electrical charges. We are familiar with many examples of electrostatics from our ordinary lives, from sparks which may occur from our clothes when undressing, to the large discharges of electricity which occur during lightning strikes. Much of the early experimentation with electricity involved electrostatics. It was discovered at a fairly early stage that there were *two* types of electrical charge, one of which was called *negative* and the other *positive*. While it is mathematically convenient to regard charge in this way, it does not explain what electrical charge actually is and how it behaves. This will be the subject of this chapter.

9.3 PROPERTIES OF ELECTRICAL CHARGES

The general properties of electrical charges are as follows:

- Charges can be considered as being of two types: positive and negative.
- The smallest unit of negative charge which can exist in isolation is that possessed by an electron, and the smallest unit of positive charge which can exist in isolation is that possessed by the proton.
- Electrical charges exert forces on each other even when they are separated by a vacuum. The forces are mutual, equal and opposite as expected by Newton's Third Law (see Sect. 5.5).
- Like charges (i.e. charges of the same sign) *repel* each other while unlike charges (of opposite signs) *attract* each other.
- The magnitude of the mutual forces between the charges is influenced by:
  — the magnitude of the individual charges
  — the medium in which they are embedded, being greatest when the medium is a vacuum
  — the inverse square of the distance between the charged bodies—this is another application of the Inverse Square Law (see Sect. 3.3).
- Electrical charges may be *induced* in a body by the proximity of a charged body, leading to a force of attraction between the two bodies.
- Electrical charges may flow easily in some materials (called *electrical conductors*) and with difficulty in other materials (called *electrical insulators*). Both types of material are capable of having charges induced in them.
- When electrical charges move they produce a magnetic field.

9.4 FORCE BETWEEN TWO ELECTRICAL CHARGES IN A VACUUM

Consider two charges q_1 and q_2 separated by a distance d in a vacuum as shown in Figure 9.1.

If we assume that both charges are of the same sign, then q_1 will exert a force of repulsion (F) on q_2 and q_2 will exert the same force of repulsion on q_1. As we have already stated above, it can be shown that:

Figure 9.1 The forces between two electrical charges q_1 and q_2 separated by a distance d are equal and opposite.

a. $F \propto q_1$
b. $F \propto q_2$
c. $F \propto 1/d^2$.

Thus F is proportional to the magnitude of each charge and to the inverse square of the distance separating them.

If we combine the factors in (a), (b) and (c) above we can produce the equation:

$$F \propto \frac{q_1 q_2}{d^2} \qquad \text{Equation 9.1}$$

If q_1 and q_2 both have the same sign, then F will be positive and will represent a force of repulsion. If the charges have opposite signs, then F will be negative and will represent a force of attraction.

If we wish to replace the proportionality sign in Equation 9.1 by an equals sign then we need to introduce a constant of proportionality (see Appendix A). This equation now reads:

$$F = \frac{q_1 q_2}{4 \pi \varepsilon_0 d^2} \qquad \text{Equation 9.2}$$

This equation is often referred to as *Coulomb's Law* of force between two charges and has particular relevance when we consider the charges between subatomic particles (Chs 26 and 27).

The constant of proportionality is $1/4\pi\varepsilon_0$, where ε_0 is the *permittivity of a vacuum* and has a value of 8.85×10^{-12} F·m^{-1}. The charges q_1 and q_2 are expressed in *coulombs*, the separation d is in *metres* and the force F is in *newtons*.

The *coulomb* corresponds to the charge carried by 6×10^{18} electrons or protons. An alternative (and more practical) definition of the coulomb is:

Definition

A charge of 1 *coulomb* is possessed by a point if an equal charge placed 1 metre away from it in a vacuum experiences a force of repulsion of $1/4\pi\varepsilon_0$ newton.

Insight

The influence of the Inverse Square Law on the force between charged bodies may be grasped if we assume that charged bodies emanate *lines of force* in all directions similar to the light emission from a point source of light obeying the Inverse Square Law. The number of such lines of force is proportional to the magnitude of the charge (analogous to the brightness of the light source). This is shown diagrammatically in Figure 9.2 where the arrows point in the direction of the force experienced by a positive charge if placed at that point. There will be further discussion of lines of force in the section of this chapter dealing with electrical field strength (see Sect. 9.6).

(a)　　　　　　　　(b)　　　　　　　　(c)

Figure 9.2 Electric 'lines of force' associated with (a) a weak positive charge, (b) a weak negative charge and (c) a strong positive charge.

9.5 PERMITTIVITY AND RELATIVE PERMITTIVITY (DIELECTRIC CONSTANT)

Equation 9.2 holds true only when the charges are in a vacuum as ε_0 is the permittivity of a vacuum. In any other medium the equation requires to be modified to:

$$F = \frac{q_1 q_2}{4\pi\varepsilon d^2} \qquad \text{Equation 9.3}$$

where ε is the permittivity of the medium.

It is, however, often convenient to compare the permittivity of the medium relative to that of a vacuum, e.g. if the permittivity of the medium is twice that of a vacuum, then the *relative permittivity* (K) is 2. This can be obtained from the simple formula:

$$K = \frac{\varepsilon}{\varepsilon_0}$$

or by cross-multiplying:

$$\varepsilon = \varepsilon_0 K \qquad \text{Equation 9.4}$$

so Equation 9.3 may be rewritten as:

$$F = \frac{q_1 q_2}{4\pi\varepsilon_0 K d^2}$$
Equation 9.5

K is known as the *dielectric constant* of the medium and so we can see that the relative permittivity and the dielectric constant are the same. Note that as the dielectric constant is a comparative number it does not have any units. (The dielectric constant is further discussed in Ch. 16 where we consider its importance in capacitors.)

9.6 ELECTRICAL FIELD STRENGTH

We have already seen that an electric charge is capable of influencing other charges placed at a distance from it. This influence on other charges at a distance is known as a *field* and, for the purpose of comparing electrical charges, E is measured as the force on a unit positive charge. E is therefore measured in units of newton/coulomb. Consider the electric field around a point charge. If we wish to know the field strength at a point we simply place a unit positive charge at that point and measure the magnitude and direction of the force exerted upon it. If we consider Equation 9.5 and have $q_2 = 1$ (unit charge) then we can say that:

$$E = \frac{q_1 \times 1}{4\pi\varepsilon_0 K d^2}$$

$$E = \frac{q_1}{4\pi\varepsilon_0 K d^2}$$
Equation 9.6

We have already considered a diagrammatic representation of the field around a point charge (Fig. 9.2). The arrows represent the direction of the force acting on a unit positive charge (if placed at that point) and the line density represents the intensity of the electrical field.

9.7 ELECTROSTATIC INDUCTION OF CHARGE

As mentioned earlier, a charge may be induced on an electrical conductor or on an insulator. Each will now be considered.

9.7.1 Induction of a conductor

The situation which exists if an electrically charged body (B) is placed close to a conductor (A) is shown in Figure 9.3. A conductor is a body which will

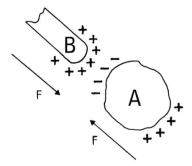

Figure 9.3 Induction of a charge on a conducting body, A, results in a force of attraction (*F*) with the inducing body.

allow a flow of electrons. The positive charge on B attracts electrons to it and leaves equal numbers of positive charges on the opposite surface of A. Notice that the opposite charge is induced on the surface of the conductor closest to the inducing charge. Also note that equal numbers of positive and negative charges are induced. There is eventually a state of equilibrium where the electrons on the surface of A experience an equal force of attraction from the two sets of positive charge. When this happens, no further electron flow takes place.

The charge distribution results in a net force of attraction as the unlike charges are closer to the charged body than the like charges.

Withdrawal of the charged body results in uniform distribution of the charges in A.

9.7.2 Induction of an insulator (dielectric)

If we bring a charged body close to an insulator, a similar force of attraction occurs—this can be demonstrated by running a comb through your hair and holding it close to a small piece of paper which will be attracted to it. This result is somewhat surprising as electrons cannot move as freely through an insulator as a conductor. Some insulators are more efficient at producing induced charges than others and it is found that this varies with the dielectric constant (see Sect. 9.5) of the material. There are two explanations of the induced charge in an insulator, *molecular distortion* and *polar molecules*.

Molecular distortion

A body is composed of atoms or molecules. These contain equal numbers of protons (+ve) and electrons (−ve) thus making the body electrically neutral. As can be seen in Figure 9.4(a), the electrons normally form symmetrical orbits around the nucleus so that the average position of the

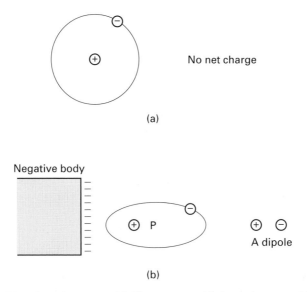

(a)

(b)

Figure 9.4 The effect of an external field on an atom: (a) shows the atom with no external field applied; (b) shows the polarisation of the atom to form a dipole caused by the proximity of a negatively charged body.

electron is over the nucleus, and so the two sets of charges cancel each other out. If a charged body is placed close to the atom (see Fig. 9.4(b)), then the electron orbits are distorted relative to the atomic nucleus. The average position of the electrons is now displaced to one side of the atom, and so the atom has been *polarised* into an *electrical dipole*.

Polar molecules

Some molecules exist in which the atoms are so arranged that the average position of the electrons is not coincident with that of the nuclei even when the atoms are not subject to an electrical field. These molecules are polarised even when not subject to an electric field. The effect of an external electric field is to rotate these molecules such that they tend to become aligned with the field. This means that the structure now has a definite positive end and a definite negative end as shown in Figure 9.5. Within the body, the dipoles are so close together that the positive and negative ends of adjacent dipoles cancel each other's effects. Practical dielectrics use such materials as they produce a much stronger effect than molecular distortion alone.

9.8 ELECTRICAL POTENTIAL

There are a number of similarities between electrical potential and potential energy. In the case of potential energy this represents the work done in

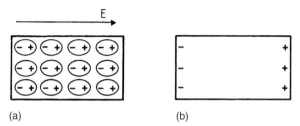

Figure 9.5 The induction of charge on an insulator containing polar molecules: (a) shows the alignment of the polar molecules; (b) shows the net charges at the ends of the body.

raising the body through a height h with reference to zero level. Similar concepts will now be discussed for electrical potential.

9.8.1 Zero electrical potential

The most convenient point to choose as having zero electrical potential is the point at which the force exerted by the charged body on a unit positive charge would be zero. This point is *infinity* and all work performed on a unit charge is measured from there. Obviously infinity is chosen for its mathematical convenience rather than its practicality!

Insight

It is often stated that 'the earth is at zero potential'. The earth is assumed to be electrically neutral in that it contains equal numbers of positive and negative charges. Thus there is no force between neutral earth and a unit positive charge and so no effort is needed to move the latter towards earth. Hence no work is done and the electrical potential of earth, or any other neutral body, is zero.

9.8.2 Absolute potential and potential difference

From the discussion so far, we may define the *absolute electrical potential* at a point as follows:

Definition

The *absolute electrical potential* at a point is the work done in moving a unit positive charge from infinity to that point.

In practice it is often more convenient to compare the potential at one point relative to another rather than know its absolute potential. If the potential at point A is V_A and the potential at a point B is V_B then the potential difference (PD) between A and B is $V_A - V_B$ and represents the difference in the work done in moving a unit positive charge from infinity to point A and from infinity to point B. It can be seen that this is the same as the work which would be required to move a unit positive charge from point A to point B. This leads to the definition of *potential difference*:

> **Definition**
>
> The *potential difference* between two points is the work done on a unit positive charge in moving it from one point to the other.

9.8.3 The volt

The volt is the SI unit of potential and is defined as:

> **Definition**
>
> *1 volt* of *potential* exists at a point if *1 joule* of work is performed in moving *1 coulomb of positive charge* from infinity to that point.

Similarly for potential difference we have:

> **Definition**
>
> *1 volt* of *potential difference* exists between two points if *1 joule* of work is done in moving *1 coulomb of positive charge* from one point to the other.

These definitions can be shown in the form of an equation:

$$\text{volts} = \frac{\text{joules}}{\text{coulombs}}$$

Equation 9.6

9.8.4 Electrical potential due to a point charge

Consider a point charge Q as shown in Figure 9.6 where a unit positive charge has been moved from infinity to a distance r from Q. The nearer the unit charge comes to Q the greater the force of repulsion (if Q is positive) or attraction (if Q is negative). Thus the *potential is positive if Q is positive and negative if Q is negative* since the potential is the *work done on* the unit positive charge. If we consider that the work done on all unit positive charges which are equidistant from Q will be the same, then it is logical to assume that *equipotential surfaces* will be concentric spheres with Q as the centre—this is similar to the concentric spheres concept of the Inverse Square Law (see Sect. 3.4.1). It is also worth noting that the particular path chosen to bring a unit positive charge from infinity to the point r is of no importance and so paths (1) and (2) give exactly the same electrical potential.

Electrical potential is usually given the symbol V and so we can produce the equation:

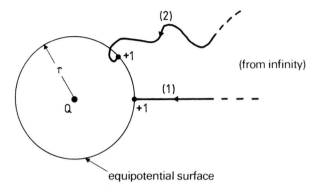

Figure 9.6   The electrical potential energy of a point charge Q.

work = force × distance

$$V = \frac{Q \times r}{4\pi\varepsilon_0 r^2}$$

$$V = \frac{Q}{4\pi\varepsilon_0 r}$$ Equation 9.7

where V is in Volts, Q is in coulombs and r is in metres.

The electrical potential due to a point charge is given the term *Coulomb potential* and the force between two charges is the *Coulomb force* (see Sect. 9.4).

9.8.5 Electrical potential due to a conducting sphere

If we place a charge Q on a conducting sphere, then the charged particles will mutually repel each other and so the charges will be evenly distributed on the outer surface of the sphere—this is true whether the sphere is hollow or is solid. Thus no potential difference exists between any points either on the surface or within the sphere (if a potential difference did exist the charge would redistribute in such a way that the whole body was at a constant potential). When we consider the potential which exists outside the sphere, it may be shown mathematically that the sphere behaves as though all the charge Q is placed at its centre. This is shown in the graph in Figure 9.7. Thus Equation 9.7 can be used to calculate the potential of points outside the sphere where r is the distance from the centre of the sphere.

9.9 DISTRIBUTION OF ELECTRICAL CHARGE ON AN IRREGULARLY SHAPED CONDUCTOR

Having considered the charge distribution on a sphere, it is now useful to consider the distribution of charge on a conducting body of irregular

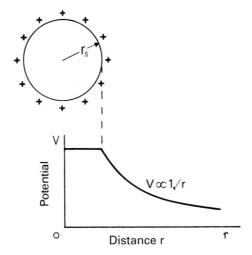

Figure 9.7 The electrical potential of a conducting sphere of radius r_s. The potential is constant within the sphere and reduces outside it ($V \propto 1/r$).

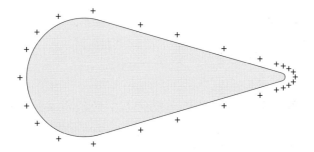

Figure 9.8 The distribution of positive charge on an irregularly shaped conductor. *Note* the high intensity of charge at the area of low radius of curvature.

shape. Such a body is shown in Figure 9.8. Again the charge is distributed so that no potential difference exists between any points *within the body*. This gives the charge distribution shown in the diagram. Note that there are large collections of charge at parts of the body which have a small radius of curvature. This is important in the design of the X-ray tube both in prevention of *coronal discharge* (where electrons are forcibly removed from their orbits to create an electrical spark) from sharp corners and also in the use of a sharp-edged focusing cup for electron focusing (see Ch. 22).

Summary

In this chapter you should have learnt:

- The properties of electrical charges (see Sect. 9.3)
- The force between two electrical charges in a vacuum (see Sect. 9.4)
- The meaning of permittivity and relative permittivity (dielectric constant) (see Sect. 9.5)
- The concept of electrical field strength (see Sect. 9.6)
- The meaning of electrostatic induction (see Sect. 9.7)
- Electrostatic induction of a conductor (see Sect. 9.7.1)
- Electrostatic induction of an insulator or dielectric (see Sect. 9.7.2)
- The concept of electrical potential (see Sect. 9.8)
- The meaning of zero electrical potential (see Sect. 9.8.1)
- The meaning of absolute potential and potential difference (see Sect. 9.8.2)
- The definition of the volt (see Sect. 9.8.3)
- Electric potential due to a point charge (see Sect. 9.8.4)
- Electric potential due to a conducting sphere (see Sect. 9.8.5)
- Electrical charge distribution on an irregularly shaped conductor (see Sect. 9.9).

SELF-TEST

a. List the properties of electrical charges.

b. List the factors which determine the force between two point charges in a vacuum.

c. Discuss the induction of charge on:
   (i) a conductor
   (ii) an insulator
   when a positively charged body is brought into close proximity with it.

d. Discuss the statement 'Earth is at zero potential'.

e. Describe the distribution of charge on a conducting:
   (i) sphere
   (ii) irregularly shaped body.

FURTHER READING

Ball J L, Moore A D 1986 Essential physics for radiographers, 2nd edn. Blackwell Scientific Publications, London, ch 3
Gifford D 1984 A handbook of physics for radiologists and radiographers. John Wiley & Sons, Chichester, ch 5
Hay G A, Hughes D 1983 First year physics for radiographers. Baillière Tindall, London, ch 3

10

Electricity (DC)

10.1 AIM

The aim of this chapter is to introduce the reader to the concept of electron flow as a means of conducting electricity. Factors affecting the resistance to this flow will be explored and Ohm's Law will be discussed. The consequences of resistance in terms of electrical 'power loss' will be discussed and the practical implications of this in the design of X-ray generating apparatus will be considered.

10.2 INTRODUCTION

In the previous chapter we considered the behaviour of static electrical charges. This chapter considers the behaviour of electrical charges which are unidirectional in their movement—*direct current* or *DC electricity*. In a vacuum, gas or liquid (e.g. in an air ionisation chamber; see Ch. 33) both positive and negative charges move with relative freedom. These charges are called *ions*. In a solid, however, the atomic nuclei are relatively tightly bound to other atoms and so take no part in the flow of charge. The electrical properties of a given solid are thus determined by the way in which the orbiting electrons behave. This behaviour will form the initial discussion in this chapter.

10.3 SIMPLE ELECTRON THEORY OF CONDUCTION

To explain why some materials readily allow a flow of electrons (i.e. are good electrical conductors) and other materials will only allow electron flow in extreme conditions (i.e. are good insulators) we need to look more closely at the structure of the atom. This chapter will only look at atomic structure in terms of explaining the electrical properties of the material and there will be a fuller description of the atom in Chapter 26.

The nucleus of the atom contains protons (+ve charge) and around this in orbitals are electrons (−ve charge). If we consider a single atom (see Fig. 10.1), we can appreciate that electrons near the nucleus experience a high level of attraction (unlike charges attract) and are thus said to be *tightly bound*. Electrons in the more remote orbitals experience less force of attraction from the nucleus (remember $F \propto 1/d^2$) and are also repelled by

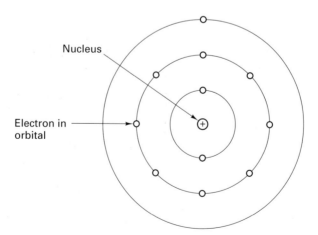

Figure 10.1 Diagrammatic representation of the sodium atom. Note the positive charge on the nucleus and that the electrons occupy specific orbitals.

other electrons which lie between them and the nucleus and so are said to be more *loosely bound*. Because the electrons in a given single atom are influenced only by that atom, the electrons lie at discrete energy levels as shown in Figure 10.2(a).

When electrons are brought closer together, as in a solid, the orbitals of the electrons are strongly influenced by the proximity of neighbouring atoms. This means that electrons are no longer at discrete energy levels but that they are now within a band of energies. This situation is shown in Figure 10.2(b).

For the purpose of this discussion, only the outer two energy bands are of interest to us: the *valence band* and the *conduction band*. The valence band is that band which contains the outermost electrons of the atom and may be partially or completely full of its permitted maximum number of electrons. The configuration of electrons in this band determines the *chemical properties* of the atom, i.e. its ability to form *chemical bonds* with other atoms. If electrons exist further away from the nucleus than the valence band, then their energies lie in the conduction band. This band is populated with electrons which have, for some reason, become free from their original atoms. Because of this, once an electron is in the conduction band of a solid, it is able to move relatively freely and hence may take part in electrical conduction through the material. Thus a material with a large number of electrons in the conduction band is a *good electrical conductor* whereas a material with no electrons in the conduction band is a *perfect electrical insulator*. Whether or not a material is a conductor, an insulator or a semiconductor is thus determined by the number of electrons in the conduction band. This number is in turn determined by the size of the *forbidden energy gap (E)* which exists between the top energy of the valence

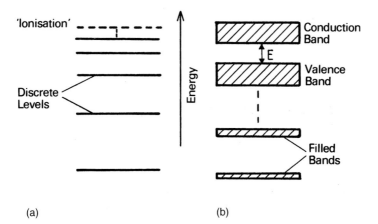

(a)   (b)

Figure 10.2   (a) Electron energy levels in a solitary atom. (b) Electron energy bands in an atom of a solid.

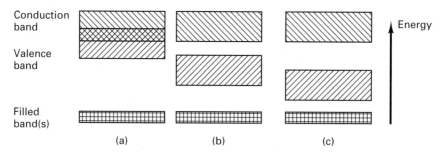

Conduction band

Valence band

Filled band(s)

(a) (b) (c)

Energy

Figure 10.3 Energy bands for (a) a conductor, (b) a semiconductor and (c) an insulator.

band and the bottom energy of the conduction band. The arrangement of the valence and conduction bands for conductors, semiconductors and insulators is shown in Figure 10.3. Each of the above will now be considered individually.

10.3.1 Electron arrangements in a conductor

As can be seen from Figure 10.3(a), the conduction band and the valence band of energies overlap in a conductor. This means that there is a ready exchange of electrons between the bands and so a large number of electrons always exist in the conduction band. This means that these electrons can be moved through the solid with *little resistance* to their flow. The main impedance to their flow is because of collisions with other electrons or atoms. If the temperature of the conductor is increased, this results in an increase in the vibrational energy of the atoms and so increases the likelihood of collision with moving electrons. Thus we can see that *the resistance to the flow of electrons in a conductor will increase with an increase in its temperature.*

Insight

As mentioned above, the main cause of resistance to the flow of electrons in a conductor is collisions with other atoms. It would therefore seem logical to suggest that, if the vibrational energy of the atoms could be reduced, or even stopped, then the resistance of the conductor could be reduced. This is done by cooling the conductor to temperatures close to absolute zero. At these temperatures, atomic vibration virtually ceases to exist and so flow of electrons through the conduction band is virtually unimpeded. Materials operating in this mode are known as *superconductors* and this technique is used to produce the large magnetic field required for magnetic resonance scanning.

10.3.2 Electron arrangements in a semiconductor

In a semiconductor there is a gap between the maximum energy of the valence band and the minimum energy of the conduction band (see Fig. 10.3(b)) and so electrons need to be given energy to bridge this gap and so flow through the material (this will be discussed in more detail in Ch. 18 which deals with semiconductors). Thus *semiconductors have a greater resistance to the flow of electrons than conductors.* If we increase the temperature of the semiconductor, we will increase the energy of the electrons in the valence band and so make it easier for them to transfer to the conduction band and so move through the solid. Thus *increasing the temperature of a semiconductor will reduce its resistance to the flow of electrons.*

10.3.3 Electron arrangements in an insulator

In an insulator there is a significant gap between the maximum energy of the valence band and the minimum energy of the conduction band (see Fig. 10.3(c)). This means that electrons cannot readily bridge this energy gap, and so the conduction band contains no electrons, making conduction impossible. If the material is heated, then the electrons in the valence band gain energy, and so the gap between the valence and the conduction bands is narrowed, making it more likely that electrons can 'jump' the gap. Thus *increasing the temperature of an insulator reduces its resistance.*

The effect on the resistance to the flow of electrons of increasing the temperature is shown in Figure 10.4.

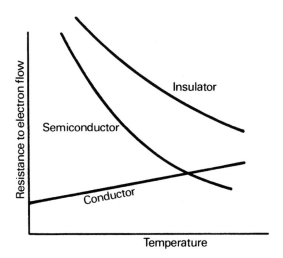

Figure 10.4   Effect of temperature on the electrical resistance of a conductor, a semiconductor and an insulator.

10.4 ELECTRIC CURRENT

Electricity is the flow of electrons in a material. The rate of flow of electrons is a measure of the *electric current.* In order to produce a current the following conditions must be satisfied:

- There must be a source of electric *potential difference* (see Sect. 9.8.2).
- There must be a *complete circuit* around which the electrons are able to travel.

These two points are illustrated in Figure 10.5. The battery (B) is a source of potential difference but if the switch (S) is open (as in Fig. 10.5(a)), no electric current flows and the bulb does not light up. When the switch is closed (see Fig. 10.5(b)), a complete circuit exists around which electrons are able to flow and so the bulb lights up. The *potential difference* may be thought of as the *driving force* which causes electrons to flow, while the *current* is the rate of flow of electrons, i.e. the number of electrons passing a given point in unit time.

Definition

An *electric current of 1 ampere* (A) flows at a point if a charge of *1 coulomb* (C) flows past that point *per second*.

Thus we can say mathematically:

$$\text{amperes} = \frac{\text{coulombs}}{\text{seconds}} \qquad \text{Equation 10.1}$$

From Section 9.4 we know that a charge of 1 coulomb is equivalent to approximately 6×10^{18} electrons so 1 ampere is simply this number of electrons passing a point in 1 second.

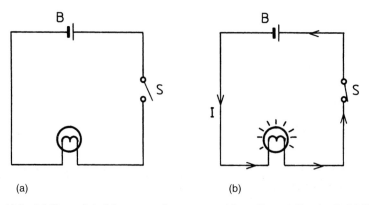

(a)   (b)

Figure 10.5 (a) The switch S is open and so no current flows through the circuit. (b) When the switch is closed, current will flow through the circuit and the bulb will light. This shows that a continuous circuit is necessary for electrical current to flow.

> **Insight**
>
> We are accustomed to an instant response when we close an electrical switch and so it is surprising to discover that the average velocity of electrons in a circuit is only in the order of 0.5 mm·s^{-1}. When the switch is closed, electrons start to flow through the whole circuit and so the bulb in Figure 10.5 will light up even if the electrons from the battery have not yet reached it—this is similar to the situation where water enters a pipe from a reservoir when a tap is opened; water leaves the tap immediately although it might be some time before the water from the reservoir reaches it.

10.5 mA, mAs AND MILLICOULOMBS

The electric current through an X-ray tube is a small one and so it is measured in *milliamperes* (mA) rather than in amps—1 mA = 10^{-3} A. This measures the rate of flow of electrons through the tube. If we wish to measure the number of electrons which have travelled across the tube during a given radiographic exposure, then we need to multiply the rate of flow by the time of the exposure. This unit is in *milliampere-seconds* (mAs) where:

$$mAs = mA \times seconds \qquad\qquad \text{Equation 10.2}$$

Now the total number of electrons which have crossed the X-ray tube is just a measure of the charge—measured in *coulombs*. From Equation 10.1:

$$amps = \frac{coulombs}{seconds}$$

By cross-multiplying (see Appendix A):

$$coulombs = amps \times seconds$$

so:

$$millicoulombs = milliamps \times seconds \qquad\qquad \text{Equation 10.3}$$

So we can say that:

$$1\ mAs = 1\ millicoulomb \qquad\qquad \text{Equation 10.4}$$

10.6 POTENTIAL DIFFERENCE AND ELECTROMOTIVE FORCE (EMF)

We have already considered potential difference in Section 9.8.2 and defined the potential difference in volts:

Definition

The potential difference in volts is the work done in moving 1 coulomb of positive charge from one point to another.

Thus:

$$\text{volts} = \frac{\text{joules}}{\text{coulombs}} \qquad \text{Equation 10.5}$$

In electricity we are concerned with moving charges and, as mentioned previously, we can regard the potential difference as the 'driving force' which moves the electron along a conductor.

Electromotive force (EMF) is also expressed in *volts* and is a measure of electrical potential energy developed across a *source* of electricity (e.g. a battery or a generator). Thus the EMF is the 'driving force' behind the electron flow in the circuit.

It is therefore possible to speak about the potential difference (PD) across any part of the circuit including the source of electricity, whereas the term electromotive force (EMF) is reserved solely for the latter. It would not therefore be correct to use the term 'EMF across a resistor' as a resistor is not a *source* of electricity—the appropriate terminology would be 'PD across a resistor'.

Insight

It is interesting to note that the *PD* across the terminals of a battery is less than the *EMF* when a current flows. This is due to the internal resistance of the battery. The effect is known as *regulation*. A similar effect is observed with transformers and will be discussed more fully in that section (Ch. 17).

10.7 RESISTANCE

The elementary theory of conduction discussed earlier in this chapter refers to two mechanisms which impede electron flow:

- lack of 'free' electrons in the conduction band—as in an insulator
- collisions between flowing electrons with other vibrating electrons in the material.

This impedance to the flow of electrons is given the term *electrical resistance* or simply *resistance* and is measured in *ohms*. Obviously, from the earlier discussion, insulators have much higher resistance than conductors of the same shape and size. The resistance of a conductor can vary depending on a number of factors which will be discussed below.

10.7.1 **Factors affecting resistance**

The resistance of a substance will be affected by:

● the *shape* of the substance
● the *type* of the substance
● the *temperature* of the substance.

Note that the resistance of the substance is not affected either by the potential difference across it or by the current flowing through it.

a. Shape

The shape of a body is capable of infinite variation so for simplicity we shall consider circular conductors of constant cross-sectional area.

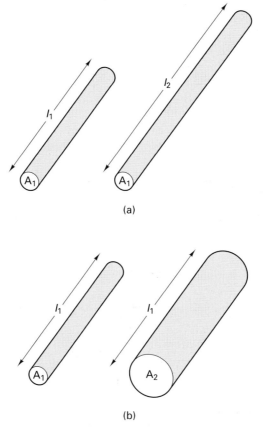

Figure 10.6   Factors affecting resistance of a conductor. In (a) the conductors are of different lengths and the resistance increases with the length. In (b) the conductors have differing cross-sectional areas and the resistance is inversely proportional to the cross-sectional area.

Figure 10.6 illustrates such a body and the effect on the resistance R of altering its length l and its cross-sectional area A.

The resistance is proportional to the length of the conductor ($R \propto l$). If we consider a situation where the length of the conductor is doubled, then electrons travelling along the conductor have twice as many vibrating atoms to get past so the resistance to their flow will be doubled.

The resistance is inversely proportional to the cross-sectional area ($R \propto 1/A$). If the area is doubled, there are twice as many electrons capable of conducting charge. The number of atoms each electron must get past for the length of the conductor remains the same and so doubling the area will halve the resistance.

b. Type of substance

By definition, good electrical conductors will have a lower resistance than insulators. Different metals also have different values of resistance. As we have just seen, the shape of the substance also affects its resistance, so that a standard shape and size must be used when comparing the resistance of different materials. The standard used is a cube of side 1 metre and the resistance is measured when a current is passed between opposing faces of the cube. The value of the resistance so obtained is called the *resistivity* or the *specific resistance* of the material and is measured in ohm-metres. Resistivity is given the symbol ρ (Greek 'rho') and it is clear that the resistance of the material will be directly proportional to its resistivity— $R \propto \rho$.

If we now consider all the factors discussed in (a) and (b), we have:

$$R \propto \frac{\rho l}{A}$$
Equation 10.6

In the SI system ρ is defined so that the constant of proportionality in the above equation is unity and so we can say:

$$R = \frac{\rho l}{A}$$
Equation 10.7

The resistivities of insulators are about 1 million times greater than those of semiconductors, which in turn are about 1 million times greater than those of metallic conductors.

c. Temperature

As we have described at the beginning of this chapter, a change in temperature affects the resistance of a body. This effect is different for conductors, semiconductors and insulators as shown in Figure 10.4.

Because of these variations, resistance is usually quoted at a particular temperature (e.g. 20°C). The *temperature coefficient of resistance,* α, is defined as *the fractional change in resistance (or resistivity) per unit temperature change.*

$$\alpha = \frac{\text{change in resistivity}}{\text{original resistivity}} \, / \text{ temperature change}$$

α is different for different conductors.

10.8 OHM'S LAW

Ohm's Law applies to metallic conductors and combines, in a particularly simple and elegant way, the relationship between *current, potential difference* and *resistance.* It is found experimentally that the current flowing through a conductor is proportional to the potential difference applied across it—*as the driving force on the electrons is increased, so the number of electrons passing a point in unit time increases by a proportional amount.* Thus, if a potential difference of 2 volts causes a current of 1 amp to flow through a conductor, then a potential difference of 4 volts will cause a current of 2 amps to flow. Ohm's Law may be formally stated as:

> The *current* **flowing through a** *metallic conductor* **is** *proportional* **to the** *potential difference* **which exists across it provided that all** *physical conditions* **remain constant.**

The main *physical condition* which must remain constant is the temperature of the conductor, as an alteration in the temperature will cause an alteration in the resistance (see Sect. 10.7.1).
   Ohm's Law may be stated mathematically thus:

$$I \propto V \qquad\qquad\qquad\qquad \text{Equation 10.8}$$

where I and V are the magnitude of the current and the potential difference respectively.
   Note that Ohm's Law does not mention the word *resistance.* The resistance of the body (R) is introduced into Equation 10.8 as a constant of proportionality (see Appendix A) and so the equation may now be rewritten:

$$V \propto I$$
$$\therefore V = R \times I$$

$$\therefore V = I \times R \qquad\qquad\qquad\qquad \text{Equation 10.9}$$

As we have already established, R is a *constant* for a given conductor at a given temperature and *does not depend on V or I*.

R is measured in ohm (Ω) and we can see from Equation 10.9 that when $V = 1$ volt and $I = 1$ amp then R will be 1 ohm. The ohm may be defined as follows:

Definition

A body is said to have an electrical resistance of *1 ohm* if a potential difference of *1 volt* across it produces an electrical current through it of *1 ampere*.

(*Note* that a potential difference always occurs *across* a body *never through it*. Likewise an electrical current always flows *through* a body and *does not exist across it.*)

Although Ohm's Law is simple in its formulation it has far-reaching implications which can be applied to radiological physics. The most important of these will now be discussed.

10.8.1 Resistors in series

If we join resistors *in series* (end-to-end) and apply a potential difference of V volts across the unit, then a current of I amps flows through it. This is shown in Figure 10.7. Note that the same current flows through each resistor since the whole unit may be regarded as a continuous circuit and so electrons are neither lost nor gained throughout the circuit. Also note that the potential difference across the ends of the unit is equal to the sum of the potential differences across each resistor ($V = V_1 + V_2 + V_3$). We wish to calculate the effective resistance of the unit (R), i.e. *what would be the value of a single resistor which would behave in exactly the same way as the whole unit?*

If we apply Ohm's Law to each resistor in turn then we get:

$$V_1 = IR_1; V_2 = IR_2; V_3 = IR_3$$

We already know that:

$$V = V_1 + V_2 + V_3$$
$$V = IR_1 + IR_2 + IR_3$$
$$V = I(R_1 + R_2 + R_3)$$

Figure 10.7 Combining resistors in series to produce a total resistance, R.

$$\frac{V}{I} = R_1 + R_2 + R_3 \qquad\qquad \text{Equation 10.10A}$$

If we apply Ohm's Law to the total unit then:

$$V = I \times R$$
$$R = \frac{V}{I}$$

By substitution this value of V/I into Equation 10.10A we get:

$$R = R_1 + R_2 + R_3 \qquad\qquad \text{Equation 10.10}$$

Thus, when resistors are connected in series the total resistance may be obtained simply by adding together the values of each separate resistor.

10.8.2 Resistors in parallel

A potential difference of V exists across points A and B in Figure 10.8 and, since each resistor is connected to A and B, the potential difference across each resistor is also V volts. Electrons flow into the circuit at point A and then some will pass through each resistor to meet again at point B. Since electrons are neither gained nor lost in the circuit:

$$I = I_1 + I_2 + I_3 \qquad\qquad \text{Equation 10.11A}$$

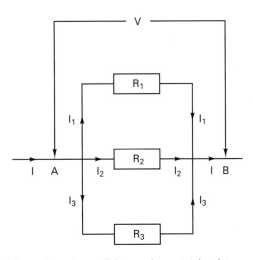

Figure 10.8   Combining resistors in parallel to produce a total resistance, R.

If we apply Ohm's Law to each of the resistors we get:

$$V = I_1 R_1; \; V = I_2 R_2; \; V = I_3 R_3$$

or $I_1 = \dfrac{V}{R_1}; \; I_2 = \dfrac{V}{R_2}; \; I_3 = \dfrac{V}{R_3}$

By substituting these values in Equation 10.11A:

$$I = \frac{V}{R_1} + \frac{V}{R_2} + \frac{V}{R_3}$$

or $I = V\left(\dfrac{1}{R_1} + \dfrac{1}{R_2} + \dfrac{1}{R_3} \right)$

so

$$\frac{I}{V} = \frac{1}{R_1} + \frac{1}{R_2} + \frac{1}{R_3} \qquad \text{Equation 10.11B}$$

If we apply Ohm's Law to the whole unit (assuming it has a resistance R), then we get:

$$V = IR$$

or $\dfrac{I}{V} = \dfrac{1}{R}$

If we now substitute this value in Equation 10.11B we get:

$$\frac{1}{R} = \frac{1}{R_1} + \frac{1}{R_2} + \frac{1}{R_3} \qquad \text{Equation 10.11}$$

10.8.3 Calculations using Ohm's Law

a. A 30 Ω resistor is connected into a circuit and has a PD of 10 V across its ends. What is the current flowing through the resistor?
By Ohm's Law:

$$V = IR$$
$$I = \frac{V}{R}$$
$$= \frac{10}{30} \, \text{A}$$
$$= 0.33 \, \text{A}$$

b. A 6 V battery is connected across a 10 Ω and a 20 Ω resistor connected in series. What current flows in the circuit and what is the potential difference across each resistor?

When resistors are connected in series:

$$R = R_1 + R_2$$
$$= 10 + 20 \ \Omega$$
$$= 30 \ \Omega$$

By Ohm's Law:

$$V = IR$$
$$I = \frac{V}{R}$$
$$= \frac{6}{30} \ A$$
$$= 0.2 \ A$$

We know that the same current flows through each resistor and so we can apply Ohm's Law to each.

$$V_1 = IR_1 \qquad \text{and} \qquad V_2 = IR_2$$
$$\quad = 0.2 \times 10 \ V \qquad\qquad\qquad = 0.2 \times 20 \ V$$
$$\quad = 2 \ V \qquad\qquad\qquad\qquad = 4 \ V$$

Note that the sum of the PDs across the resistors is equal to the PD across the battery terminals (6 volts).

c. A 6 V battery is connected across a 10 Ω and a 20 Ω resistor connected in parallel. What is the total resistance of the circuit, the current flowing through the whole circuit and the current flowing through each resistor?

For resistors in parallel:

$$\frac{1}{R} = \frac{1}{R_1} + \frac{1}{R_2}$$
$$= \frac{1}{10} + \frac{1}{20}$$
$$= \frac{3}{20}$$
$$R = \frac{20}{3} \ \Omega$$
$$= 6.67 \ \Omega$$

From Ohm's Law:

$$V = IR$$

$$I_1 = \frac{V}{R_1} \qquad \text{and} \qquad I_2 = \frac{V}{R_2}$$

$$= \frac{6}{10} A \qquad\qquad\qquad = \frac{6}{20} A$$

$$= 0.6 \text{ A} \qquad\qquad\qquad = 0.3 \text{ A}$$

The total current flowing in the circuit is the sum of the current values for each resistor:

$$I = I_1 + I_2$$
$$= 0.6 + 0.3 \text{ A}$$
$$= 0.9 \text{ A}$$

10.9 ELECTRICAL ENERGY AND POWER

To get an electric current to flow through a conductor the electrons must be driven by a potential difference. As the electrons move through the conductor they are involved in collisions with the atoms of the conductor and so *work* must be done to keep all the electrons moving in the same direction. The electrons dissipate energy to the atoms of the material which they pass through and so heat is produced in the material—this is the mechanism by which the filament of the X-ray tube is heated to produce electrons by thermionic emission (see Chs 22 and 28).

10.9.1 The joule

As already discussed (Sect. 6.3) the joule is the SI unit of energy. The key to the method of calculating electrical energy lies in the definition of potential difference. As we discovered in Section 9.8.3, *the potential difference between two points is 1 volt when 1 joule of work is done in moving 1 coulomb of positive charge from one point to the other.* Thus we can say:

$$\text{volts} = \frac{\text{joules}}{\text{coulombs}} \qquad\qquad \text{Equation 10.12}$$

or:

$$\text{joules} = \text{volts} \times \text{coulombs} \qquad\qquad \text{Equation 10.13}$$

Since the ampere is a rate of flow of charge of 1 coulomb per second, then we can say:

$$joules = volts \times amperes \times seconds \qquad \text{Equation 10.14}$$

10.9.2 The watt

We also saw in Section 6.3 that the SI unit of power is the watt where 1 watt = 1 joule per second. Thus we can say that:

$$\frac{joules}{seconds} = \frac{volts \times amperes \times seconds}{seconds}$$

or:

$$watts = volts \times amperes \qquad \text{Equation 10.15}$$

This is a general equation used in the calculation of electrical power which applies to any electrical system. It is, however, particularly useful to apply this formula to a metallic conductor which obeys Ohm's Law.

10.9.3 Power in a resistor

Consider a current I passing through a metallic resistor of resistance R when a potential difference V is applied across its ends. As previously discussed:

$$W = V \times I$$

However, we can apply Ohm's Law to the resistor:

$$V = I \times R$$

so $\quad W = I \times I \times R$

or $\quad W = I^2R$

By similar manipulations of Ohm's Law we can get three possible equations for the electrical power in a resistor:

$$W = VI$$
$$W = I^2R$$
$$W = \frac{V^2}{R} \qquad \text{Equation 10.16}$$

The second of the three equations is probably the most useful one in radiography. Some calculations may clarify the use of these equations.

Examples

a. 10 amps flows through a 2 ohm resistor. What power is generated in the resistor?

Using the equation:

$W = I^2R$
$= (10)^2 \times 2$ watts
$= 100 \times 2$ watts
$= 200$ watts

b. If a potential difference of 20 volts is applied across a 2 ohm resistor, what power is generated in the resistor?

Using the equation:

$W = \dfrac{V^2}{R}$
$= \dfrac{(20)^2}{2}$ watts
$= \dfrac{400}{2}$ watts
$= 200$ watts

c. If a potential difference of 20 volts is applied across a resistor and this causes a current of 10 amps to flow through the resistor, what will be the power generated in the resistor?

Using the equation:

$W = VI$
$= 20 \times 10$ watts
$= 200$ watts

10.10 POWER LOSS IN CABLES

If we consider electricity in the form of a current I passing through a cable with a resistance R, it becomes apparent that some of the available electrical power will be 'lost' in the cable. The term lost does not imply that there is a breach of the Law of Conservation of Energy but that the power is not available for the user at the far end of the cable—the 'lost' energy is in fact converted into heat.

It is obviously desirable that the power which is lost in the cables be kept to a minimum as this is not available to the user. If we consider that the power loss is given by the equation $P = I^2R$, then it can be seen that the power loss can be kept to a minimum in one of two ways:

a. reducing the current flowing within the cable
b. reducing the resistance of the cables.

a. Reducing the current flowing within the cable

Electrical power is a combination of the potential difference (V) across the cables and the current (I) flowing through them, i.e. $P = VI$. Thus, if we wish to transmit a given amount of electrical power with the minimum loss in the cables, this can be done by using a high voltage and a low current. This is shown in Figure 10.9 where a power of approximately 100 watt is required to heat the filament of the X-ray tube. This power is transmitted from the autotransformer to the filament transformer (see Ch. 17) in the form of a relatively high voltage and low current. At the filament we wish to use this power to generate heat, so it is converted to a relatively low voltage and high current at the filament transformer. Similar techniques are used in transmitting power from the generating stations to our homes.

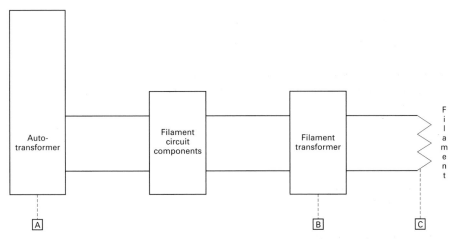

Figure 10.9   Transmission of electrical power from the autotransformer to the X-ray tube filament. Between points A and B, power is in the optimum form for transmission with minimum power loss—high voltage and low current. Thus 100 watt of power would be transmitted in the form of 100 volts and 1 ampere. Between points B and C, power is in the optimum form for heat generation at the filament. Thus 100 watt of power would be transmitted in the form of 10 volts and 10 amperes.

b. Reducing the resistance of the cables

This is achieved in two ways—making the cables of a material with a low resistivity (usually copper) and making the cables as thick (large cross-sectional area) as possible. Because the cables are required to transmit power from one point to another there is little scope for the third possibility—reducing the length of the cables.

10.10.1 Mains cable resistance and X-ray exposures

As we have previously discussed, there is a potential difference across any resistor which is related to the current through the resistor ($V = IR$). This volt drop is removed from the EMF available when a current flows to an X-ray unit. This can be seen in Equation 10.17 below:

$$V = \text{EMF} - IR_c \qquad\qquad \text{Equation 10.17}$$

where R_c is the resistance of the mains cables and V is the PD available at the mains supply when the unit is 'on load'. It is also worth noting that this volt drop is related to the resistance of the cables and the current to the X-ray unit.

In practice, with static X-ray units, the resistance of the mains cables is fairly constant so it is possible to compensate for this volt drop using a *static mains voltage compensator*. For mains-dependent mobile units the volt drop can vary for different parts of the hospital—obviously, the mains cables that reach the tenth floor are longer than the cables to the ground floor. This means that this type of mobile unit has an *adjustable mains voltage compensator*. Usually, the plug for the unit in the ward is coded in some way so that we know the correct setting for the compensator.

Insight

Many modern mobile X-ray units overcome this problem by being 'mains independent'. Such units remove power from the mains in small amounts *between exposures* (they require to be plugged in to the mains when not in use) and then release this power through the X-ray tube during the exposure. The electrical power may be stored in special batteries or in capacitors (see Ch. 16).

Summary

In this chapter you should have learnt the following:

- A simple electron theory of conduction (see Sect. 10.3)
- The requirements for a flow of electric current (see Sect. 10.4)
- The relationships between mA, mAs and millicoulombs (see Sect. 10.5)
- The meaning of potential difference and EMF (see Sect. 10.6)
- The meaning of electrical resistance (see Sect. 10.7)
- The factors affecting electrical resistance (see Sect. 10.7.1)
- Ohm's Law (see Sect. 10.8)
- The effect of connecting resistors in series (see Sect. 10.8.1)
- The effect of connecting resistors in parallel (see Sect. 10.8.2)
- How to undertake calculations using Ohm's Law (see Sect. 10.8.3)
- The meaning of electrical energy and power (see Sect. 10.9)

- The meaning of the joule (see Sect. 10.9.1)
- The meaning of the watt (see Sect. 10.9.2)
- Power in a resistor (see Sect. 10.9.3)
- Power loss in cables (see Sect. 10.10)
- Mains cable resistance and X-ray exposures (see Sect. 10.10.1).

SELF-TEST

a. Explain what is meant by the terms *electrical conductor* and *electrical insulator* and show how their electrical behaviour may be described by the simple electron theory of conduction.

b. List the factors upon which the resistance of a conductor depends.

c. 1 metre of wire of a given cross-sectional area is found to have the same resistance as a length of wire of the same material but of double the cross-sectional area. How long is the second wire?

d. Define Ohm's Law and the unit of resistance.

e. Resistors are connected as shown in the diagram below:

Calculate the total resistance of the unit, I, I_1, I_2, V_1 and V_2.

f. A current of 5 A flows through a 10 Ω resistor for 2 minutes. Calculate the energy used in the resistor and the power used.

g. The EMF from the mains supply to an X-ray set is 400 V. The resistance of the mains cables is 0.5 Ω. When a certain exposure is made, a current of 40 A is drawn from the mains. Calculate the volt drop in the cables and the potential difference available across the X-ray set during the exposure.

FURTHER READING

Ball J L, Moore A D 1986 Essential physics for radiographers, 2nd edn. Blackwell Scientific
Publications, London, ch 7
Foster E 1985 Equipment for diagnostic radiography. MTP Press, Lancaster, ch 1
Hay G A, Hughes D 1983 First year physics for radiographers. Baillière Tindall, London, ch 4
Stockley S M 1986 A manual of radiographic equipment. Churchill Livingstone, Edinburgh,
chs 1, 2, 3

Magnetism

11.1 AIM

The aim of this chapter is to explore the phenomenon of magnetism and to consider briefly its application to radiographic science. This chapter will act as a foundation for Chapters 12, 13, 14 and 17, which consider further applications of magnetism in technology relevant to radiography.

11.2 MAGNETIC POLES

If a magnetic compass is suspended freely, it will align itself in a north–south direction. Such a compass contains a *permanent* magnet (i.e. a magnet which is not easily demagnetised). Such a magnet contains two *poles*; the end pointing to the north is called the north pole of the magnet and the end pointing to the south, the south pole. Thus we see that there are two types of magnetic pole (north and south) in the same way as there are two types of electrical charge (positive and negative).

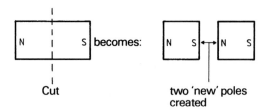

Figure 11.1 The effect of cutting a bar magnet in two. Magnetic poles always exist in pairs so there are now two bar magnets.

Many of the properties of magnetism are similar to those of electrical charges as may be seen by comparison of this chapter with Chapter 9. However, there is one fundamental difference between magnetic poles and electrical charges: electrical charges may exist in isolation (e.g. a single electron) whereas poles always exist in *pairs*. Consider the situation shown in Figure 11.1. If we take a permanent magnet and cut it in half, when the two halves are separated we get two magnets with both north and south poles. Further subdivisions of the magnet will produce further smaller bar magnets each with a north and a south pole. This would lead us to suspect that individual *atoms* of the material behave like small bar magnets with a north and a south pole and there is evidence that this is the case. As we shall see in Chapter 12, magnetism is caused by moving electrical charges, so magnetic atoms are produced by the circulation in their orbitals of the charged electrons of the atoms. When the orbitals of the electrons of an atom tend to be in the same direction, then the total effect is to produce a very magnetic atom (e.g. iron), whereas if the orbitals are in opposite directions they tend to cancel out each other's effect and so a very weak magnetic atom exists.

11.2.1 Force between two magnetic poles

The effect of two magnetic poles on each other is very similar to the effect of electrical charges on each other (see Sect. 9.3) and may be stated as:

Like poles repel while unlike poles attract.

Calculating the magnitude of the force between two poles in a vacuum is likewise a similar argument to that between two charges. For the purpose of such calculations, a north pole is considered to be positive and a south pole is considered to be negative. Thus if poles of strength m_1 and m_2 are separated by a distance d (see Fig. 11.2) then a mutual force F exists between them, where:

$$F \propto \frac{m_1 m_2}{d^2}$$

Equation 11.1

Figure 11.2 The mutual force of repulsion between two like poles, m_1 and m_2, separated by a distance, d. Note the similarities between this and Figure 9.1.

In the SI system of units the constant of proportionality in this equation is $1/4\,\pi\mu_0$ so that Equation 11.1 can now be rewritten:

$$F = \frac{m_1 m_2}{4\pi\mu_0 d^2}$$
Equation 11.2

where F is in newtons, d is in metres and m_1 and m_2 are in webers (Wb). μ_0 is the 'permeability of free space' and has a value of $4\pi \times 10^{-7}$ henry per metre (H·m^{-1}). The henry is further discussed in Chapter 13.

Again the similarities between Equation 11.2 and Equation 9.2 emphasise the close link which exists between magnetism and electricity. This similarity is further extended if the poles are embedded in a medium:

$$F = \frac{m_1 m_2}{4\pi\mu d^2}$$
Equation 11.3

where μ is the 'permeability' of the medium. The term d^2 in the equations shows that the force between magnetic poles (like that between electrical charges) obeys the Inverse Square Law (see Ch. 3).

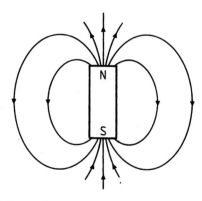

Figure 11.3 Magnetic lines of force due to a bar magnet. The arrows point in the direction a north pole would move if placed in that position.

11.3 MAGNETIC FIELDS

A magnetic field is said to exist at a point if a force would be experienced by a magnetic pole placed at that point. Thus the term *magnetic field* is used to indicate the extent of the magnetic effect around (and within) a magnetised body.

Figure 11.3 illustrates the concept of magnetic lines of force around a bar magnet. The arrows on the lines of force indicate the direction of the force exerted on a north pole placed at that point. If this north pole were free to move it would thus travel along the line of force. The total number of lines of force are referred to as the *magnetic flux* and this will be considered in more detail in the following section.

Insight

Although there are many similarities between electrical and magnetic lines of force, there are some fundamental differences. One such difference is that magnetic lines of force are *continuous*, as can be seen in the diagram. Electrical lines of force always begin on a positive charge and end on a negative charge.

11.4 MAGNETIC FLUX AND FLUX DENSITY

Consider Figure 11.4. The total number of lines of force passing through the area A is defined as the *magnetic flux* (N) passing through (or linked

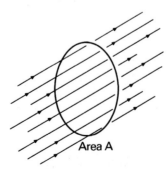

Figure 11.4 Lines of magnetic flux through an area A.

with) A. The *magnetic flux density* (B) is the number of lines of flux in a unit area placed at right angles to the lines of flux. If we assume that the area A in Figure 11.4 is at right angles to the parallel lines of magnetic flux, then the relationship can be stated thus:

$$B = \frac{N}{A}$$

Equation 11.4

As already mentioned, the unit of magnetic flux is the weber (Wb) and the unit of flux density is the tesla (T) so:

$$1\,T = 1\,Wb \cdot m^{-2}$$

The definition within the SI system relates the electrical units and the units of magnetic flux density through the motor principle.

We shall use the concepts of magnetic flux and magnetic flux density in Chapter 13 when we consider electromagnetic induction and in Chapter 15 when we consider the motor principle.

11.5 MAGNETIC INDUCTION

When discussing electrostatics we saw that a charge could be induced in a material and we now find that a similar situation exists for magnetism, i.e. magnetism may be induced in a suitable material. This is achieved by placing the substance within a magnetic field and so subjecting it to a *magnetising force* (H). If the substance contains magnetic atoms, these will tend to rotate to align with the direction of the magnetising force. Figure 11.5 illustrates this principle where an unmagnetised sample (Fig. 11.5(a)) initially has its atoms pointing in random directions. When it is subjected to a magnetising force, then these tend to line up with the direction of the force. This process produces a north pole at one end of the sample and a south pole at the other and so magnetism is said to have been induced in the sample. *Note* the similarity between magnetic induction and the

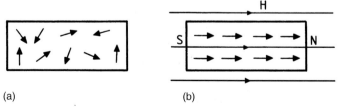

(a)   (b)

Figure 11.5 Inducing magnetism in a sample (the arrows represent the north end of a molecular magnet): (a) shows the randomised distribution of molecular magnets when no magnetic field is applied; (b) shows that the molecular magnets align with a magnetic field.

induction of charge in a sample caused by the rotation of polar molecules (see Sect. 9.7.2(b)).

The effect of aligning atoms is to produce a total flux density, B, within the sample which is greater than that in the air alone, such that:

$$B = \mu H \qquad\qquad \text{Equation 11.5}$$

where μ is the permeability of the medium (see Sect. 11.2.1). Here the magnetising force, H, is regarded as the *cause* of the magnetic flux density, B, in a medium of permeability μ.

Different substances respond to different extents. A sample containing very magnetic atoms has a large value of μ so that, once the whole sample is magnetised, a correspondingly large magnetic flux density results. Table 11.1 shows the *relative permeabilities* of some common materials—the relative permeability (μ_r) is found by comparing the permeability of the substance (μ) with that of a vacuum (μ_0). This is stated mathematically thus:

$$\mu_r = \frac{\mu}{\mu_0} \qquad\qquad \text{Equation 11.6}$$

As can be seen from the table, there is a wide variety of relative permeabilities in different substances ranging from just under unity for bismuth (difficult to magnetise) to 80 000 for mumetal (easily and strongly magnetised).

Table 11.1 Relative permeabilities of materials

Material	Relative permeability μ_r	Comments
Vacuum	1.0	By definition
Air	1.0000004	Usually taken as 1.0
Water	0.99999	Diamagnetic
Bismuth	0.999985	Diamagnetic
Platinum	1.0001	Paramagnetic
Cobalt	240	Ferromagnetic
Nickel	660	Ferromagnetic
Iron	5500	Ferromagnetic
Stalloy	6700	Ferromagnetic alloy
Mumetal	80 000	Ferromagnetic alloy

11.5.1 Intensity of magnetism

The total magnetic flux density, B, obtained by applying a magnetising force, H, to a substance is composed of two factors:

- the magnetic flux density due to the air around the sample ($\mu_0 H$)
- the magnetic flux density due to the induced magnetism in the material.

The total flux density is given by the equation $B = \mu H$ (see Equation 11.5). However, it is sometimes desirable to separate these two factors so that the magnetism induced in the sample may be considered separately. This is known as the *intensity of magnetism, I,* of the sample and measures the extent to which the sample itself has become magnetised.

Insight

The intensity of magnetism is defined as *the magnetic moment per unit volume of the magnetised sample.* This is the turning force which will be applied to a field perpendicular to its axis. If a pole strength p per unit area is induced in a sample of cross-sectional area A and length l, then the magnetic moment is pAl.

$$\text{Thus the intensity of magnetism} = \frac{\text{magnetic moment}}{\text{volume}} = \frac{pAl}{Al} = p$$

i.e. the intensity of magnetism is equal to the induced pole strength per unit area (in $Wb \cdot m^{-2}$).

11.6 TYPES OF MAGNETIC MATERIALS

We are all probably aware that some materials are easily and strongly magnetised while others appear to be unaffected by the presence of an external magnetic field. Thus we may confidently expect to pick up some steel pins using a bar magnet but would not expect to pick up wooden matches using the same magnet. Such differences in magnetic behaviour of different materials result in there being three basic types of magnetic substance. These are called *diamagnetics, paramagnetics* and *ferromagnetics.* In radiography it is ferromagnetic materials which are put to most use in transformers etc. (see Ch. 17) so this section will concentrate mainly on this type of material. However, diamagnetic and paramagnetic materials are used in *magnetic resonance imaging* (MRI) and so will also be considered.

11.6.1 Diamagnetism

Diamagnetism is the term which is given to the influence of the applied magnetic field on the electrons orbiting the nuclei within any substance. As we shall see in Chapter 13, Lenz's Law of electromagnetic induction describes the opposing effect between the induced currents and the varying magnetic fields applied to a conductor. Electrons orbiting a nucleus may be considered as conductors with zero electrical resistance. They thus suffer changes in their orbitals when an external magnetic field is applied. These changes in the orbitals of the electrons caused by the magnetic field interacting with them result in the orbitals opposing the external magnetic field (similar to Lenz's Law for a conductor). They remain in this condition until the magnetic field is removed and then they revert to their original orbitals. Two conclusions follow:

- *All* materials are diamagnetic.
- Magnetic induction is produced within the sample which *opposes* the direction of the applied magnetic field, so the relative permeability is always less than unity. Bismuth (see Table 11.1) has a relative permeability of 0.999985 and is an example of a diamagnetic material.

Diamagnetism is normally a very weak phenomenon and is usually completely obscured by paramagnetism and ferromagnetism when these exist in a material. Diamagnetism is not affected by the temperature of the material.

11.6.2 Paramagnetism

The cause of magnetism in individual atoms is the spinning and orbiting of electrons around their nuclei. If the effect of each electron is cancelled out by the effect of another electron, as outlined above, then the material is diamagnetic. If the resultant effect, however, allows us to consider the atom as an elementary bar magnet then the material is *paramagnetic*. In such materials the atoms will align with an external magnetic field as previously shown in Figure 11.5.

Temperature is a measure of the kinetic energy of the atoms of a material (see Sect. 8.3) and so is a factor which tends to destroy the ordered alignment of atoms within the sample. For this reason, a paramagnetic sample rapidly becomes demagnetised at room temperature after the external magnetic field has been removed—the demagnetisation is caused by the disruption that results from collisions between the atoms. As the temperature is increased, it becomes more difficult to magnetise a paramagnetic sample and there is a point at which it may not be possible to magnetise the material at all. At this point it is solely a diamagnetic since this effect is not influenced by the temperature.

Platinum (see Table 11.1) has a relative permeability of 1.0001 and is an example of a paramagnetic material. Note that the figure of the relative permeability is composed of a *positive* effect due to paramagnetism and a *negative* effect due to diamagnetism.

11.6.3 Ferromagnetism

Diamagnetism and paramagnetism are extremely weak magnetic phenomena compared to *ferromagnetism*. Ferromagnetic materials (see Table 11.1) have relative permeabilities which are measured in hundreds or thousands. Because of this the magnetic flux density of magnetised ferromagnetic materials may be sufficiently large to allow us to put it to practical uses—ferromagnetic materials are used in transformer cores.

The reason for the strong magnetic induction of ferromagnetic materials lies in the behaviour of so-called *magnetic domains* within them. Such a

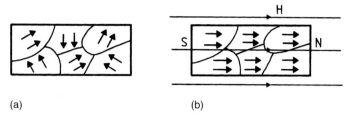

(a)   (b)

Figure 11.6 The 'domains' within a ferromagnetic material (the arrows represent the north end of each molecular magnet): (a) shows the material in its unmagnetised state; (b) shows how the domains align with the external magnetic field in a magnetised sample.

domain is a small volume within the material where all the atoms are pointing in the same direction. The random alignment of these domains in an unmagnetised sample is shown in Figure 11.6(a).

If an external magnetic field is applied to this material, it will apply a rotating force to each domain causing the atoms in the domain to turn. If the force is sufficiently strong, all the domains will align with the magnetic field. In this condition the sample is said to have reached *magnetic saturation* since no further magnetisation is possible.

It is because of the alignment of the atoms within each domain that a ferromagnetic material shows such a strong induced magnetisation to an applied magnetic field—each domain behaves like a team of atomic magnets working together. In a paramagnetic material the atoms behave as individual magnets and so it is much more difficult to align them to an applied magnetic field because of the disruptive effect of interatomic collisions.

Ferromagnetic materials change their properties with temperature. At a particular temperature, known as the *Curie temperature*, the atoms can no longer overcome the disrupting effect of the increased interatomic collisions and so the domains disappear. Thus, below the Curie temperature the material is ferromagnetic and above the Curie temperature the material is paramagnetic. Because of the resulting atomic disorder, the relative permeability is greatly reduced.

Examples of ferromagnetic materials and their relative permeabilities are given in Table 11.1. We are probably most familiar with the magnetic properties of iron, but stalloy, because of its use in transformer cores, is also important in radiographic science. The Curie temperature for iron is 1043 K (770°C).

An important phenomenon in the magnetisation of a ferromagnetic material is the effect known as *hysteresis* and this will now be considered briefly. Because hysteresis is of great importance in the choice of materials for a transformer core, the full discussion of hysteresis will be in Chapter 17 which deals with the AC transformer.

11.7 HYSTERESIS

For diamagnetic and paramagnetic materials, the intensity of magnetisation within the sample, I, is proportional to the magnetising force, H. Thus if H is doubled then I is also doubled. However, this is not the case with ferromagnetic materials due to the effect of the domains on each other. Two types of forces exist between the domains:

• An *elastic* or *reversible* force caused by the movement of the domain boundaries—some domains get larger at the expense of others when an external magnetic field is applied. This is reversible when the field, H, is removed.

• A *frictional* or *irreversible* force corresponding to the rotation of the domains as they attempt to align themselves with the external magnetic field in a series of minute *jerks*.

This jerking movement between the domains means that the applied magnetic field increases before some of the domains respond to it by rotating. Thus the orientation of the domains and hence the induced magnetism (I) *lags behind* the magnetising force (H). If the magnetising force is now removed, some magnetism will remain in the sample and requires a magnetising force in the opposite direction to remove it. This effect of the magnetism lagging behind the magnetising force is known as *hysteresis* and will be discussed further in Chapter 17 where its effect on the efficiency of an AC transformer will be considered.

Insight

The effect described for hysteresis is exactly the same as the situation which exists if you try to rotate a book on a table top. The rotational force applied must increase to a point where it is greater than the frictional forces between the book and the table top before rotation of the book will occur. If the book is to be returned to its original orientation a rotational force, in the opposite direction, larger than the frictional forces, must now be applied.

Summary

In this chapter you should have learnt:

• Magnetic poles always exist in *pairs* because the atoms of a magnetic substance behave like small bar magnets (see Sect. 11.2).
• The force between two magnetic poles is given by the equation $F = m_1 m_2 / 4\pi\mu d^2$ where F is in newtons, m_1 and m_2 are in webers, d is in metres and μ is in henry per metre (see Sect. 11.2.1).
• If μ_0 is the permeability of a vacuum, and μ is the permeability of a substance, then the *relative permeability* μ_r is given by $\mu_r = \mu/\mu_0$ (see Sect. 11.2.1).
• A *magnetic field* exists at a point if a force would be experienced by a magnetic pole placed at that point (see Sect. 11.3).
• The *magnetic force H* is the magnitude of the magnetic field (or field strength) (see Sect. 11.3).

- The *magnetic flux density B* is a measure of the amount of magnetic flux per unit area (Wb·m^{-2}) and has the special unit the tesla (T) where 1 T = 1 Wb·m^{-2}. It is dependent on the medium through which it passes (see Sect. 11.4).
- The relationship between the magnetising force, H, and the magnetic flux density, B, is given by the equation $B = \mu H$ where μ is the permeability of the medium (see Sect. 11.5).
- If:
  — μ_r is less than unity then the material is *diamagnetic*
  — μ_r is just greater than unity then the material is *paramagnetic*
  — μ_r is much greater than unity then the material is *ferromagnetic* (see Sect. 11.6).
- All materials are *diamagnetic*, but the effect is usually negligible compared to the *paramagnetism* or *ferromagnetism* in the same sample (see Sect. 11.6.1).
- At high temperatures, paramagnetic materials become diamagnetics. Ferromagnetics become paramagnetics above the *Curie temperature* (see Sects 11.6.2 and 11.6.3).
- The reason for the relatively high permeabilities of ferromagnetic materials is the internal ordered arrangement of atoms into *magnetic domains*. Within each domain the atoms point in the same direction but the direction of the domains is randomised in the non-magnetised material (see Sect. 11.6.3).
- The application of a magnetising force, H, to a ferromagnetic material results in two types of forces within the material:
  — one which allows the expansion of some domains at the expense of others and which will disappear when the magnetising force, H, is removed
  — one which rotates the domains in the same direction as H but which will not disappear completely when H is removed (see Sect. 11.7).
- The fact that the domains are 'sticky' in their movement means that the magnetisation of the sample (I) lags behind the magnetising force H. This is known as *hysteresis* (see Sect. 11.7).

SELF-TEST

a. Give the equation which can be used to calculate the force between two magnetic poles m_1 and m_2 separated by a distance d in a vacuum.

b. Draw the magnetic field around a bar magnet (for simplicity, the influence on this field by the earth's magnetic field can be ignored).

c. Materials may be either diamagnetic, paramagnetic or ferromagnetic. Discuss the differences between the three types of materials.

d. Discuss the meaning of the term *hysteresis*.

FURTHER READING

Ball J L, Moore A D 1986 Essential physics for radiographers, 2nd edn. Blackwell Scientific Publications, London, ch 8

Gifford D 1984 A handbook of physics for radiologists and radiographers. John Wiley & Sons, Chichester, ch 6

Hay G A, Hughes D 1983 First year physics for radiographers. Baillière Tindall, London, ch 6

Ohanian H C 1994 Principles of physics. W W Norton, London, ch 21

Thompson M A 1994 Principles of imaging science and protection. W B Saunders, London, ch 5

12

Electromagnetism

12.1 AIM

The aim of this chapter is to consider the basic properties of magnetism discussed in Chapter 11 and show how these can be applied to a current-carrying conductor thus giving an electromagnet.

12.2 INTRODUCTION

In the previous chapter it was shown that magnetism is a phenomenon associated with atoms, and is due to the spinning and orbiting of electrons around those atoms. Electrons are negatively charged particles (Sect. 9.3), and so we may conclude that magnetism is caused by moving electric charges. It is thus reasonable to ask whether an electric current in a wire (for example) may also produce a magnetic field, since an electric current is just the flow of electrons in a conductor (Sects 10.2 and 10.3). This is found to be so in practice and the term *electromagnetism* is used to describe this effect (i.e. *electricity* producing *magnetism*).

12.3 ELECTRON FLOW AND 'CONVENTIONAL' CURRENT

When electricity was first discovered, it was assumed that it was the *positive* charges which flow in a conductor, and not the negative charges. This concept is now known as the 'conventional' current. However, it is now known that the *positive* charges in a solid material *do not have any net movement* (although they vibrate with heat energy; Ch. 8), since they form the protons in the nuclei of atoms (Ch. 26). Thus it is the *electrons* which move in a solid, as explained by the elementary electron theory of conduction (Sect. 10.2).

In gas or liquid, any positive and negative charges present may take part in current flow, since the positive charges are free to move, unlike in a solid. In radiography and many other subjects, however, it is the *electron* flow in conductors which is most frequently under consideration, and herein lies a difficulty, for many rules (or conventions) in electromagnetism and electromagnetic induction (Ch. 13) are based upon the totally erroneous assumption of the 'conventional' current, which in a mathematical sense is supposed to flow in the opposite direction to that of the electrons.

This and further chapters will therefore discuss both electromagnetism and electromagnetic induction on the basis of *electron flow only*, in an attempt to eliminate much of the confusion which undoubtedly exists at present in many people's minds. Some caution is therefore required when studying these subjects from other books, as they may invoke the 'conventional' current for their rules. Differences in the two approaches are explained in the 'Insights' where appropriate.

12.4 MAGNETIC FIELD DUE TO A STRAIGHT WIRE

Historically, the presence of a magnetic field around a current-carrying conductor was first discovered by Oersted when passing a current through a straight wire placed near a magnetic compass, as illustrated in Figure 12.1.

If the wire is aligned in a north–south direction (i.e. along the direction of the compass needle), then an electric current through the wire causes deflections of the compass as shown: *clockwise* when the wire is above the compass (a), and *anticlockwise* when the wire is below the compass (b). This is possible only if the lines of magnetic force (Sect. 11.3) are circular and in an anticlockwise direction when viewed along the same direction as the movement of the flowing electrons. We may therefore use the following convention:

Convention

Each moving electron produces an *anticlockwise* magnetic field about itself when viewed along the direction of its motion.

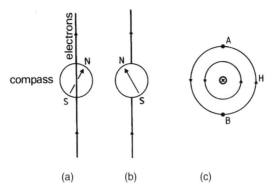

Figure 12.1   (a) and (b) show the effect of the magnetic field produced by the electrons flowing in the wire upon a magnetic compass; (c) shows that if we look along the wire in the direction of electron flow, then the field is in an anticlockwise direction (⊗ means that the electrons are flowing away from the eye of the observer).

This convention is illustrated in Figure 12.1(c), where the symbol '⊗' means that electron flow is away from the eye (' ⊙ ' is towards the eye). The arrows on the lines of force are in an anticlockwise direction, in accordance with our convention, and give the direction in which a north pole would move if placed in that position (Sect. 11.3). Thus, a weightless north pole would, if released, travel round and round the wire indefinitely in an anticlockwise circle.

12.5 MAGNETIC FIELD DUE TO A CIRCULAR COIL OF WIRE

Figure 12.2(a) shows a circular coil of wire in which an electric current is made to flow. Now, each individual moving electron produces anti-clockwise magnetic lines of force about itself (Sect. 12.4) as illustrated in

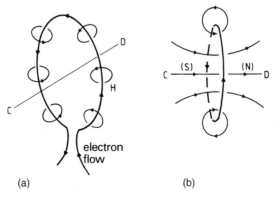

Figure 12.2   The magnetic field around a coil of wire carrying a current. Note the similarity to the field around a small bar magnet.

Figure 12.2(a). The closeness of the lines of force to each other represents the total magnetic effect, (i.e. the magnetic flux density, as described in Sect. 11.4). The addition at a point of all the magnetic flux densities represented by the lines of force produces the total magnetic flux density at that point. Note that, within the coil, the lines of force all tend to be in the direction C to D, while outside the coil, they are from D to C. A top view of the coil (Fig. 12.2(b)) shows the pattern of the overall lines of force so obtained. It is interesting to note the similarity of these lines of force to those of a short bar magnet (see Fig. 11.3), where they emerge from the north pole end and travel around the magnet to the south pole end and back again. Here we have the reason for the 'atomic magnets', where (on a tiny scale) the coil would be equivalent to the net flow of electrons around a particular atomic nucleus, producing lines of force as in Figure 12.2(b) and hence the magnetised atom.

12.6 MAGNETIC FIELD DUE TO A SOLENOID

A solenoid consists of several coils joined together, and so produces magnetic lines of force, as shown in Figure 12.3(a), similar to a bar magnet. The effect of a piece of soft iron within the solenoid is to increase the magnetic flux density many times because of the induced magnetism within the soft iron (Sects 11.5 and 11.6.3). This effect is reflected by an increase in the number of lines of force in Figure 12.3(b) compared to Figure 12.3(a). The combination of solenoid and soft iron in this manner is known as an electromagnet.

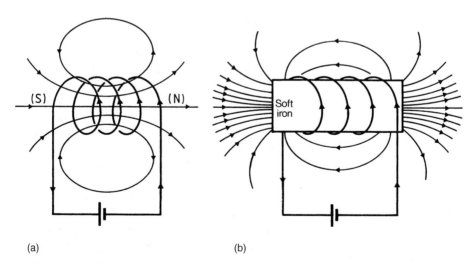

(a)   (b)

Figure 12.3   (a) shows the magnetic field produced by a current-carrying solenoid; (b) shows the large increase in the magnetic field produced when using a soft-iron core in the solenoid.

Insight

A general method of calculating the magnetic flux from any general shape of current-carrying conductor is due to Biot and Savart. The formula shown in Figure 12.4 may be used to calculate the magnetic flux density from any general shape of wire. (Table 12.1 shows some of these examples.)

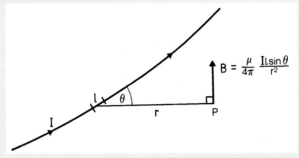

$$B = \frac{\mu}{4\pi} \frac{I L \sin \theta}{r^2}$$

Figure 12.4 Biot and Savart's Law for determining the magnetic flux density due to any shape of current-carrying conductor.

Now, $B = \mu H$ (from Equation 11.5)

$$H = \frac{B}{\mu} = \text{constant} \times \frac{Il}{r^2}$$ (from rearranging the equation in Fig. 12.4)

so that the units of the magnetic field strength (or magnetising force) H are in ampere/metre.

12.7 THE ELECTROMAGNETIC RELAY

The electromagnetic relay is a very useful electrical device for switching electrical circuits on and off by remote control. It makes possible the switching of large currents and/or voltages to remote devices (e.g. an X-ray tube) by the application of a small current to the solenoid of the electromagnetic relay. The great advantage of the use of an electromagnetic relay for this purpose lies in the increased safety factor to the operator, since no large voltages or currents need to be connected to any of the controls on the operating console. Such controls on the X-ray panel (e.g. 'X-ray tube changeover switch') supply power to electromagnets which switch on the appropriate part of the X-ray electrical circuit. This may be verified by hearing the 'clonking' noise which occurs at the high-tension transformer when a different tube is selected. Many of the functions which were formerly carried out by relays are now carried out by solid-state switches (see Ch. 18).

The general structure of the electromagnetic relay is as shown in Figure 12.5.

Conductor	Magnetic flux density, B. (Tesla)
Infinite straight wire	$B = \dfrac{\mu_o I}{2\pi r}$
Circular coil	$B = \dfrac{\mu_o I}{2 r}$
Infinite solenoid	$B = \mu_o n I$ (air only) $B = \mu n I$ n is no. turns/metre

Table 12.1 The magnetic flux density from different shapes of current-carrying condutors

Operation

When switch S is open, no current flows through the solenoid and so the soft iron piece M is held in the position shown by the spring P. Contacts C_1 and C_3 are in contact, while C_1 and C_2 are 'open'. When S is closed, the current passing through the solenoid magnetises the soft iron core (Sect. 11.5) which attracts M by induced magnetism. M pivots about O so

Figure 12.5   The electromagnetic relay (see text for details of operation).

that the arm L lifts C_1 away from C_3 and into contact with C_2. Thus, if the external circuit is joined, current will flow between C_1 and C_2 but no current will flow between C_1 and C_3. Opening S reduces the current in the solenoid to zero and hence restores the system to its original condition, since M loses its magnetism and is pulled quickly away under the action of the spring P (C_1 and C_3 are closed and C_1 and C_2 are open).

Summary

In this chapter you should have learnt:

- Atomic magnetism is caused by electrons orbiting atomic nuclei. Electromagnetism is caused by 'isolated' moving particles (e.g. 'free' electrons) (see Sect. 12.2).
- Negative and positive charges may flow in a vacuum, gas or liquid, but only negative charges (electrons) may flow in a solid. This is because the atomic nuclei (which contain the positively charged protons) are not free to move in a solid (see Sect. 12.3).
- Circular magnetic fields exist around moving charges:
  —anticlockwise around negative charges
  —clockwise around positive charges
  when viewed along the direction of motion (see Sect. 12.4).
- The magnetic flux density due to a current-carrying solenoid may be increased many times by inserting within it a material of high permeability, e.g. soft iron, since $B = \mu H$ (see Table 11.1). The magnetic domains become aligned with the direction of H, so adding to the overall magnetic flux density (see Sect. 12.6).
- The electromagnetic relay is a device used for switching a circuit on and off under remote control, depending upon whether a solenoid is energised or not. The advantage of such a system is that a low current may be used to switch a high current or voltage at a remote location, thus increasing the safety factor against electrical shock for the operators of the equipment (see Sect. 12.7).

SELF-TEST

a. Compare the similarities between the atomic magnets within a bar magnet and the magnetic field produced by an electric current in a coil of wire.

b. Why does a piece of soft iron within a solenoid increase the magnetic effect of the solenoid when an electric current is passed through it? Explain why this increase does not continue indefinitely as the current through the solenoid is increased. (*Hint:* see Sect. 11.6.3)

c. What is an electromagnetic relay? Draw a simple diagram of its construction and hence explain how it operates.

FURTHER READING

Ball J L, Moore A D 1986 Essential physics for radiographers, 2nd edn. Blackwell Scientific Publications, London, ch 8
Hay G A, Hughes D 1983 First year physics for radiographers. Baillière Tindall, London, ch 6
Ohanian H C 1994 Principles of physics. W W Norton, London, ch 21

13

Electromagnetic induction

13.1 AIM

The aim of this chapter is to consider the laws of electromagnetic induction. The direction of the induced current will be identified. The concepts of mutual induction and self-induction will be discussed in preparation for Chapter 17 where the application of these will be considered in transformer design.

13.2 INTRODUCTION

In the previous chapter we covered the topic of *electromagnetism* and in this chapter we will deal with the topic of *electromagnetic induction*. As can be seen from the definitions below, one is just the reverse of the other. They may each be defined as follows:

> **Definitions**
>
> *Electromagnetism* is the production of a magnetic field by the passage of an electrical current (see Ch. 12).
>
> *Electromagnetic induction* is the production of electricity by the interlinking of a conductor with a changing magnetic field, or moving a conductor relative to a stationary magnetic field (also known as the generator effect).

13.3 CONDITIONS NECESSARY FOR ELECTROMAGNETIC INDUCTION

Consider the simple experiment depicted in Figure 13.1. A solenoid L is joined to a meter which can measure both the magnitude and the direction of the current flowing through the solenoid. The following effects are observed:

- No current flow is observed on the meter if the magnet is *stationary* with respect to the solenoid (Fig. 13.1(a) and (c)).

Figure 13.1 An example of electromagnetic induction. A current flows only when there is relative movement between the bar magnet and the solenoid.

- A current flows through the meter whenever the magnet is *moved* towards or away from the solenoid (Fig. 13.1(b) and (d)).
- The *magnitude* of the induced current is *greater* if the magnet is moved *faster*.
- Reversing the direction of the movement of the magnet reverses the direction of the induced current (Fig. 13.1(b) and (d)).
- Reversing the pole of the magnet which is closer to the solenoid reverses the direction of the induced current for a given movement.

From this simple experiment we can conclude that *only a changing magnetic field relative to the conductor* is able to induce electricity in the conductor. Also we can see that the amount of electricity produced is in some way related to the *rate of change of the magnetic field* relative to the conductor. Finally we can conclude that the *direction of movement of the magnetic field* influences the direction of the induced current. These concepts will be discussed in more detail in the following sections of this chapter.

13.4 FARADAY'S LAWS OF ELECTROMAGNETIC INDUCTION

Faraday produced two laws of electromagnetic induction which cover some of the observations we made in the previous section. These may be defined as follows:

1. A change in the magnetic flux linked with a conductor induces an EMF in the conductor.
2. The magnitude of the induced EMF is proportional to the rate of change of the magnetic flux linkage.

In order to understand Faraday's Laws we need to have a clear understanding of *EMF* and *magnetic flux linkage.*

EMF (electromotive force) was considered in Section 10.6 and can be considered as the force which is capable of causing electrons to flow (i.e. EMF will cause a current to flow in a complete circuit). It is important to note that Faraday's Laws do not specify whether or not the conductor is connected to an external circuit, but in either case, an EMF will be induced in it.

In Section 11.4 *magnetic flux* and *magnetic flux density* were discussed. The magnetic flux through a volume V may be visualised as being proportional to the number of lines of flux passing through that volume (see Fig. 13.2). Thus if a magnetic flux of 10 weber (Sect. 11.4) passes through V, then the magnetic flux linkage with V is also said to be 10 weber. If the magnet in Figure 13.2 is moved to the left of the page, then the number of lines of flux (or the flux linkage) in the volume V will be reduced.

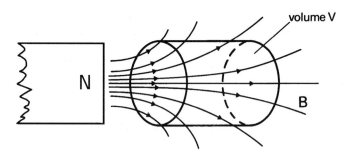

Figure 13.2 The magnetic flux linkage associated with a volume *V*.

We now see that moving the magnet relative to the solenoid will alter the flux linkage between the magnet and the solenoid and so an EMF will be induced—Faraday's First Law. Also, a rapid movement of the magnet increases the rate of change of flux linkage and so increases the size of the induced EMF—Faraday's Second Law.

Changing the magnetic flux linkage associated with a particular conductor may be achieved in two ways:

- by moving the conductor relative to a stationary magnet—this principle is used in the AC generator or dynamo (Sect. 13.9)
- by varying the magnitude of the magnetic flux while the conductor is stationary—this principle is used in the AC transformer (see Ch. 17).

13.5 LENZ'S LAW

In our initial observations regarding the induced current (Sect. 13.3) we noted the direction as well as the size of the current. Faraday's Laws apply to *open* or *closed* circuits but, as Lenz's Law concerns the direction of the induced current, it can only be applied to *closed* circuits. The law can be stated as follows:

> **The *direction* of the induced *current* in a conductor caused by a changing magnetic flux is such that its own magnetic field *opposes* the changing magnetic flux.**

Insight

Lenz's Law is an example of the application of the Law of Conservation of Energy (Sect. 5.3). If the direction of the induced current was such that its magnetic field *helped* the changing magnetic field, then we would be getting something for nothing so we could establish perpetual motion of the conductor and the magnetic field. This would be in defiance of the Law of Conservation of Energy.

When the north pole of a bar magnet is moved towards a solenoid (see Fig. 13.1(b)), the current will flow in the solenoid in such a direction that it produces a north pole at the end closest to the magnet. This has the effect of producing a force of repulsion between the bar magnet and the solenoid and so *work* must be done against this force in order to keep the magnet moving towards the solenoid. Thus *mechanical energy* is transformed to *electrical energy* and the Law of Conservation of Energy is maintained. The reverse occurs when the magnet is withdrawn.

13.6 SIGN CONVENTION FOR THE INDUCED CURRENT

When current flow was considered as the flow of positive charge, this was determined using Fleming's Right Hand Rule. As we now know that

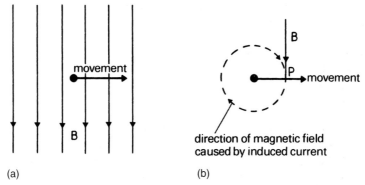

(a)   (b)

Figure 13.3   An example of the use of the convention described in the text for establishing the direction of the induced current.

current flow is a flow of electrons, Fleming's hand rules are liable to cause confusion and so the direction of current flow will be determined using the convention shown below:

Convention

Consider a situation similar to that shown in Figure 13.3(a) where a conductor is moved at right angles to a magnetic field—the direction of the movement and the direction of the magnetic field are as shown in the diagram. We wish to determine whether the induced electron flow along the conductor will be either into the page or out of the page. This can be determined as follows:

1. Mark the position of the conductor and draw a line to indicate the direction of movement.
2. Draw a second line to represent the permanent magnetic field direction to intersect the first line at the point P (see Fig. 13.3(b)).
3. Now draw a circle with the conductor at its centre such that its circumference passes through the point P.
4. This circle represents the magnetic field which will be caused by the current induced in the conductor. The direction of this magnetic field is the same as the direction of the permanent magnetic field at the point P—the field is in a clockwise direction.
5. As we learnt in Section 12.4 *the magnetic field around a current-carrying conductor is anticlockwise when the electrons are travelling away from us*. Thus, because of the

clockwise magnetic field we can conclude that the electrons (of the induced current) are travelling towards us.

13.7 MUTUAL INDUCTION

If a changing current is passed through one conductor, then this will produce a changing magnetic field around this conductor (see Ch. 12). If a second conductor is placed within this changing magnetic field, then (by Faraday's Laws) an EMF will be generated in the conductor and a current will flow in it if the conducting loop is complete (see Fig. 13.4). By Lenz's Law this current will be in the opposite direction to the original current. The size of this secondary current will vary with the magnetic field—it will be a current of changing magnitude as there is a changing magnetic field. This changing secondary current will produce its own changing magnetic field which will induce an EMF and current in the first conductor. Thus *each conductor induces electricity in the other* and the effect is known as *mutual induction*.

Consider Figure 13.4. When the switch SW is closed, electrons will flow from the negative pole of the battery to its positive pole via the coil P. During the time while the rate of flow of electrons builds up, there is a changing magnetic field around P. This is linked to S via the iron core (the iron core greatly enhances the flux linkage) and so an EMF and current flow will occur in S. The direction of the pointer on the ammeter M indicates that this flow of electrons in S is in the opposite direction to that in P, thus verifying Lenz's Law. After a short time, the current in P is

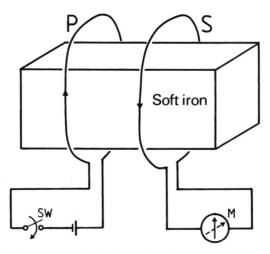

Figure 13.4 Principles of mutual induction. A changing current in coil P (the primary coil) induces a current in coil S (the secondary coil) and vice versa. The soft iron core magnifies the effect by improving the magnetic flux linkage between the coils.

constant and so S is no longer influenced by a *changing* magnetic field. As a result no EMF is generated in S (Faraday's First Law). If the switch SW is now opened, the magnetic field around P collapses and so an EMF is again generated in P, but this time it is in the opposite direction. If a more powerful battery is now used, this will produce a greater current in P, thus a greater magnetic field and consequently a greater EMF in S (the magnitude of the induced EMF is proportional to the rate of change of the magnetic flux). Finally, if we undertake the experiment with the iron bar present, and then with the iron bar removed, we find that the EMF produced in the coil S is greatest when the iron bar is present. This is because of improved magnetic flux linkage (Faraday's Second Law).

From this experiment we can show that the EMF induced in the secondary winding E_s is:

a. proportional to the rate of change of the current in P (the primary)
b. dependent on the detailed design of the two conductors and the flux linkage between them. This is called the *mutual inductance (M)*.

Thus:

$$E_s = M \times \text{rate of change of primary current} \qquad \text{Equation 13.1}$$

The greater the mutual inductance, M, the greater the mutual effect between the two conductors. M is measured in henry and may be defined as:

Definition

A mutual inductance of 1 *henry* exists between two conductors if 1 volt is induced in one conductor where there is a current change of 1 ampere per second in the other.

As will be explained in Chapter 17, an AC transformer works on the principle of mutual induction.

13.8 SELF-INDUCTION

Consider the solenoid in Figure 13.5(a). If the switch SW is closed, current flow starts to build up in the solenoid. As this current increases, *each turn* of the solenoid produces a changing magnetic flux which is linked to the *other turns* of the solenoid (the flux from one turn is shown in Fig. 13.5(a)). Thus from Faraday's and Lenz's Laws an EMF in the opposite direction to the EMF from the battery will be induced in the solenoid—this is known as a *back EMF*. This effect is known as *self-induction* and, if the self-induction is large, the current in the coil will take an appreciable time to build up to its maximum value. The self-induction in an electrical system is defined

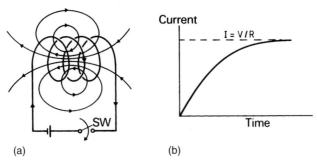

(a)   (b)

Figure 13.5 Principles of self-induction. The changing magnetic flux produced by the current flow through the solenoid links with all the turns of the coil. This produces a back EMF which slows down the rate of growth of current in the coil.

in a very similar manner to the mutual induction and is given by the equation:

$$E_B = L \times \text{rate of change of current} \qquad \text{Equation 13.2}$$

Here E_B is the back EMF and L is the self-inductance measured in henry. Thus we can say that:

Definition

A conductor has a *self-inductance* of 1 *henry* if a back EMF of 1 volt is induced when the current flowing through it changes at 1 ampere per second.

A graph of the current flowing through the solenoid is shown in Figure 13.5(b). As can be seen, the induced back EMF slows down the rate of growth of the current and so it takes an appreciable time to reach its maximum value determined by Ohm's Law (Sect. 10.8). If the wire of the solenoid were unwound to become a straight conductor, then there would be no magnetic flux linkage and consequently no back EMF. Thus the current would rise to its maximum value very quickly.

As in the case of mutual induction, a soft iron bar placed in the solenoid will enhance the self-induction as the magnetic flux linkage between the coils is improved.

As will be explained in Chapter 17, an autotransformer works on the principle of self-induction.

13.9 THE AC GENERATOR

Electric power is produced from an AC generator. This is an example of a situation where mechanical energy is converted to electrical energy. The basic components of such a generator are shown in Figure 13.6(a). A permanent magnetic field exists between the poles of the magnet, and coils

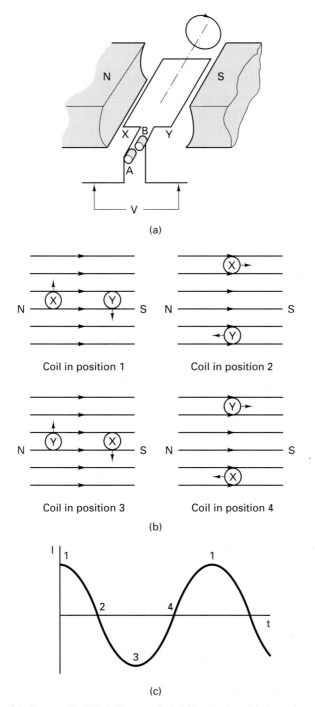

(a)

Coil in position 1

Coil in position 2

Coil in position 3

Coil in position 4

(b)

(c)

Figure 13.6 (a) shows a simplified diagram of an AC generator; (b) shows four positions of the coil relative to the magnetic field; (c) shows the current waveform produced when the coil moves through positions 1, 2, 3, 4 and returns to 1. A complete turn of the coil will produce one cycle of current.

of copper wire are made to rotate through this field—for simplicity, only one coil is shown in the diagram. The EMF generated in the device is collected at *brushes* positioned at A and B.

Consider the situation where the coil shown is rotated in a clockwise direction. Thus, from the initial position, side X of the coil will move upwards through the magnetic field and side Y will move downwards (see Fig. 13.6(b)). At this point in its movement, the coil is cutting the maximum number of lines of flux as it is moving at right angles to the flux lines, and so the maximum EMF will be generated. If we use the convention discussed earlier (see Sect. 13.6) to establish the direction of electron flow, we can see that electrons will travel towards us on side X and away from us on side Y. Thus an excess of electrons will exist at brush A and a shortage of electrons will exist at brush B—brush A is negative and brush B is positive. This situation is shown as position 1 on the graph in Figure 13.6(c). Now consider the situation when the coil has turned in a clockwise direction from its initial position through 90°—this is the second position of the coil shown in Figure 13.6(b). In this position both side X and side Y of the coil are moving parallel with the lines of magnetic flux and so no current is generated—this is again shown as position 2 in Figure 13.6(c). In position 3 the coil has rotated through 180° from its original position. Side X of the coil is now moving downwards through the magnetic field and side Y is moving upwards. As in position 1, a maximum number of lines of flux are being cut as the conductor is moving at right angles to the flux, and so, again, the maximum EMF will be generated. The polarity of A and B is now the reverse of position 1. In position 4 the conductor is again moving parallel to the lines of flux so no EMF is generated. The conductor then returns to position 1 and so one cycle is complete. The process is then repeated. The type of current shown in Figure 13.6(c) is known as an *alternating current* and will be the subject of the next chapter.

In cases where there is no external circuit connected, then no current is able to flow and only sufficient work to overcome the frictional resistance is necessary to keep the rotational movement at the same speed. As soon as an external circuit is connected, then a current is able to flow in the circuit and in the winding. It should come as no surprise to discover that this current will flow in such a direction as to oppose the motion of the coil (remember Lenz's Law). This means that mechanical work must be performed to overcome this resisting force, i.e. mechanical energy is converted into electrical energy.

The effect of suddenly increasing the electrical load demanded from the generator (e.g. when making an X-ray exposure) is to suddenly increase the opposition to its rotation. Hence, the generator slows down momentarily and the induced EMF (which depends on the speed of rotation) is reduced. Thus we find that, in times of increased demand on the generators, there is a drop in the voltage they supply. In X-ray units this is taken into account by the inclusion of a *mains voltage compensator* on the unit.

Summary
In this chapter you should have learnt: • That an EMF is induced in a conductor if it is linked with a changing magnetic field (see Sect. 13.3)   • Faraday's First and Second Law of electromagnetic induction (see Sect. 13.4)   • Lenz's Law which determines the direction of the current flowing as the result of the induced EMF (see Sect. 13.5)   • The sign convention for the direction of the induced current (see Sect. 13.6)   • The meaning and a simple application of mutual induction (see Sect. 13.7)   • The meaning and a simple application of self-induction (see Sect. 13.8)   • The mode of operation of an AC generator (see Sect. 13.9).

SELF-TEST

a. What is meant by the term *electromagnetic induction* and how does it differ from the term *electromagnetism*?

b. State and explain Faraday's and Lenz's Laws of electromagnetic induction. List the factors on which the magnitude of the induced EMF depends.

c. In what circumstances is it possible to have an induced EMF without an induced current?

d. If a wire is moved as indicated by the arrow across a magnetic field, *B*, what will be the direction of the EMF induced in the wire? In what direction would the wire be moved relative to the magnetic field to produce:
   (i) the maximum EMF
   (ii) zero EMF?

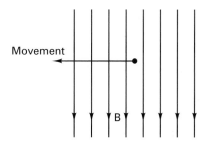

e. A bar magnet having its north pole pointing downwards is dropped through a horizontal loop of wire. What is the direction of the induced current in the wire when the magnet is moving downwards:
   (i) above the wire
   (ii) below the wire?

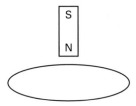

f. What is meant by *mutual induction* and *self-induction*? Define the unit in which each is measured.

g. Explain the generation of an EMF in an AC generator. What is the effect on this generator of a sudden increase in the load drawn from it? Explain how this affects the output from the generator.

FURTHER READING

Ball J L, Moore A D 1986 Essential physics for radiographers, 2nd edn. Blackwell Scientific Publications, London, ch 9
Hay G A, Hughes D 1983 First year physics for radiographers. Baillière Tindall, London, ch 7
Ohanian H C 1994 Principles of physics. W W Norton, London, ch 22
Thompson M A 1994 Principles of imaging science and protection. W B Saunders, London, ch 5

14

Alternating current flow

14.1 AIM

The aim of this chapter is to introduce the reader to alternating current flow. The various parameters used to measure such a current will be discussed. Simple AC circuits will be considered as will three-phase power supplies.

14.2 INTRODUCTION

Direct current (DC) electricity (Ch. 10) is representative of a flow of electrons in one direction only. This chapter deals with the situation where electrons flow through a circuit first in one direction and then in the other—this is known as an *alternating current* (AC) flow.

14.3 TYPES OF DC AND AC

Figure 14.1 shows some different types of DC and AC in graphical form.

• Figure 14.1(a) is a case where the number of electrons passing a point per second in the circuit is constant and so we get a horizontal straight line. This is an example of the type of DC described in Chapter 10.
• Figure 14.1(b) is a case where the electrons always move in the same direction but the number of electrons passing a point varies with time—the electrons move as a series of pulses and so this is known as a *pulsatile* or *pulsating* DC.

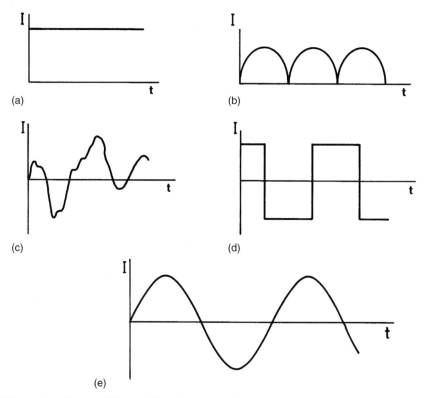

Figure 14.1 Types of DC and AC: (a) constant DC; (b) pulsatile DC; (c) irregular AC; (d) square wave AC; (e) sinusoidal AC.

- In Figure 14.1(c) there is no discernible pattern in the flow of the electrons except to say that they flow in both directions at different times. This is an example of an *irregular AC* waveform.
- Figure 14.1(d) shows a situation where the number of electrons travelling in one direction is constant for a short period of time and then the same number of electrons travel in the opposite direction for the same period of time. This is an example of a *square wave AC* waveform.
- Lastly, Figure 14.1(e) shows an example of a *sinusoidal AC* waveform. This is the most common type of AC waveform and will be discussed in detail in the rest of this chapter.

14.4 SINUSOIDAL AC

The sinusoidal AC waveform is illustrated in more detail in Figure 14.2 together with some of the quantities used to measure it. These are defined below:

Definitions	
One cycle:	One complete waveform, starting at any point and continuing until we reach the same point on the pattern. This is usually measured from zero to zero (ABCDE) or from peak to peak (BCDEF).
Period (T):	The time taken to complete one cycle, measured in seconds.
Frequency (f):	The number of cycles which occur in 1 second, measured in cycles per second or hertz (Hz).
Amplitude:	The maximum value of positive or negative current (or voltage) on the waveform. This may be referred to as the peak value.

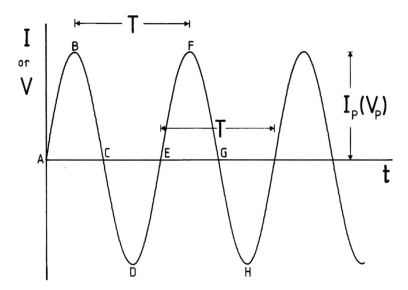

Figure 14.2   A sinusoidal current or voltage waveform.

There is a simple relationship between the *period* (*T*) and the *frequency* (*f*) which can be seen if we consider the following situation. Suppose we have a frequency of 10 Hz (10 cycles per second). Since the waveform is regular, each cycle must last for 0.1 second. Thus we can say:

$$f = \frac{1}{T}$$ Equation 14.1

For a sinusoidal current this equation may be rewritten as:

$$I_t = I_p \sin 2\pi ft$$

where I_t is the current at a time t and I_p is the amplitude or the *peak value* of the current. A similar equation can be produced for the voltage.

14.4.1 Peak current (or voltage)

The peak current is the same as the amplitude, i.e. *it is the maximum positive or negative value of the current*. Similarly, the peak voltage is the maximum value of the voltage. In radiography, the peak voltage across the tube, when the anode is positive and the cathode is negative, is usually quoted. If an X-ray tube is operating at 75 kV_p then the peak potential difference between the anode and the cathode is 75 kV. The reasons for quoting the tube voltage as kV_p will be considered later in this chapter.

14.4.2 Average current (or voltage)

As we can see from the graph in Figure 14.2, the average current flowing in one cycle of a sinusoidal waveform is *zero*, as the current flowing in one direction during the positive half-cycle has the same overall value (but opposite sign) as the current flowing in the opposite direction during the negative half-cycle. The same conclusion applies to any number of complete cycles. A similar argument suggests that the average voltage for a sinusoidal waveform is also zero. Thus for a sinusoidal waveform:

$$I_{AV} = 0$$
$$V_{AV} = 0$$ Equation 14.2

However, if the waveform is *rectified* (or made unidirectional) (Ch. 19) then a value of the average current (or voltage) is obtained. The voltage waveform produced for *half-wave rectification* is shown in Figure 14.3(a). This results in a pulsating voltage which (assuming a complete external circuit) results in a net electron flow in one direction—this allows us to consider average values of voltage and current which are not zero.

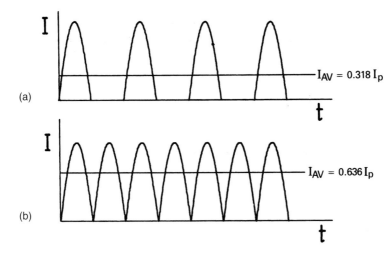

Figure 14.3 Forms of rectified sinusoidal AC: (a) shows half-wave rectification and (b) shows full-wave rectification.

The voltage waveform for a *full-wave rectified circuit* is shown on the same scale in Figure 14.3(b). Again a pulsating voltage is produced where the average value is twice that for the half-wave rectified circuit as there are twice as many peaks in unit time.

Thus we can say for half-wave rectification:

$$I_{AV} = 0.318I_P$$
$$V_{AV} = 0.318V_P$$

Equation 14.3

and for full-wave rectification:

$$I_{AV} = 0.636I_P$$
$$V_{AV} = 0.636V_P$$

Equation 14.4

14.4.3 Effective (or RMS) current or voltage

If an AC supply is connected across a resistor, then electrons will flow in one direction during the first half-cycle and in the opposite direction during the second half-cycle. As there is no net movement of electrons for any given number of complete cycles, the average current is zero. This does not mean, however, that the net *heating effect* is zero. Electrons will produce heat within a resistor irrespective of their direction of travel. The *average current* is therefore a quantity which is not suitable for determining the *energy* or *power* expended in a circuit which is connected to an AC supply. The quantity of importance is the *effective* or *RMS value* of the current and may be defined as:

Definition

The *effective current* is that value of constant current which, flowing for the same time, would produce the same expenditure of electrical energy in a circuit as the alternating current.

The effective value of the current is also known as the *root mean square (RMS) value* for reasons which we will consider below.

The effective or RMS *voltage* is defined in a very similar manner

---

Definition

The *effective voltage* is that value of constant voltage which, being present for the same time, would produce the same expenditure of electrical energy in a circuit as the alternating voltage.

Insight

Consider the graphs shown in Figure 14.4. The alternating current *I* has an average value of zero because each positive value is matched with an equal and opposite negative value.

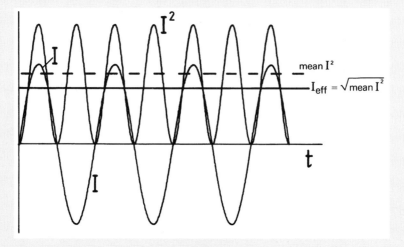

Figure 14.4 Graphic representation of an effective (RMS) value of current.

Thus the peak positive value is matched with a peak negative value. If we take these peak values and square them, this allows us to get rid of the negative sign and so it is possible to get an average value of the peak current squared. If we now take the square root of this value we have the *root* of the *mean* of the *square* of the peak value of the current. This is the effective value of the current, i.e.:

$$I_{RMS} = \frac{I_P}{\sqrt{2}}$$

In Section 10.9.3 it was shown that the general equation for DC electrical power was $W = VI$ where W is expressed in watts, V in volts and I in amperes. In an AC circuit both V and I are continually changing and so it is the effective or RMS value of each which must be taken into account when using the above equation:

$$W = V_{RMS} \times I_{RMS} \qquad \text{Equation 14.5}$$

Here W is the *average* power generated in the circuit taking into account at least one half-cycle of AC.

We can manipulate Equation 14.5 in a similar way to Equation 10.16 to get:

$$W = I_{RMS}^2 \times R$$

$$W = \frac{V_{RMS}^2}{R} \qquad \text{Equation 14.6}$$

Note that we can apply Ohm's Law (Ch. 10) to AC circuits provided the same types of units for voltage or current (e.g. RMS) are used throughout the equation.

The RMS values of current or voltage can be related to the peak relationships by the following equations:

$$I_{RMS} = 0.707 I_P$$
$$V_{RMS} = 0.707 V_P \qquad \text{Equation 14.7}$$

and:

$$I_P = 1.414 I_{RMS}$$
$$V_P = 1.414 V_{RMS} \qquad \text{Equation 14.8}$$

Thus, for an alternating current, the effective value is just over 70% of the peak value.

14.5 AC AND THE X-RAY TUBE

In order to produce X-rays, an X-ray tube requires a high potential difference (voltage) across it and a current flowing through it. The voltage available from the mains supply is far too low for use directly across the X-ray tube so a means of increasing it to the high values of thousands of volts is required. This is relatively easy to accomplish using an AC transformer (Ch. 17). Because this transformer increases the voltage, it is known as a *step-up transformer*. The filament of the X-ray tube requires a fairly low voltage supply so that it can produce the electrons which form the mA through the tube, and so the mains voltage passes through a *step-down transformer* before being applied to the filament. Thus an alternating voltage may either be *increased using a step-up transformer* or *decreased using a step-down transformer.*

In AC circuits the voltages or currents are usually expressed in terms of their effective values unless otherwise stated. When considering the X-ray circuit, the following convention applies:

- The voltage across the tube (kV) is expressed in terms of the *peak* voltage, i.e. kV_p.
- The current flowing through the tube (mA) is expressed in terms of the *average* current.
- The mains voltage and current to the X-ray set are expressed as *effective* or *RMS* values.

14.5.1 Voltage across the X-ray tube (kV_p)

The potential difference across the X-ray tube is expressed in terms of the peak value for the following reasons:

- The maximum energy of X-ray photons emitted by the anode is the same value in keV, i.e. an X-ray tube operated at 100 kV_p will emit X-ray photons with a maximum energy of 100 keV. (This will be explained in more detail in Ch. 28.)
- The voltage rating of the HT cables must be able to withstand the maximum voltage applied to them. This occurs during the peak value of the voltage.

If the voltage applied to the X-ray tube is a constant potential (Ch. 19), then this is effectively a DC supply so the peak and the effective values are the same.

14.5.2 Current through the tube (mA)

The mA meter is designed to measure the *average* current flowing through the X-ray tube during an exposure. The intensity of the radiation beam is proportional to the average current. If we take the average current (mA) and multiply this by the exposure time in seconds we get the mAs for that exposure. This represents the total charge which has passed through the X-ray tube during the exposure. The quantity of X-rays produced during the exposure is proportional to the mAs.

14.5.3 The mains voltage and current

The electrical mains is the source of power and so it makes sense to quote the mains supply in terms which make the calculations of power most convenient—the effective or RMS values. The mains voltage in the UK has a nominal value of 230 volts$_{RMS}$ and so this gives us a peak value for this voltage of approximately 325 volts (Equation 14.7).

14.6 BASICS OF AC CIRCUITS

Having considered the different measures which can be made of an alternating current or voltage, we are now ready to look at the consequences of passing this current through some basic circuits.

14.6.1 Phase difference

So far in this chapter we have only considered the case where the peak voltage occurs at the same time as the peak current. The current and voltage are then said to be *in phase*. This is not necessary for all types of AC circuits and we can get situations where a *phase difference* exists between the current and the voltage. Examples of such phase differences are shown in graphical form in Figure 14.5. In Figure 14.5(a) the current (I) lags behind the voltage (V)—a waveform displaced to the right occurs later than and therefore lags behind the waveform with which it is being compared. Also in Figure 14.5(b) we have a situation where the I leads V.

The angle between the two waveforms is expressed as the *phase angle* where 360° is equivalent to one cycle. This situation is often represented using a *vector diagram* (see Fig. 14.6(a)). (If you are not familiar with vector diagrams and vector addition, refer to Appendix A.) A phase angle of θ exists between the current and the voltage where OC is the current vector and OA is the voltage vector both of which rotate anticlockwise at a rate of f revolutions per second, where f is the frequency of the AC supply. In this example the voltage vector leads the current vector by θ. The magnitude

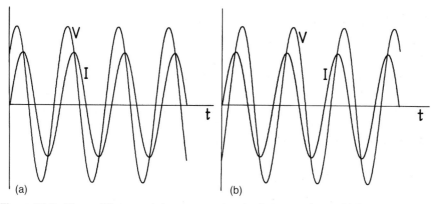

Figure 14.5   Phase differences between current and voltage waveforms: (a) I lags behind V; (b) I leads V.

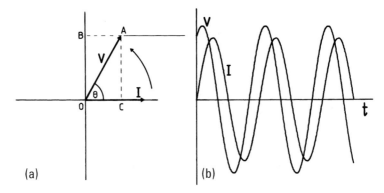

Figure 14.6 (a) A vector diagram for voltage and current. The vectors *V* and *I* rotate anticlockwise and the vertical height of each gives the instantaneous values of voltage and current. The angle *θ* is maintained throughout the rotation. *I* lags behind *V* on this diagram. (b) shows a plot of the voltage and the current against time for the vector diagram shown in (a).

of the voltage and the current at any stage during the cycle can be given by the *vertical distance* of the tip of each vector—the length OB for the voltage vector OA as shown in the figure. The angle *θ* between the vectors is maintained throughout the rotation of both vectors.

14.6.2 Reactance and impedance

When we considered the opposition to the flow of direct current in a circuit we found that this opposition consisted of *resistance* and was measured in ohms (see Ch. 10). There are two additional measures of 'AC resistance' of a circuit—the *reactance* and the *impedance*. Both are measured in ohms as in DC resistance but measure different quantities as explained below.

Consider Figure 14.7 where a phase difference of *θ* exists between the voltage across the circuit and the current flowing through it.

The *reactance*, *X*, is defined as the ratio OB/OC where OB is measured in volts and OC in amperes. The important point to note is that the measurements of the voltage and of the current taken are at right angles to each other. As will be shown later in this chapter, reactance is produced by capacitors and inductors, but not by resistors.

The *impedance*, *Z*, is defined as the ratio OA/OC where OA is measured in volts and OC is measured in amperes.

To summarise: Resistance, reactance and impedance all represent opposition to the flow of current and are all measured in ohms. They are expressed by the ratio of volts to amps but the voltage vector is different in each case—it is *in phase* with the current for *resistance*, at *right angles* to the current for *reactance* and at the *phase angle* to the current for *impedance*.

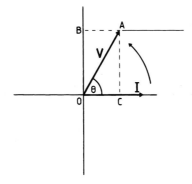

Figure 14.7   A vector diagram for voltage and current separated by a phase angle of θ.

Impedance is thus the general term for opposition to current flow, and *reactance* and *resistance* form separate components of this. The examples shown in Section 14.7 will help to further clarify these concepts.

14.6.3 Power in AC circuits

If an instantaneous voltage V causes an instantaneous current I to flow through a circuit, then the power W at that instant can be calculated from the equation $W = VI$ (see Sect. 10.9.3). However, in most cases we are not concerned with the instantaneous power during a point in the cycle but with the average power over one or more cycles. To get this value we use the effective (or RMS) values of the voltage and current (see Equation 14.5):

$$W = V_{RMS} \times I_{RMS}$$

This formula only holds true when there is no phase difference between V and I, i.e. $\theta = 0°$. It will be shown in the next section that reactance does not contribute to the power drawn from a supply—hence only the power produced in the resistance in the AC circuit needs to be considered. The latter is obtained by resolving V along I (i.e. $V \cos \theta$) so that the final expression of the power in an AC circuit is:

$$W = V_{RMS} \times I_{RMS} \times \cos \theta \qquad\qquad \text{Equation 14.9}$$

The *power factor* is the value of $\cos \theta$. This is unity for a circuit containing only resistors as there is no phase difference between voltage and current. If the circuit contains components which cause a phase difference between current and voltage, the value of the power factor will be less than unity.

The *wattless component* of the voltage V is $V \sin \theta$ and represents the component of V which produces no average power because it is in phase with the reactance. Likewise, the current flowing through a reactance is termed *wattless current*.

The power rating of high-tension transformers used in radiographic equipment is often quoted in *kVA*—kilovolts times amperes. This specifies the maximum output of the transformer when running continuously into a resistive load, i.e. *V* and *I* are in phase. The RMS values of the kV and current are used to calculate the values of kVA.

14.7 SIMPLE AC CIRCUITS

In Section 14.6 we considered a general account of *phase, reactance, impedance*, etc. and how they apply in general to AC circuits. In this section these concepts are applied to individual circuit components and their combined effect in a simple circuit is considered.

14.7.1 Resistors in AC circuits

Figure 14.8 shows the connection of an AC supply across a resistor. In this case there is no phase difference between the voltage and the current and

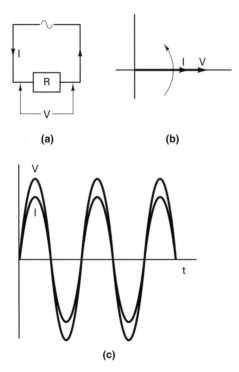

Figure 14.8 (a) A circuit diagram of an alternating current passing through a pure resistance; (b) shows the voltage and current vector diagram; (c) shows the voltage and current plotted against time for the vector diagram in (b). Note that *V* and *I* are in phase.

so the vector diagram shows both pointing in the same direction. They both rotate together giving sinusoidal voltage and current wave forms which peak at the same times and cross the axis at the same times.

As already explained, the average power generated in the resistor is given by the equation $W = V_{RMS} \times I_{RMS}$.

14.7.2 Capacitors in AC circuits

The detailed construction of capacitors and their functions in radiography will be discussed in Chapter 16. In this section we are purely interested in the effect caused when a capacitor is introduced into an AC circuit.

As can be seen from Figure 14.9, this results in a phase difference between the voltage and the current. The vector diagram indicates that the voltage across the capacitor *lags behind* the current flowing in and out of the capacitor by 90°. Thus a perfect capacitor in an AC circuit is considered as having reactance but no resistance.

The value of the *capacitance reactance* (X_C) is given by:

$$X_C = \frac{1}{2\pi fC} \qquad\qquad \text{Equation 14.10}$$

where *f* is the frequency of the AC supply (in Hz) and *C* is the capacitance of the capacitor in farads (see Ch. 16 for definitions of *capacitance* and the *farad*). Thus the capacitance reactance is inversely proportional to the frequency of the supply and the capacitance of the capacitor.

If we apply Equation 14.9 to the capacitor we can calculate that the average power generated in the capacitor is *zero* (cos 90° = 0). This is because in one half-cycle power is being supplied to the capacitor and in the other half-cycle the capacitor is giving the power back to the circuit.

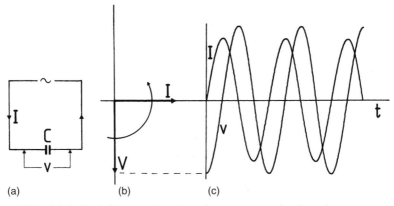

Figure 14.9 (a) A circuit diagram of an alternating current passing through a pure capacitance; (b) shows the voltage and current vector diagram; (c) shows the voltage and current plotted against time for the vector diagram in (b). Note that *I* leads *V* by 90°.

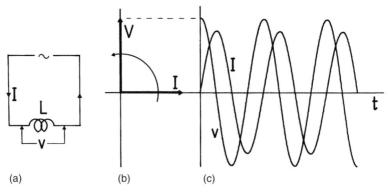

(a) (b) (c)

Figure 14.10 (a) A circuit diagram of an alternating current passing through a pure inductor; (b) shows the voltage and current vector diagram; (c) shows the voltage and current plotted against time for the vector diagram in (b). Note that *I* lags behind *V* by 90°.

14.7.3 Inductors in AC circuits

If we consider Figure 14.10 we can see that, when an inductor is placed in an AC circuit, the current and voltage are again out of phase. In this case the voltage *leads* the current by 90°. Thus a perfect inductor in an AC circuit is considered as having reactance but no resistance.

The reactance of an inductor (X_L) is given by the equation:

$$X_L = 2\pi f L \qquad\qquad \text{Equation 4.11}$$

where *f* is the frequency of the AC supply and *L* is the value of the inductance in henry. Thus the inductive reactance is directly proportional to the frequency (opposite to the capacitor; see Equation 14.10).

Because the current and voltage are 90° out of phase the net power drawn from the circuit is *zero*.

We have now seen that both capacitors and inductors which have only reactance consume zero power and so we can say that reactance consumes no power. Resistance, as mentioned earlier (see Equation 14.5) does consume power.

14.7.4 RLC in series—resonance circuits

Consider Figure 14.11(a) where a resistor (R), an inductor (L) and a capacitor (C) are connected in series with an AC supply. From the previous sections where we considered the effect of each on the circuit we can now draw a vector diagram of the inductive reactance (X_L), the capacitance reactance (X_C) and the resistance (R). Such a vector diagram is shown in Figure 14.11(b). (*Note* that the vectors for the reactance and the resistance are separated by the same phase angle as the voltages across each of the

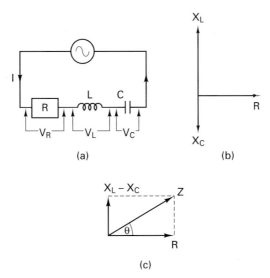

Figure 14.11   (a) A circuit diagram of an alternating current passing through a resistor (R) an inductor (L) and a capacitor (C). A vector diagram (b) shows the vectors of each of the components and (c) shows the net reactance and the overall impedance (Z) of the RLC circuit.

components.) We can now do vector addition to calculate the impedance (Z). As the capacitance reactance and the inductive reactance are in opposite directions, the net reactance is $(X_L - X_C)$. The diagram for the vector addition is shown in Figure 14.11(c). This shows that the impedance Z will have a phase difference of θ with respect to the current. (*Note* that the voltage and impedance vectors will be coincident and so the voltage and current will also have a phase difference of θ between them.)

We can now use Pythagoras' theorem as applied to Figure 14.11(c) to calculate the impedance thus:

$$Z^2 = R^2 + (X_L - X_C)^2$$

$$Z = \sqrt{[R^2 + (X_L - X_C)^2]} \qquad \text{Equation 14.12}$$

We can also calculate the phase angle as follows:

$$\tan \theta = \frac{(X_L - X_C)}{R}$$

$$\therefore \theta = \tan^{-1} \frac{(X_L - X_C)}{R} \qquad \text{Equation 14.13}$$

Finally, if we know the supply voltage, we can calculate the current flowing through the circuit:

$$Z = \frac{V}{I}$$

$$\therefore I = \frac{V}{Z}$$

$$= \frac{V}{\sqrt{[R^2 + (X_L - X_C)^2]}}$$

Equation 14.14

It is important to remember that if V is expressed in terms of peak voltage then the current calculated will be the peak current; if V is in RMS units so will be I.

A sample calculation may help to consolidate your understanding.

Example

A resistor of resistance 26 Ω is connected in series with an inductor of inductance 100 mH and a capacitor of capacitance 50 μF in an AC circuit with a frequency of 100 Hz. If the voltage has a peak value of 400 V, calculate the *impedance,* the *phase angle* and the *peak current.*

$$
\begin{aligned}
X_L &= 2\pi fL && \text{(from Equation 14.11)}\\
&= 2\pi \times 100 \times 100 \times 10^{-3}\\
&= 2\pi \times 10\\
&= 62.8\ \Omega
\end{aligned}
$$

$$
\begin{aligned}
X_C &= \frac{1}{2\pi fC} && \text{(from Equation 14.10)}\\
&= \frac{1}{2\pi \times 100 \times 50 \times 10^{-6}}\\
&= \frac{10^6}{2\pi \times 100 \times 50}\\
&= 31.8\ \Omega
\end{aligned}
$$

$$
\begin{aligned}
\text{net reactance} &= (X_L - X_C)\\
&= (62.8 - 31.8)\ \Omega\\
&= 31\ \Omega
\end{aligned}
$$

We can now calculate the impedance (Z):

$$
\begin{aligned}
Z &= \sqrt{[R^2 + (X_L - X_C)^2]} && \text{(from Equation 14.12)}\\
&= \sqrt{[(26)^2 + (31)^2]}\\
&= \sqrt{[676 + 961]}\\
&= \sqrt{1637}\\
&= 40.5\ \Omega
\end{aligned}
$$

The phase angle can now be calculated:

$$\theta = \tan^{-1} \frac{(X_L - X_C)}{R} \qquad \text{(from Equation 14.13)}$$

$$= \tan^{-1} (31/26)$$
$$= \tan^{-1} 1.19$$
$$= 50°$$

Finally the peak current may be calculated thus:

$$I = \frac{V}{Z}$$
$$= \frac{400}{40.5}$$
$$= 9.9 \text{ A}$$

Resonance

In Figure 14.11(c), Z is always greater than R because it is the hypotenuse of the triangle. Since $I = V/Z$ the current becomes greater as Z decreases or smaller as Z increases. The smallest possible value of Z is when $X_L = X_C$, so that $\theta = 0°$ and the impedance is composed solely of the resistance R. The current is then at a maximum for the circuit. This effect is called *resonance* and depends on the values of L, C and f as shown below.

Resonance occurs when:

$$X_L = X_C$$
$$2\pi f L = \frac{1}{2\pi f C} \qquad \text{(by cross-multiplication)}$$
$$\therefore f^2 = \frac{1}{4\pi^2 LC}$$
$$\therefore f = \frac{1}{2\pi\sqrt{LC}} \qquad \text{Equation 14.15}$$

For given values of L and C, the value of f obtained from this equation is that frequency at which *resonance* or maximum current occurs. Higher or lower frequencies than this *resonance frequency* produce lower currents so that a resonance curve similar to Figure 14.12 is obtained. This principle of resonance in AC circuits is used in the receiver section of the *magnetic resonance imager* (see Appendix D) where a capacitor is used in series with an inductor to produce a resonant frequency of the same value as the signal from the patient which we wish to record. Thus the receiver is relatively insensitive to other frequencies. This allows us to collect the signal from a specific area within the patient. (A similar principle is also used to allow us to tune a radio to a specific station frequency.)

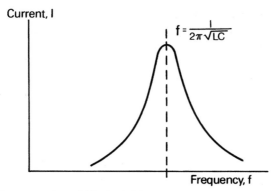

Figure 14.12 Resonance in an RLC circuit. The current is at a maximum at the resonance frequency.

14.8 THREE-PHASE AC

The basis of the generation of electricity was explained in Section 13.9. The requirements for electrical power vary widely dependent on the piece of machinery used. Thus any national electrical supply must be able to cope with a wide variation in the demand for electrical power. This is done by making available one or more *phases* of AC. This is made possible by the winding geometry of three-phase AC generators. These have three symmetrical windings (W_1, W_2 and W_3 in Figure 14.13(a)) on a rotor. These windings are separated by an angle of 120° and, when the rotor is rotated, each in turn moves through a magnetic field.

Each set of windings has a sinusoidal alternating voltage induced in it (see Sect. 13.9) but these voltages are out of phase with each other because of the different times they encounter the strongest regions of the magnetic

Figure 14.13 Three-phase electrical generation: (a) diagrammatic representation of the three sets of windings in the AC generator.

field within the generator. These voltages (V_1, V_2 and V_3 from the windings W_1, W_2 and W_3) are known as *phase voltages* and are separated by 120° from each other as shown in Figure 14.13(b). Thus a phase difference of 120° exists between each phase voltage. These voltages are now stepped up for transmission over long distances and are then stepped down for use in homes, hospitals, etc. This is accomplished using *star* and *delta* connections of the phase voltages as outlined below.

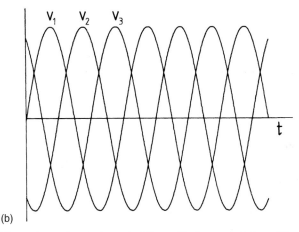

(b)

Fig. 14.13   Three-phase electrical supply; (b) graphical representation of the three voltage phases against time showing the 120° separation between each phase.

14.8.1 Star and delta connections

Star and delta connections of the phase voltages are shown in Figure 14.14. If we assume that an RMS voltage of 230 volts is induced in each winding of the generator, then three sets of 230 volt supply are available from the delta connection. The centre of the star connection is called the neutral and is kept as near earth potential as possible by equalising the power outputs from the three phases. This allows the possibility of six voltages from the star connection:

- three phase voltages of 230 volts are possible if a connection is made to the neutral and to one end of a winding
- three line voltages of 398 volts are possible by making connections to the ends of two of the windings—one such connection is shown between W_1 and W_3.

Note that the line voltage is 398 volts and not 460 volts as would be expected as each phase voltage is 230 volts. This is because of the phase difference between the phase voltages. It may be shown (see 'Insight' below) that the line voltage is also sinusoidal and has a magnitude which is a factor of √3 greater than the phase voltage.

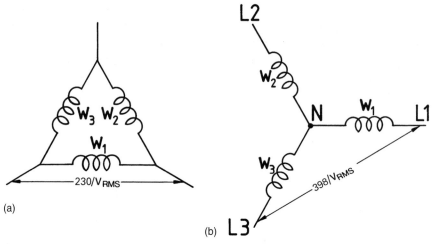

(a)

(b)

Figure 14.14 Three-phase connections: (a) delta connection; (b) star connection.

Insight

The voltage across L_1 and L_3 in Figure 14.14 is the *difference* between the voltages across L_1–N and L_3–N. If we consider a situation where the potential of N is zero, L_1–N is 10 volts and L_3–N is 4 volts, then the potential difference between L_1 and L_3 is $10 - 4 = 6$ volts. Thus we may use the vector diagram shown in the figure below to calculate the line voltage (L) across V_1–V_3.

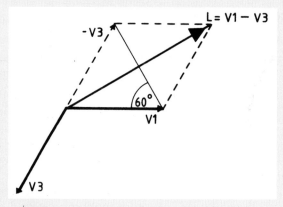

Now $\sin 60° = \sqrt{3}/2$

$$= \frac{(L/2)}{V_1} \quad \text{from the figure}$$

$$\therefore L = \sqrt{3}V_1$$

Thus the *line voltage* is $\sqrt{3}$ times the *phase voltage*. In the UK the phase voltage is 230 volts (RMS) and so the line voltage is 398 volts (RMS).

The transfer of power from the generating station to a city is shown diagrammatically in Figure 14.15. The four wires L_1, L_2, L_3 and N are distributed to domestic, hospital and industrial users and the appropriate voltages (phase or line) are available, i.e. phase voltages for domestic use and both phase and line voltages for hospital and industrial use. The star connection is often referred to as a *three-phase four-wire supply* for obvious reasons.

Figure 14.15   Generation and distribution of three-phase supplies. The consumer has a choice of three 'phase' voltages (e.g. L1–N) or three 'line' voltages (e.g. L1–L2).

14.8.2 Three-phase circuits in radiography

Three-phase supplies are used in radiography for three main purposes:

● The line voltage from a three-phase supply is used to ensure that a 398 volt supply is available for most static X-ray sets. This means that the turns ratio (see Ch. 17) required in step-up transformers is less than that required for a 230 volt supply.

● The three-phase X-ray generator uses all three phases to produce an almost constant voltage across the X-ray tube during an X-ray exposure. This will be further discussed in Chapter 19.

● The induction motor used to rotate the anode of the X-ray tube uses three phases. This is further discussed in Chapter 22.

Summary

In this chapter you should have learnt:

● Sinusoidal AC is described mathematically by the formula $I = I_p \sin 2\pi ft$ and $V = V_p \sin 2\pi ft$ where I_p, V_p are the peak current and voltage and f is the frequency of the AC supply in hertz (see Sect. 14.4).

- One *cycle* is one complete waveform; the *period* is the time for one cycle; the *frequency* is the number of cycles per second; and the *amplitude* is the maximum value of voltage or current (see Sect. 14.4).
- The *frequency* (f) and the *period* (T) are related by the following equation $f = 1/T$ (see Sect. 14.4).
- For *sinusoidal waveform* the average current (or voltage) is = 0. For *half-wave rectified AC* the average current (or voltage) is = 0.318 × peak current (voltage). For *full-wave rectified AC* the average current (or voltage) is = 0.636 × peak current (voltage) (see Sect. 14.4.2).
- The definition of the RMS current as *that value of constant current which, acting over the same time, would produce the same expenditure of electrical energy in a circuit as the alternating current*. All AC voltages and currents are quoted in RMS values unless otherwise stated. $I_{RMS} = 0.707 \times I_p$; $V_{RMS} = 0.707 \times V_p$ (see Sect. 14.4.3).
- Voltages across the X-ray tube are expressed in peak voltages (kV_p); current through the tube is expressed in average value (mA), and mains supply is expressed in RMS values (see Sect. 14.5).
- The *power* used in a circuit is given by the equation $W = V_{RMS} \times I_{RMS} \times \cos \theta$ where $\cos \theta$ is the *power factor*. $V \sin \theta$ is the *wattless voltage* and $I \sin \theta$ is the *wattless current* (see Sect. 14.6).
- AC circuits involving the use of capacitors and/or inductors produce a *phase difference* between the current and voltage waveforms. This may be represented by rotating vectors (see Sect. 14.6.1).
- *Resistance, reactance* and *impedance* are all measured in ohm and are the ratio of voltage to amperes (both peak or RMS) at $0°$, $90°$ and θ to the current respectively. θ is the phase difference between the current and voltage waveforms (see Sect. 14.6.2).
- *Inductors* have reactance of $2\pi fL$ which *leads* the current by $90°$. *Capacitors* have reactance of $1/2\pi fC$ which *lags behind* the current by $90°$ (see Sect. 14.7).
- Reactance consumes no net power from an AC supply (see Sect. 14.7.3).
- *Resonance* occurs in an AC circuit when the current is greatest at a particular frequency. For a series RLC circuit the resonance frequency (f) is given by the equation $f = 1/2\pi\sqrt{LC}$ (see Sect. 14.7.4).
- Three-phase circuits consist of three sinusoidal waveforms $120°$ apart. These may be connected by *star* or *delta* configurations (see Sect. 14.8).
- The *phase voltage* is that across individual windings; the *line voltage* is that obtained across each of the three connections of the star and delta connections. For a delta connection, the line and phase voltages are equal; for a star connection, the line voltage is $\sqrt{3} \times$ the phase voltage (see Sect. 14.8.1).

SELF-TEST

a. What is meant by *sinusoidal alternating current*? Illustrate your answer with a graph of current against time.

b. Explain what is meant by *peak*, *average* and *RMS* (*or effective*) values of a sinusoidal alternating current. What is the relationship between these values of the current? How will these relationships change if the current is full-wave rectified?

c. A 10 V RMS supply is connected across a 100 Ω resistor. What is:
   (i) the RMS current in the circuit
   (ii) the peak current in the circuit
   (iii) the average current in the circuit
   (iv) the average power produced in the resistor?

d. If a resistor of resistance 40 Ω, an inductor of inductance 200 mH and a capacitor of capacitance 80 μF are connected in series to an AC supply of frequency 50 Hz and peak voltage 300 V, what is the net impedance in the circuit, the phase angle and the peak current through the circuit?

e. What is meant by the *resonance frequency* of an RLC circuit? What will be the resonance frequency of a circuit which contains an inductor of inductance 200 mH and a capacitor of capacitance 80 μF connected in series?

f. A UK hospital is connected to a three-phase four-wire mains supply. What are the RMS values of the line voltages and phase voltages available?

FURTHER READING

Ball J L, Moore A D 1986 Essential physics for radiographers, 2nd edn. Blackwell Scientific Publications, London, ch 10

Foster E 1985 Equipment for diagnostic radiography. MTP Press, Lancaster, ch 1

Hay G A, Hughes D 1983 First year physics for radiographers. Baillière Tindall, London, ch 8

Ohanian H C 1994 Principles of physics. W W Norton, London, ch 23

Stockley S M 1986 A manual of radiographic equipment. Churchill Livingstone, Edinburgh, ch 2

Thompson M A 1994 Principles of imaging science and protection. W B Saunders, London, ch 4

15

The motor principle

15.1 AIM

The aim of this chapter is to consider the motor principle. The application of this principle to the DC motor and the AC induction motor will be considered as will the magnetic deflection of electrons. Finally, the relevance of these to radiography will be discussed.

15.2 INTRODUCTION AND DEFINITION OF THE MOTOR PRINCIPLE

In Chapter 12 we considered the topic of electromagnetism where a magnetic field was produced by an electric current. This chapter considers what happens when an electromagnetic field is created *in the presence of* another magnetic field. If we consider two bar magnets lying in close proximity one to another, then (depending on their orientation) a force of repulsion or attraction will exist between them (see Ch. 11). If one of the bar magnets is now replaced by a *solenoid* (see Sect. 12.6), we would expect a force between the solenoid and the bar magnet when an electric current is passed through the solenoid, since it behaves like a bar magnet under these circumstances. This force will cause the solenoid to move if it is free to do so. When the current is switched off, the magnetic field due to the solenoid disappears and so does the force between it and the magnet. This interaction between electromagnetism and another magnetic field is known as the *motor principle* (or motor effect) and may be formally defined:

Definition

A current-carrying conductor will experience a force when placed within a magnetic field.

The principle of the electric motor is that it converts electrical energy into kinetic energy (mechanical energy) through the interaction of the two magnetic fields.

15.3 DIRECTION AND MAGNITUDE OF THE FORCE ON THE CONDUCTOR

Consider a length l of straight wire which is carrying an electric current I, the whole wire being placed in a uniform magnetic flux density B as shown in Figure 15.1. In this diagram it is assumed that the direction of B and of

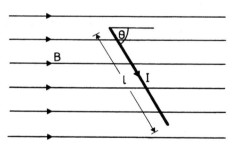

Figure 15.1 The interaction of the permanent magnetic field, B, with the magnetic field caused by the current flowing through the wire causes a force to act on the wire—the motor principle.

the wire are both in the plane of the paper. Experimentally the following results are observed:

a. The *direction* of the force on the wire is always into or out of the paper, i.e. at *right angles* to the direction of B and I.
b. The *direction* of the force on the wire is *reversed if the current is reversed*.
c. The *magnitude* of the force is proportional to:
   —the magnetic flux density, B
   —the magnitude of the electric current, I
   —the length of the wire, l

—the sine of the angle between the direction of B and I, i.e. $\sin \theta$ in Figure 15.1. Thus the force on the wire is at its maximum when the wire is at right angles to the field ($\sin 90° = 1$) and zero when the wire is parallel to the field ($\sin 0° = 0$).

Combining the factors in (c) above we have:

$$F = BIl \sin \theta \qquad\qquad \text{Equation 15.1}$$

where F is in newton, B in tesla, I in ampere and l in metre.

The findings discussed above may be used to define the *tesla* as follows:

Definition

A magnetic flux density of *1 tesla* (*T*) exists if the force on a straight wire of length *1 metre* is *1 newton* when the wire carries a current of *1 ampere* and is placed at *right angles* to the direction of magnetic flux.

The *direction* of the force on the current-carrying conductor may be obtained using the appropriate rule or convention. As we saw before, in Chapter 13, Fleming's Right and Left Hand Rules were produced to deal with 'conventional current' and not electron flow. To avoid confusion, a different convention will be presented to calculate the direction of the force on the current-carrying conductor.

15.4 CONVENTION FOR THE DIRECTION OF THE FORCE

Consider the situation shown in Figure 15.2(a) where a wire is carrying an electric current such that the electrons are flowing away from the eye of the observer into the paper. The magnetic field, H, produced by this current is in an anticlockwise direction as shown. If an external magnetic field, B, is

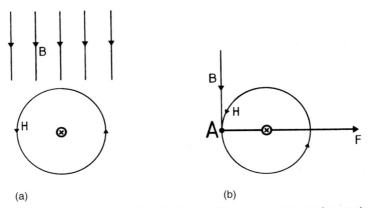

(a)   (b)

Figure 15.2 Convention for establishing the force acting on a current-carrying conductor placed in a magnetic field. For an explanation of how to use the convention see the text.

applied to the wire as shown, it is found that the wire experiences a force which pushes it to the right. Figure 15.2(b) shows the convention which will be used to determine the direction of the force—this is similar in many way to the convention used in Section 13.6 to determine the direction of the induced current. The direction of the force can be determined as follows:

1. Mark the position of the wire, and draw the direction of electron flow and the magnetic field around it. In Figure 15.2(b) this is an anticlockwise magnetic field as the electrons are flowing away from us.

2. Align one of the lines of force from the external magnetic field (B) so that it touches the field around the wire at the point where both fields are in the same direction. This occurs at point A in Figure 15.2(b).

3. Now draw a line from this point through the wire (AF). The direction in which you draw this line indicates the direction of the force acting on the wire. This line is drawn from left to right in this case agreeing with the previous findings.

This procedure can be applied to any direction of current and any orientation of the wire and the magnetic field. In some cases, however, the applied magnetic field is not exactly perpendicular to the wire and so cannot be made to line up to the field produced by it as described so far. In this situation, the applied magnetic field may be split into two components: one parallel to the wire (which produces no force on the wire) and one perpendicular to the wire (which will produce a force on the wire according to the above convention). The following examples should help to clarify the above points.

Examples

a. The situation of the wire and the external magnetic field is shown in the left-hand diagram. In the right-hand diagram the observer is looking along the wire (as if looking from the bottom of the page). The convention described previously can now be applied giving an upward direction of force. If we now reconsider the left-hand diagram it can be seen that the force will be out of the paper towards the observer.

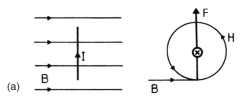

b. In this case, when we draw the right-hand diagram, the electrons will be flowing towards the observer and so the magnetic field around the wire will be in a clockwise direction. By applying the convention it can be found that the force is downwards into the paper (the opposite of the previous situation).

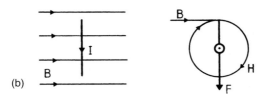

(b)

c. In diagram (c) the wire and the lines of flux are parallel and so no force will be experienced by the wire when current flows through it.

(c)

d. In the situation shown in diagram (d) the wire is not at 90° to the lines of flux and so these must be split into two components, B_0 which is parallel to the wire and B_{90} which is at right angles to it. This is shown in the right-hand diagram. As described in the previous example, the field which is parallel to the wire (B_0) will have no effect on it and so can be ignored. Application of the convention now shows that the force acting on the wire will be in an upwards direction as in the first example.

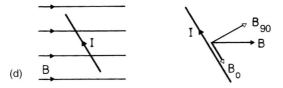

(d)

15.5 INTERACTION OF TWO ELECTROMAGNETIC FIELDS

So far in this chapter we have seen that a force exists on a current-carrying conductor when it is in the presence of a magnetic field and that this is known as the motor principle. It is immaterial whether the magnetic field interacting with the conductor is from a permanent magnet or whether it is produced electromagnetically. In this way, if two current-carrying solenoids are held close together, they behave in the same way as two bar magnets with a north pole at one end of the solenoid and a south pole at the other. Thus the solenoids will attract or repel each other dependent on the orientation in which they are placed—like poles repel; unlike poles attract (see Sect. 11.2.1).

15.5.1 Two parallel wires of infinite length

This rather improbable situation is used in the SI system to define the ampere and so will be considered here. Figure 15.3 shows two parallel wires C and D carrying currents I_C and I_D respectively. Figure 15.3(a) shows the plan view of the wires while Figure 15.3(b) is the view obtained by looking along the wires towards C and D where the electron flow is into the paper for both wires. The magnetic field around each wire will consist of a series of concentric circles with the field being in an anticlockwise direction. We will now consider how the magnetic field of one wire will interact with the magnetic field of the other. The magnetic field from wire C (B_C) is 'upwards' at wire D while the field from wire D (B_D) is 'downwards' at wire C. If we now apply our convention to this situation we can see that we get forces F_C and F_D as shown in Figure 15.3(b). Thus there is a mutual force of attraction between the wires. This situation is used as the basis of the definition of the ampere in the SI system:

Definition

A current of 1 *ampere* flows in one infinite straight wire if an equal current in a similar wire placed 1 metre away in a vacuum produces a mutual force of 2×10^{-7} newton per metre.

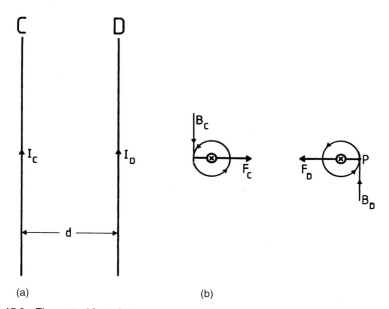

(a)   (b)

Figure 15.3 The mutual force between two parallel current-carrying wires of infinite length; (b) shows the same wires rotated through 90° so that the flow of electrons is into the paper. This arrangement is used for the definition of the ampere.

15.6 THE DC ELECTRIC MOTOR

The electric motor is, of course, the prime example of the motor principle in that it converts electrical energy into mechanical energy. To understand the workings of the electric motor we need to understand the motor principle and also electromagnetic induction (see Ch. 13). A simplified DC electric motor is shown in Figure 15.4 where a battery is connected to a coil of wire KLMN via brushes B at a commutator C. The coil of wire is in the magnetic field of a permanent magnet, the direction of whose field is from left to right in the figure.

When the current is switched on, the electron flow is in the direction indicated in the diagram, and the coil is affected by a clockwise force due to the motor principle (i.e. an *upward* force on KL and a *downward* force on MN as may be verified using the convention in Sect. 15.4). The commutator C turns with the coil KLMN so that the current always flows in the same direction relative to the permanent magnet. Hence the coil always experiences a clockwise force and keeps turning. Without the commutator, KLMN would eventually stop at right angles to the permanent magnetic field.

Since a clockwise force is being continuously applied to the coil, it would seem logical to assume that the speed of rotation would continuously increase. This does not, in fact, happen. The speed of rotation increases up to a certain rate and then remains constant. To understand why this happens we need to look at electromagnetic induction. We have a conductor KLMN which is moving relative to a magnetic field—i.e. undergoing a change of magnetic flux—so an EMF and current must be induced according to Faraday's and Lenz's Laws (see Sects 13.4 and 13.5). The faster the coil rotates, the greater is the induced EMF and current because the rate

Figure 15.4   The DC electric motor.

of change of flux linkage increases (Faraday's Second Law). The direction of the induced EMF is in the opposite direction to the applied EMF so this opposes the motion of electrons along KLMN. Thus the faster the coil rotates the smaller is the net current which flows. Thus for a free-moving frictionless motor the rotational speed becomes such that no current at all flows because the forward and back EMFs cancel each other out. It is for this reason that an electric motor does not rotate more and more quickly; it achieves a steady speed of rotation due to the back EMF induced in the windings.

When the motor is under load—performing mechanical work—then the rotational speed reduces so that a net current may flow and electrical energy may be transformed into mechanical and other types of energy.

15.7 THE AC INDUCTION MOTOR

The type of motor commonly used in an AC circuit is an AC induction motor, so called because it works on the principle of electromagnetic induction (particularly Lenz's Law). The principle of such a motor may be understood by considering the simple experiment depicted in Figure 15.5(a) where a bar magnet is moved around the rim of a supported copper disk. It is found that the disk follows the movement of the magnet. The sequence of events is as follows:

- A moving magnetic flux from the magnet is linked with the conductor—the copper disk.

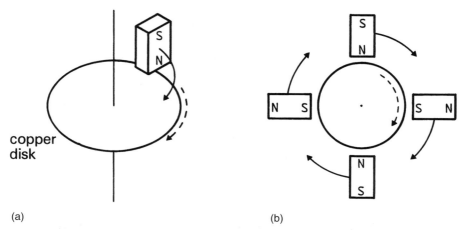

(a)   (b)

Figure 15.5 An elementary explanation of the induction motor. Rotating the magnets in (a) and (b) will cause the disk to rotate in the same direction because of eddy current formation in the copper.

- From Faraday's Laws we know that an EMF will be induced in the disk. From Lenz's Law we can deduce that a current will be induced in the disk in such a way as to oppose the change producing it.
- The disk thus moves in the same direction as the magnet in order to reduce the relative motion between them, so opposing the change producing the current as required by Lenz's Law. In a frictionless system, the disk would eventually move at the same speed as the magnet so that there would be no relative motion and no induced currents.

A rather more efficient system is shown in Figure 15.5(b) where more magnets are used and so a higher magnetic flux linkage is obtained. The copper disk follows the direction of rotation of the magnets for the reasons outlined above. It is not necessary to use permanent magnets since current-carrying solenoids will act as magnets.

The arrangement of the coils for such a motor are shown in Figure 15.6. The current through AB will be 90° out of phase with the current through CD. This produces a magnetic field which appears to rotate at the same frequency as the AC mains supply (50 Hz) and so the disk will also rotate at the same speed (50 revs per second (r.p.s.) = 3000 revs per minute (r.p.m.)).

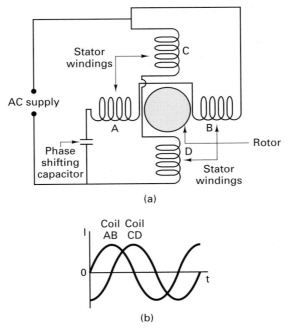

(a)

(b)

Figure 15.6 (a) A cross-section to show the typical arrangement of stator coils and rotor in an induction motor; (b) shows the current waveform produced by the two pairs of coils because of the influence of the phase-shifting capacitor. *Note* that the current from one pair of coils is at its maximum when the current from the other pair is at zero.

15.8 MAGNETIC DEFLECTION OF AN ELECTRON BEAM

There are a number of situations in radiography where we wish to deflect a beam of electrons, e.g. a beam of electrons is made to scan the face of a television monitor to produce an image. Figure 15.7 shows an electron beam travelling in a vacuum and passing through such a magnetic field. It can be seen that the path taken by the electron beam when it passes through the magnetic field is circular since the direction of the deflecting force is always at right angles to the direction of travel. Thus the electrons are deflected when they pass through the magnetic field. After leaving the magnetic field, the beam again travels in a straight line.

The angle of deflection increases as the magnetic flux density increases so that the direction of the beam can be controlled by varying the magnetic flux density. Thus by placing magnetic deflection coils on either side of a television monitor we can scan the electron beam in a pattern (known as a *raster*) across the face of the monitor.

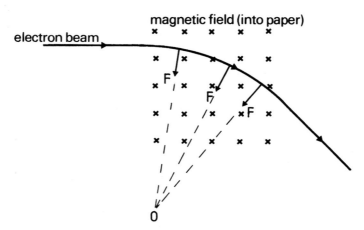

Figure 15.7 The deflection of an electron beam due to a magnetic field. The electrons enter the magnetic field from the left and are deflected on a circular path with O as the centre of the circle. The electrons continue on a straight path when they leave the influence of the magnetic field.

15.9 THE MOTOR PRINCIPLE IN RADIOGRAPHY

The motor principle is relevant to radiography whenever electrical energy is transformed into mechanical energy via magnetic energy. Obvious examples of this include the use of electric motors to drive mobile X-ray machines and the use of motors to tilt or elevate X-ray tables. The motor principle is also utilised in rotating the anode of the rotating anode X-ray tube. Finally, the motor principle is applied to allow scanning of the electron beam in television cameras and monitors.

Summary

In this chapter you should have learnt:

- The definition of the motor principle (see Sect. 15.2)
- The factors affecting the direction and magnitude of the force acting on a current-carrying conductor in a magnetic field (see Sect. 15.3)
- A convention to establish the direction of the force on a current-carrying conductor in a magnetic field (see Sect. 15.4)
- The interaction between two electromagnetic fields and how this is applied to two parallel wires (see Sect. 15.5)
- The operation of the DC motor (see Sect. 15.6)
- The operation of the AC induction motor (see Sect. 15.7)
- The factors influencing the magnetic deflection of an electron beam (see Sect. 15.8)
- The applications of the motor principle in radiography (see Sect. 15.9).

SELF-TEST

a. Define the motor principle.

b. List the factors which determine the magnitude of the force experienced by a current-carrying conductor placed in a magnetic field and give an equation to calculate this force.

c. Describe the operation of a DC induction motor.

d. List three uses of the motor principle in radiography.

FURTHER READING

Ball J L, Moore A D 1986 Essential physics for radiographers, 2nd edn. Blackwell Scientific Publications, London, ch 8
Foster E 1985 Equipment for diagnostic radiography. MTP Press, Lancaster, ch 5
Hay G A, Hughes D 1983 First year physics for radiographers. Baillière Tindall, London, ch 6
Ohanian H C 1994 Principles of physics. W W Norton, London, ch 21
Stockley S M 1986 A manual of radiographic equipment. Churchill Livingstone, Edinburgh, ch 6
Thompson M A 1994 Principles of imaging science and protection. W B Saunders, London, ch 5

16

Capacitors

16.1 AIM

The aim of this chapter is to introduce the reader to the subject of capacitors and capacitance. The chapter then considers the factors which influence the performance of a capacitor, how capacitors can be linked on to other components and how capacitors are used in radiography. Finally it aims to give the reader a brief list of the factors which influence the choice of capacitor and the types of capacitors available.

16.2 INTRODUCTION

In Chapter 14 we considered the influence of a capacitor on the current and the voltage in an AC circuit. We were able to do this without an understanding of the construction or the operation of a capacitor. However, there are other circumstances where capacitors are used where we need to understand either the construction and/or the operation of the capacitor to understand its function within the piece of equipment. This chapter deals with the physics of the capacitor and its principal applications in radiography.

16.3 ELECTRICAL CAPACITY (CAPACITANCE)

We have previously shown in Chapter 9 that when a body has a net positive or negative charge it also possesses an electrical potential, because work must be done in moving a unit positive charge from infinity to the body. This potential is positive if the charge on the body is positive and negative if the charge on the body is negative.

The *electrical capacity* or *capacitance* of the body is the relationship between the charge put on the body and its potential:

$$\text{capacitance} = \frac{\text{charge}}{\text{potential}}$$

or $\quad C = \dfrac{Q}{V}$
Equation 16.1

16.3.1 Definitions and unit of capacitance (farad)

The definition of capacitance varies slightly depending on the type of body holding the charge. When a body consists of **one surface** only (e.g. a sphere) the following definition applies:

> **Definition**
>
> The *capacitance* of a body is the ratio of the total charge on the body to its potential.

If the body consists of **two surfaces** close together we must consider the *potential differences* between the surfaces rather than the potential on each. This leads to the following alternative definition of capacitance:

> **Definition**
>
> The *capacitance* of a body is the ratio of the total charge of one sign on the body to the potential difference between its surfaces.

It is important to remember that capacitance involves both charge and potential and so it is not correct to think of capacitance as 'the amount of charge a body can hold' unless we add the phrase 'per unit potential difference'.

The SI unit of capacitance is the *farad* and may be defined as:

Definition

An electrical system has a capacitance of 1 *farad* if a charge of 1 coulomb held by the body results in a potential (or potential difference) of 1 volt.

Thus Equation 16.1 may be expressed as:

$$\text{farads} = \frac{\text{coulombs}}{\text{volts}} \qquad \text{Equation 16.2}$$

Insight

An alternative definition of capacity, and one which is often more useful in radiography, is to consider capacity in terms of the *change* of charge divided by the corresponding *change* in potential.

If a capacitor starts with a charge Q and a potential difference V then by definition:

$$C = \frac{Q}{V} \qquad \text{Equation A}$$

If an extra charge, ΔQ, is added to the plates and an extra potential difference, ΔV, results, then:

$$C = \frac{(Q + \Delta Q)}{(V + \Delta V)}$$

i.e. *capacitance is the total charge divided by the total potential difference.*

By cross-multiplying the above equation we get:

$$CV + C\Delta V = Q + \Delta Q \qquad \text{Equation B}$$

But we can say from Equation A that:

$$CV = Q$$

Thus Equation B can be rewritten:

$$C\Delta V = \Delta Q$$
$$\therefore C = \frac{\Delta Q}{\Delta V}$$

This gives the alternative definition of capacitance which can be used in radiography for calculations involving capacitor discharge circuits etc.

For practical purposes, the farad (F) is rather a large unit in which to measure capacitance and so it is more commonly expressed in units of *microfarads* (μF) or *picofarads* (pF), where:

$$1\,\mu F \;=\; 10^{-6}\,F$$
and $\quad 1\,pF \;=\; 10^{-12}\,F$

16.4 CAPACITANCE OF A PARALLEL-PLATE CAPACITOR

Figure 16.1 shows a parallel-plate capacitor with two plates of equal area, A, separated by a distance, d. The plates are made of electrical conductors so that charge may flow in and out of each plate. If the capacitor is *charged*—e.g. by connecting it across a battery as shown—then a charge of $+Q$ will exist on one plate and a charge of $-Q$ on the other. If the battery is disconnected, the charge will continue to be stored on the plates of the capacitor as the positive charge on one plate attracts the negative charge on the other. This is why a capacitor is often described as a device for storing charge. (*A large capacitor will retain this charge for a long period of time after it has been disconnected from the source of EMF. For this reason it should be treated with extreme care as severe electric shock may result from touching the plates or the electrical connections to the capacitor.*)

When the capacitor is fully charged, a potential difference equal to that of the battery exists across the plates. Thus, the capacitance of the parallel-plate capacitor is given by the equation $C = Q/V$ where Q is the charge of one sign on one of the plates and V is the potential difference between the plates.

Certain characteristics of the capacitor will affect its capacitance and these will now be considered.

Area of the plates

If the area of the plates (A) is increased, then more charge will be able to flow on to the plates from the battery until the charge per unit area is the same as before. It can be seen that if the area of the plates is doubled then the amount of charge which they will hold to give the same charge per unit area will also be doubled. In this situation V remains unaltered as it is the

Figure 16.1   A parallel-plate capacitor charged by a battery.

same as the potential difference from the battery and $Q \propto A$. Since $C = Q/V$ we can say that:

$$C \propto A$$

Note: If the plates are not directly opposite each other, then the area taken for this calculation of capacitance is the area of the plates which are in direct opposition.

Separation of the plates

If the rest of the capacitor remains unaltered but the plates are brought closer together, then the charges on opposite plates will experience a greater force of attraction so that the battery will be able to 'push' more charge on to the plates. Once again V is constant, but $Q \propto 1/d$. Since $C = Q/V$ we can then say that:

$$C \propto \frac{1}{d}$$

Dielectric constant of material between the plates

A material with a high dielectric constant is an insulator where it is relatively easy to induce a charge on its surface (see Sect. 9.7.2). The effect of placing such a material between the plates of a charged capacitor is shown in Figure 16.2. The close proximity of the charges on the plates and on the dielectric results in some 'cancellation' of charges (as shown ringed in Fig. 16.2(b)). If this capacitor is now reconnected to the battery, it will be seen that more charge will flow on to the capacitor. Thus, once again, V is the same value but Q has increased and so the capacitance of the capacitor increases with the dielectric constant (K) so we can say:

$$C \propto K$$

This leads to the definition of the *dielectric constant*.

(a)   (b)

Figure 16.2   (a) shows a parallel-plate capacitor with no dielectric between its plates; (b) shows the action of the dielectric. The induction of charge in the dielectric cancels some of the charges stored on the plates (shown as ringed). This means that the battery can now put more charge on to the plates of the capacitor.

Definition

The *dielectric constant* of a material is the ratio of the capacitance of the capacitor with the dielectric, to the capacitance without the dielectric (i.e. with a vacuum between the plates of the capacitor).

From this it can be seen that the dielectric constant of a vacuum is unity. If we take the above three components together we get:

$$C \propto \frac{KA}{d}$$

By the addition of a constant of proportionality (ε_0) this now becomes:

$$C = \frac{\varepsilon_0 KA}{d}$$
Equation 16.3

16.5 CAPACITORS IN PARALLEL

If capacitors are connected in parallel (see Fig. 16.3) then they behave together like one capacitor of a particular value. The value of this *total* or *equivalent* capacitance may be calculated as follows.

The total capacitance, C, is defined as $C = Q/V$. The total charge, Q, is the sum of all the charges on the individual capacitors (q_1, q_2, etc.) while the potential difference across each capacitor is the same value, V. Thus:

$$C = \frac{Q}{V}$$
$$= \frac{(q_1 + q_2 + q_3)}{V}$$
$$= \frac{q_1}{V} + \frac{q_2}{V} + \frac{q_3}{V}$$

but $\quad C_1 = \frac{q_1}{V}; \ C_2 = \frac{q_2}{V}; \ C_3 = \frac{q_3}{V}$

$$\therefore \ C = C_1 + C_2 + C_3$$
Equation 16.4

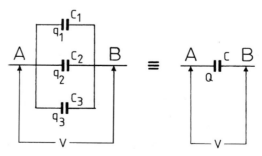

Figure 16.3 Capacitors in parallel. The capacitor C is equivalent to the effect of C_1, C_2 and C_3 connected together in parallel.

Thus the total capacitance is obtained by summing the individual capacitances. *Note* that the total capacitance must always be larger than the largest value of individual capacitance.

16.6 CAPACITORS IN SERIES

When capacitors are connected in series (see Fig. 16.4) the total or equivalent capacitance can be established as follows.

If a potential difference, V, is connected across the three capacitors, this results in charges of $+q$ and $-q$ on the plates of each individual capacitor. Thus the capacitors are now fully charged and the following relationships can be established:

$$\frac{1}{C} = \frac{V}{Q}$$

$$= \frac{(V_1 + V_2 + V_3)}{Q}$$

$$= \frac{V_1}{Q} + \frac{V_2}{Q} + \frac{V_3}{Q}$$

But: $\dfrac{V_1}{Q} = \dfrac{1}{C_1}; \dfrac{V_2}{Q} = \dfrac{1}{C_2}; \dfrac{V_3}{Q} = \dfrac{1}{C_3}$

$$\therefore \frac{1}{C} = \frac{1}{C_1} + \frac{1}{C_2} + \frac{1}{C_3} \qquad \text{Equation 16.5}$$

Note that in this case the total capacitance is less than the value of any of the individual capacitances.

Figure 16.4 Capacitors in series. The capacitor C is equivalent to the effect of C_1, C_2 and C_3 connected together in series.

16.7 CHARGING A CAPACITOR THROUGH A RESISTOR FROM A DC SUPPLY

Consider the situation illustrated in Figure 16.5(a) where a battery is connected across a resistor R and a capacitor C in series. When the switch S_1 is closed, electrons will flow on to one of the plates of the capacitor and

Figure 16.5 Charging a capacitor (C) through a resistor (R) from a DC source (V_B).

away from the other plate as shown in the illustration. The potential difference across the capacitor, V_C, therefore increases due to the charge on the plates. However, it does not increase indefinitely, but settles to a value which is the same as (but of opposite polarity to) that of the battery. To understand why this is the case, consider the forces acting on an electron at the point P. When the switch S_1 is initially closed, a complete circuit is made and, due to the EMF from the battery, a force is exerted on the electron pushing it towards the capacitor. However, as soon as the plate starts to build up electric charge, it in turn exerts a force on the electron at P in the opposite direction, which slows down the rate of flow of charge on to the plate. Eventually the two opposing forces on the electron will become equal and there is no further flow of electrons through the circuit. At this stage the potential across the capacitor is equal and opposite to the potential across the battery. This situation is shown in the graph (Fig. 16.5(b)) where there is an initial rapid rise in potential (V_C) when S_1 is closed, but this slows down and approaches V_B relatively slowly. The effect of the resistance R is to limit the electron flow rate so that V_B is approached more slowly for large values of R than for small values of R as shown on the graph.

From this it can be seen that a *capacitor does not pass DC*, for, after the short time required to charge the capacitor, all further electron movement (flow of current) ceases.

16.8 DISCHARGING A CAPACITOR THROUGH A RESISTOR

In Figure 16.6(a) a charged capacitor with a potential V_C between its plates is allowed to discharge through the resistor R when the switch S_2 is closed. When this happens, electrons travel from the negative plate of the capacitor, through the resistor R and on to the positive plate. Hence the charge on the plates and the potential between them (V_C) is reduced. The reduction in V_C means that there will be less 'push' on the electrons through the resistor so less will flow in the next time interval, resulting in a smaller drop in V_C. The situation continues as shown in the graph (Figure

Figure 16.6 Discharging a capacitor (C) through a resistor (R).

16.6(b)) until the capacitor is completely discharged and the potential difference is zero. Again, the effect of R is to slow down the current and so the rate of fall of V_C.

16.9 THE TIME-CONSTANT FOR A CAPACITOR/ RESISTOR CIRCUIT

Both of the above experiments are examples of the exponential law (Ch. 4). This can be seen by comparing the graphs in Figures 16.5 and 16.6 with those in Chapter 4. The potential difference between the plates of a discharging capacitor can be calculated from the equation:

$$V_C = V_0 e^{-t/RC}$$
Equation 16.6

where V_0 is the potential difference between the plates before discharging the capacitor, t is the time of the discharge (in seconds), R is the resistance in ohms and C is the capacitance in farads. The quantity RC is called the *time-constant* of the circuit. If R is in ohm and C is in farads then RC is in seconds. After a discharge time of 1 time-constant, i.e. $t = RC$, then the potential difference across a discharging capacitor has dropped to $1/e$ of its initial value, i.e. 0.37 of its initial value. Thus if the original potential difference is 6 V, the value after 1 time-constant is $0.37 \times 6 = 2.2$ V. After 2 time-constants the value will be reduced to a further 0.37, i.e. $0.37 \times 2.2 = 0.8$ V. Note that this is very similar to the concept of half-life discussed in Chapter 4 since both are examples of exponential decay.

If we consider a capacitor being charged then the equation for the potential across it is:

$$V_C = V_0(1 - e^{-t/RC})$$
Equation 16.7

V_0 is the charging source EMF. Again RC is the time-constant. After 1 time-constant the potential across the capacitor will be $1 - 1/e$ which is

0.63. Thus, for a charging capacitor after 1 time-constant the potential across its plates will be 0.63 of its final value (the final value will be the same as the charging source EMF).

16.10 CAPACITORS AND ALTERNATING CURRENT

We have already shown in this chapter that a capacitor will eventually possess the same potential difference as the electrical supply connected across it. If the potential difference of supply is changed, a new equilibrium will become established where, once again, the two values of potential difference are equal. Thus, if an alternating supply is connected across the capacitor, the potential of the capacitor 'follows' the potential of the supply. Thus it can be said that *a capacitor passes AC* since the PD on the capacitor changes continually in sympathy with the PD of the supply.

As we have already seen in Chapter 14, when a capacitor is introduced to an AC circuit, the PD across the plates lags 90° behind the current. The effect of this phase difference must be taken into account for many of the uses of capacitors in AC circuits.

16.11 CAPACITORS IN RADIOGRAPHY

The ability to store electrical charge on the plates of a capacitor has important practical consequences in radiography. Some of the practical uses of capacitors in radiography are listed below:

- capacitor discharge mobile units
- electronic timers
- voltage smoothing
- phase splitting for AC induction motors.

There is insufficient space in this text to describe these uses in detail and so only a brief overview of each will be given.

16.11.1 Capacitor discharge mobile units

When an exposure is made on a mains-dependent mobile unit, a large current (around 30 A) is drawn from the mains during the exposure. This large current can cause large power losses in the mains cables (remember $P = I^2R$). The capacitor discharge mobile works on the principle that a small current is drawn from the mains to charge a capacitor before the X-ray exposure, and this capacitor is allowed to discharge through the X-ray tube during the exposure. Since the electrical energy to the tube comes from the capacitor, no significant stress is applied to the mains supply during the exposure.

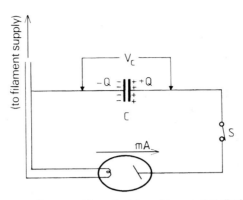

Figure 16.7 A simplified diagram of the principles of a capacitor discharge X-ray circuit.

Figure 16.7 shows the basic principles of such a circuit. With the switch S open, the capacitor is initially charged until the required potential (V_C is the same value as the kV which will be applied to the tube) is established across its plates. On closing the switch S, electrons flow from the negative plate of the capacitor to the positive plate via the X-ray tube. This means that a potential difference (kV) is applied across the tube and charge (mAs) flows through it comprising a radiographic exposure. At the end of the exposure the switch S is opened. As a result of the exposure, the capacitor loses some of the charge on its plates and so the potential difference at the end of the exposure is less than the initial potential difference. This must be taken into account when selecting exposure factors on such a unit.

16.11.2 Electronic timers

A type of electronic timer which uses a resistor and a capacitor is shown in Figure 16.8(a). This type of timer may be used to switch off the X-ray exposure after a predetermined time. The switch S is normally in position B which means that the capacitor is uncharged. The radiographer selects an exposure time by selecting a resistance at the variable resistor R—as will be explained below, a large resistance will give a long exposure time while a small resistance gives a short time. When the exposure is initiated, S is moved to position A and the capacitor is charged from the DC source (shown in the diagram as a battery, D). The potential across the plates of the capacitor is shown in Figure 16.8(b). This voltage is applied to an electronic switch and, when it reaches the trigger voltage for the switch, an *off signal* is sent, terminating the exposure.

(a)

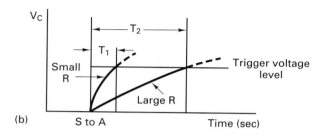

(b)

Figure 16.8   (a) shows a simplified construction diagram of a capacitor/resistance timer (for details of operation see text); (b) shows the differing times it takes the capacitor to reach the trigger voltage level for a small resistor in the line and for a large resistor in the line.

16.11.3 Voltage smoothing

When an alternating voltage is full-wave rectified (see Ch. 20) and applied to a component, the voltage waveform will be as shown in Figure 16.9(a). Thus, during each half-cycle a potential difference ranging from the peak voltage to zero volts is applied across the component. This difference between the peak and the trough in the voltage is known as the *voltage ripple*. In this case the ripple is 100%. There are some situations where it is beneficial to reduce this ripple. This is done by connecting a capacitor (or sometimes two capacitors) in parallel with the component so that the voltage supply is smoothed by the capacitor before it is applied to the component. The result of capacitor smoothing of the voltage is shown in Figure 16.9(b). The broken line shows the voltage waveform from the rectification circuit. Initially the capacitor charges so that the potential between its plates is the same as the peak potential from the rectification circuit. As this supply voltage drops, the capacitor discharges through the component so that the potential difference between its plates slowly drops. When this potential has dropped by a small amount the potential from the supply 'catches up' with it (point A on the graph) and charge will once again flow on to the capacitor so that it reaches its peak potential difference at the same time as the supply voltage. By using capacitors which are suitably matched to the component being supplied with electrical energy, the voltage ripple can be reduced to around 5–10%.

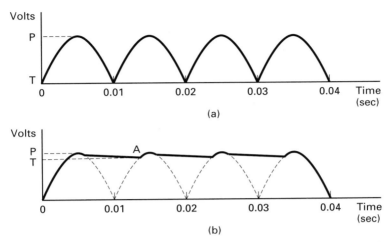

Figure 16.9 Graph (a) show the voltage from a single-phase transformer after it has been rectified. Graph (b) shows the same voltage after capacitor smoothing where P represents the peak and T the trough. The difference between the peak and the trough is known as the ripple. Note how capacitor smoothing reduces the voltage ripple.

16.11.4 Phase splitting for AC induction motors

As was discussed in Chapter 14, when a capacitor is introduced into an AC supply, it causes a phase shift between the current and voltage. This is utilised in the AC induction motor. The detail of the operation of this motor is given in Section 15.7. The role of the capacitor is to produce a current in one pair of coils which is 90° out of phase with the current in the other pair. This produces a magnetic field which appears to rotate at the same speed as the mains frequency and so produces rotation of the motor rotor.

16.12 TYPES OF CAPACITOR

Different types of capacitor are manufactured for different applications. In selecting a particular capacitor the user must be aware of various factors which influence the choice:

- the voltage rating of the capacitor—this is the maximum PD the capacitor is able to withstand and is influenced by the *dielectric strength* of the dielectric between the plates
- the *leakage* of the capacitor—this is influenced by how effective an electrical insulator the dielectric is
- whether the capacitor is to be used for AC or DC
- the physical size of the capacitor
- the price of the capacitor.

The types of capacitor available include:

- variable multi-plate 'air' capacitors
- waxed paper dielectric
- electrolytic
- tantalum
- polystyrene
- ceramic
- polycarbonate
- plastic film
- mica.

In each case the name refers to the type of dielectric material used. Further discussion on the construction and uses of these capacitors is beyond the scope of this text.

Summary

In this chapter you should have learnt:

- The meaning of the term electrical capacitance (see Sect. 16.3)
- The definition of the farad—the unit of capacitance (see Sect. 16.3)
- The factors affecting the capacitance of a parallel-plate capacitor (see Sect. 16.4)
- The definition of the term *dielectric constant* (see Sect. 16.4)
- The fact that capacitors connected in parallel have a total capacitance, C, given by the equation $C = C_1 + C_2 + C_3$ (see Sect. 16.5)
- The fact that capacitors connected in series have a total capacitance, C, given by the equation $1/C = 1/C_1 + 1/C_2 + 1/C_3$ (see Sect. 16.6)
- The consequences of charging a capacitor from a DC source through a resistor (see Sect. 16.7)
- The consequences of discharging a capacitor through a resistor (see Sect. 16.8)
- The definition and the uses of the *time-constant* for a capacitor/resistor circuit (see Section 16.9)
- The effect on the voltage and the current in an AC circuit when a capacitor is introduced to the circuit (see Sect. 16.10)
- The main uses of capacitors in radiography (see Sect. 16.11)
- The main types of capacitors available and the factors affecting the choice of capacitor (see Sect. 16.12).

SELF-TEST

a. What is meant by the term *capacitance*? Define the unit in which capacitance is measured.

b. A 1 μF capacitor is charged until the PD between its plates is 80 kV. What is the charge on the capacitor? The capacitor is then connected across an X-ray tube and an exposure of 10 mAs is made. (*Remember:* 1 mAs = 10^{-3} C.) What is the PD across the capacitor at the end of the exposure?

c. List the factors which affect the capacitance of a parallel-plate capacitor and give the equation which interlinks these factors.

d. How would you connect three capacitors to give:
   (i) the maximum capacitance
   (ii) the minimum capacitance?

e. What is the total capacitance produced by the following arrangement of individual capacitors?

(*Hint:* first calculate the total capacitance of the capacitors in parallel.)

f. A capacitor of 10 μF has a potential difference of 200 V between its plates. It is connected to a resistor of 100 kΩ for a time of 2 seconds. What will be the potential difference between the plates of the capacitor at the end of that period and how much charge will then be stored by the capacitor?

g. List four uses of capacitors in radiography.

h. List the five factors which might influence the choice of the type of capacitor to be used in a particular circuit.

FURTHER READING

Ball J L, Moore A D 1986 Essential physics for radiographers, 2nd edn. Blackwell Scientific Publications, London, ch 6
Foster E 1985 Equipment for diagnostic radiography. MTP Press, Lancaster, chs 2, 9
Gifford D 1984 A handbook of physics for radiologists and radiographers. John Wiley & Sons, Chichester, ch 5
Hay G A, Hughes D 1983 First year physics for radiographers. Baillière Tindall, London, ch 3
Johns H E, Cunningham J R 1983 The physics of radiology, 4th edn. Charles C Thomas, Illinois, USA, ch 1
Ohanian H C 1994 Principles of physics. W W Norton, London, ch 18
Stockley S M 1986 A manual of radiographic equipment. Churchill Livingstone, Edinburgh, ch 5
Thompson M A 1994 Principles of imaging science and protection. W B Saunders, London, ch 4

The AC transformer

17.1 AIM

The aim of this chapter is to discuss the main concepts which govern the operation of the step-up or the step-down AC transformer. In addition to this, two forms of 'specialist' transformers are discussed, namely the autotransformer and the constant voltage transformer. Finally there is an overview of the factors which affect transformer rating and how these factors relate to radiographic exposures.

17.2 INTRODUCTION

An AC transformer has an electrical input and an electrical output. For the transformer to function the input is an AC supply. The electrical output potential difference may either be greater or smaller than the electrical input voltage. If the output is greater than the input, then the transformer is a *step-up* transformer; if it is less, then the transformer is a *step-down* transformer. A transformer is thus a device which changes alternating currents or voltages from one level to another.

The transformer has a wide range of applications in radiography. For example the mains voltage is too small to be applied directly across the X-ray tube and so it is increased using a step-up transformer (the high-tension transformer). On the other hand, the mains voltage is too high to be connected directly across the filament and so it is reduced in the filament transformer, which is an example of a step-down transformer.

Two other types of transformer are encountered in radiography and so will also be discussed in this chapter. These are the *autotransformer* and the *saturated core* or *constant voltage* transformer.

17.3 THE IDEAL TRANSFORMER

Let us start by defining this device:

> **Definition**
>
> An *ideal transformer* is one whose output electrical power is equal to its input electrical power—there is no power 'lost' in the transformer itself.

There is, of course, no such thing as the ideal (or perfect) transformer although real transformers with efficiencies of 98% or more are not uncommon. Although it is not a practical reality, the concept of the ideal transformer is a useful one in that it simplifies the mathematics which can be used to describe the behaviour of transformers.

Consider such an ideal transformer shown in Figure 17.1 where two isolated sets of windings share a common core—there are a number of other configurations of core and windings but the one shown in the figure is the simplest. The input or *primary* side of the transformer consists of n_p turns around the core and has an alternating voltage V_p across it. The output or *secondary* side of the transformer consists of n_s turns and has a voltage V_s induced in it. This is a case of mutual induction as discussed in Section 13.7. The sequence of events is as follows:

- The alternating voltage in the primary winding, V_p, causes an alternating current to flow through the winding.
- This alternating current, I_p, produces a *changing magnetic flux density* (B) in the soft iron core.
- The *changing magnetic flux density* is linked to the secondary winding so that an EMF, V_s, is induced in it according to Faraday's and Lenz's Laws of electromagnetic induction (see Sects 13.4 and 13.5).

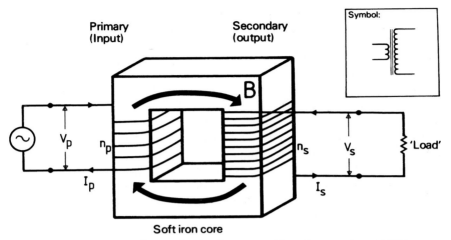

Figure 17.1 An 'ideal' transformer showing the core and the primary and secondary windings. In practice the core is laminated as shown in Figure 17.2. As there are more turns on the secondary winding than on the primary winding, this is a step-up transformer. The symbol for a step-up transformer is also shown.

As already mentioned in the introduction to this chapter, an AC supply is *essential* for the operation of the transformer since no EMF will be generated in the secondary if the magnetic flux is constant (Faraday's First Law).

The purpose of the soft iron core is to contain all the magnetic flux within it so that the magnetic flux linkage between the primary and the secondary is as near perfect as possible. The core is able to do this because of its strong induced magnetism resulting from its high magnetic permeability (see Table 11.1).

The mathematics of the ideal transformer are relatively simple if we first consider the effect of the magnetic flux on a single turn of wire around the core. Since we are assuming that the transformer is ideal, there is no magnetic flux loss and the EMF induced is independent of the position of the wire. Thus the same voltage will be induced in each turn of the primary and in each turn of the secondary. If we call this voltage v, then we can say that the total primary voltage is the voltage in each turn multiplied by the number of turns. Thus:

$$V_\mathrm{p} = v \times n_\mathrm{p} \text{ or } \frac{V_\mathrm{p}}{n_\mathrm{p}} = v$$

Similarly for the secondary:

$$V_\mathrm{s} = v \times n_\mathrm{s} \text{ or } \frac{V_\mathrm{s}}{n_\mathrm{s}} = v$$

Thus we can combine the two equations above to get:

$$\frac{V_p}{n_p} = \frac{V_s}{n_s}$$

By cross-multiplying this equation we get the formula:

$$\frac{V_s}{V_p} = \frac{n_s}{n_p} \qquad\qquad \text{Equation 17.1}$$

This equation is true for either peak or RMS values of the voltage provided V_s and V_p are both expressed in the same units.

The ratio V_s/V_p is known as the *voltage gain* of the transformer. This is greater than unity for a step-up transformer and less than unity for a step-down transformer.

The ratio n_s/n_p is known as the *turns ratio* of the transformer. Again, if this is greater than unity we have a step-up transformer and if it is less than unity we have a step-down transformer. If we have a transformer with a turns ratio of 200:1, we know that there are 200 times as many turns on the secondary as on the primary and that the voltage across the secondary is 200 times that of the primary.

The *current* flowing in the secondary of the transformer may be calculated from the power in the primary winding and secondary winding (for simplicity, in the following discussion, RMS values are assumed). In the ideal transformer the power in the primary and the power in the secondary are equal. Thus:

$$V_p \times I_p = V_s \times I_s$$
$$\therefore \frac{I_p}{I_s} = \frac{V_s}{V_p}$$

From Equation 17.1 we know:

$$\frac{V_s}{V_p} = \frac{n_s}{n_p}$$

Thus, for an ideal transformer, we can say:

$$\frac{I_p}{I_s} = \frac{n_s}{n_p} \qquad\qquad \text{Equation 17.2}$$

If we consider Equations 17.1 and 17.2 we can see that if the voltage is *increased* by a factor of n_s/n_p, then the current is *reduced* by the same factor. Thus a step-up transformer will increase the voltage but will decrease the current by the same factor.

17.4 FARADAY'S LAWS AND LENZ'S LAW APPLIED TO TRANSFORMERS

We have already considered Faraday's Laws of electromagnetic induction (Sect. 13.4) and Lenz's Law (Sect. 13.5) and we can now look at how these are applied to transformers.

As discussed in the previous section, there is a changing magnetic flux produced by the alternating supply connected to the primary and, since this is linked to both the primary and secondary windings, by Faraday's Laws, an EMF is produced in each of the windings. Assuming we have an ideal transformer, the magnitude of the EMF in each turn of the primary winding is equal to the magnitude of the EMF in each turn of the secondary.

Lenz's Law may be used to determine the direction of the induced current in the secondary. As it acts to oppose the changing magnetic flux, it will be in the opposite direction to (180° out of phase with) the current in the primary. The eddy currents induced in the core (these will be discussed later in this chapter as they are part of the transformer 'losses') will also be in the opposite direction to the primary current.

Insight

Some students find it surprising that it is the current drawn from the secondary of a transformer which determines the primary current —especially as the secondary voltage for a given transformer is determined by the primary voltage. The explanation of this fact is as follows.

Consider a situation when the secondary winding is *open circuit*—it is not connected to anything—so no current can flow through it although an EMF is induced across it. If we assume that we have an ideal transformer, then the same EMF will be induced by this magnetic flux in the primary winding and by Lenz's Law this will be in the opposite direction to the forward EMF. Thus no current flows in the primary winding when the secondary current is zero.

If the secondary is now connected across an external circuit so that some current flows through it, this current, by Lenz's Law, will oppose the magnetic flux in the core. The core flux is thus reduced and so the back EMF in the primary is reduced. The forward EMF in the primary is now greater than the back EMF and so a current flows. Thus a current in the secondary has caused a current to flow in the primary, the relative magnitudes of each being given by Equation 17.2.

17.5 TRANSFORMERS IN PRACTICE

It is not possible to construct an ideal transformer as there are always power 'losses' within the transformer itself. This means that the power in the secondary is always less than the power in the primary by an amount equal to the transformer losses. The efficiency of a transformer may be defined as follows:

Definition

The *efficiency* of a transformer is the ratio of the output power to the input power.

Note: It is often convenient to express the transformer efficiency as a percentage. For example if a transformer is 95% efficient and 100 watt of power is supplied to the primary of that transformer, then 95 watt is produced in the secondary. In this case 5% of the power is 'lost' because of power loss in the windings and core, i.e. this 5% is not available as useful electrical power.

Equation 17.1 gives a reasonable estimate of the voltage change in practical transformers but equation 17.2 no longer applies because of the power losses in practical transformers. This may be illustrated by the following example.

Example

A transformer has a turns ratio of 100:1 and an efficiency of 95%. If a current of 5 A_{RMS} flows in the primary when a voltage of 10 V_{RMS} is applied across it, what is the output RMS voltage and output RMS current?
From Equation 17.1 we get:

$$\frac{V_s}{V_p} = \frac{n_s}{n_p}$$

$$\therefore \frac{V_s}{10} = \frac{100}{1}$$

$$\therefore V_s = 1000 \ V_{RMS}$$

We also know that efficiency is the ratio of the output power to the input power. Thus:

$$\text{efficiency} = \frac{(V_s \times I_s)}{(V_p \times I_p)}$$

$$\therefore \frac{95}{100} = \frac{(1000 \times I_s)}{(10 \times 5)}$$

$$\therefore I_s = \frac{(50 \times 95)}{(100 \times 1000)} \qquad \text{(by cross-multiplication)}$$

$$= 47.5 \ mA_{RMS}$$

Note that an ideal transformer would have produced the same secondary voltage but the secondary current would be 50 mA_{RMS}.

17.6 TRANSFORMER LOSSES

A detailed analysis of the sources of transformer losses is considered in this section. These are summarised in Table 17.1 and discussed below.

Table 17.1 A summary of the losses associated with a practical transformer

Transformer loss	Comments
Copper losses	Caused by the resistance of the copper windings. Also known as 'I^2R' losses
Iron losses	Losses produced in the transformer core
Imperfect magnetic flux linkage	Very small loss
Eddy currents	Caused by electromagnetic induction within the core of the transformer—reduced by core lamination
Hysteresis	Caused by the work required to move the magnetic domains—reduced by the appropriate choice of core material (e.g. stalloy)
Regulation (a consequence of all the above losses)	Output voltage decreases with increased current load because of the increased transformer losses due to the resistance of the windings

17.6.1 Copper losses

The term *copper* refers to the copper wire of the windings of the transformer which has a small but finite resistance. If we consider a current I_{RMS} flowing through a resistance R, then there is a power of $(I_{RMS})^2R$ watt produced within the resistor. (The copper loss is often referred to as the I^2R loss of the transformer.) The copper loss produces a small heating within the coils of the transformer.

We wish to keep the copper loss as low as possible and, as it is related to I^2R, it makes sense to keep R low when I is large. As we saw in Chapter 10 the resistance of a conductor is inversely proportional to its cross-sectional area. For this reason the winding of the transformer which carries the larger current is made of the thicker wire. In the step-up transformer this is the primary winding and in the step-down transformer it is the secondary winding.

17.6.2 Iron losses

The term *iron losses* refers to the losses which occur in the soft iron core of the transformer. These take three forms as outlined below.

Magnetic flux losses

If the iron core is magnetically saturated, then all of the magnetic flux will not be contained within the core. This means that magnetic flux will be produced by the primary which is not linked with the secondary. The EMF induced in the secondary and the output electrical power will be lower than if the flux linkage were perfect. By the appropriate design of the transformer core, this loss is made very small indeed and so can be neglected for most practical purposes.

Eddy currents

From Faraday's and Lenz's Laws we know that when a changing magnetic flux is linked with a conductor an EMF and current are induced in the conductor. Also, the direction of the induced current opposes the effect of the changing magnetic flux linkage. The iron core of the transformer is an electrical conductor and so the varying flux passing through the core will induce electric currents within the core itself in such a direction as to oppose the changing magnetic flux within the core. This principle is shown in Figure 17.2(a) where the direction of the eddy currents in the core is in the opposite direction to the current in the winding. The effect of these currents is twofold:

- The flow of electrical current through the core causes heating of the core due to the electrical resistance of the core.
- The magnetic flux associated with the eddy currents is in the opposite direction to the flux from the winding and so there is a reduction in the flux interlinking with the secondary—flux which interlinks with the secondary is the flux produced at the primary minus the eddy current flux. This constitutes a power loss within the transformer core.

Eddy currents may be reduced but not entirely eliminated by *lamination* of the core as shown in Figure 17.2(b) and (c). The laminated sheets of soft iron are bolted together to produce the required cross-sectional area. Each lamination is insulated from its neighbours by the application of a thin layer of insulation (e.g. shellac varnish) to its surface. This means that the eddy currents produced in the core are now confined to the small cross-sectional area of each lamination. As resistance is inversely proportional to cross-sectional area, lamination produces an increase in resistance and a consequent reduction in the size of the eddy current. There is, however,

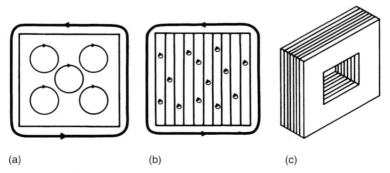

(a)   (b)   (c)

Figure 17.2 (a) shows the flow of eddy currents in an unlaminated transformer core. If the core is laminated as shown in (b) and (c), then the eddy current flow is restricted and so the eddy current losses are limited.

some eddy current present and this causes heating of the transformer core. Because of this, the transformer core requires to be cooled either by air or by immersing the transformer in oil, the latter acting as both a coolant and an insulator.

Hysteresis

We introduced the topic of hysteresis in Section 11.7 and we are now ready to look at this in more detail and also to look at its implication for transformer losses.

Hysteresis is the lagging behind of the induced magnetism in a ferromagnetic material when the applied magnetic field changes. Consider the changes which will occur in a transformer core during 1½ cycles of alternating current. The magnetising force H changes with the current (see Fig. 17.3(a)) and this produces changes in the magnetic intensity I as shown in the graph in Figure 17.3(b). This graph is referred to as a *hysteresis loop* and the shape and size of this loop is important in the function of the transformer. The shape of this loop is explained as follows.

Consider a situation where the core is initially unmagnetised. As the magnetic domains are in randomised directions there is no magnetic intensity within the core. This represents the origin O on both of the graphs. The current increases until it reaches its peak value at point A. The magnetising force increases with the current and so initially does the magnetic intensity. This, however, flattens as magnetic saturation of the sample occurs so that the line is horizontal at point A on the hysteresis graph. The current now follows the curve AB and, as the magnetising force decreases, so the magnetic intensity reduces along the curve AB on the hysteresis graph. *Note* that at point B the magnetising force is zero but there is still some magnetic intensity left in the ferromagnetic core sample. This magnetic intensity is known as the *remanence* in the core. To get rid of this remanence—so completely demagnetising the core—a *coercive force*, represented by OC, must be used. Because the current has been reversed, the magnetising force is also reversed and this continues until magnetic saturation is again produced at D. This occurs at the negative peak value of the current. As the current is reduced, the magnetising force is again reduced and it is zero when the current is at point E on the graph of current. At this point on the hysteresis graph there is again a remanence represented by OE (equal and opposite to OB) and this must be destroyed by the coercive force OF. The magnetising force now continues to its positive peak, A, and the magnetic intensity follows the curve FA. The hysteresis loop is now complete.

The *area of the hysteresis loop* is important as it represents the *work done* in taking the sample round a complete hysteresis cycle. In considering the transformer core the smaller the amount of work done the smaller the

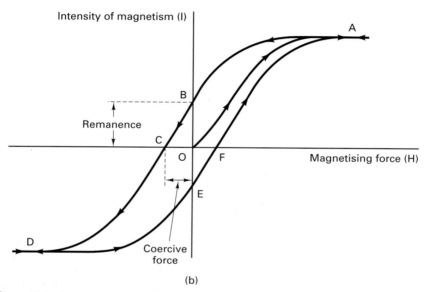

Figure 17.3 (a) shows a typical AC supply for a transformer winding; (b) shows a hysteresis loop for a ferromagnetic sample. For an explanation of the connection between the two, see the text.

iron loss from hysteresis. This should become clearer if we consider the hysteresis loops for soft iron and for steel.

Figure 17.4 shows the differences in the hysteresis loops for soft iron and steel. These differences may be summarised as follows:

● the saturation of soft iron occurs at much lower values of magnetising force than the saturation of steel

● the value of the coercive force is much greater for steel than for soft iron

● the area of the hysteresis loop is much greater for steel than for soft iron.

Soft iron is therefore suitable for situations where a strong induced magnetism is required with the minimum expenditure of energy, and

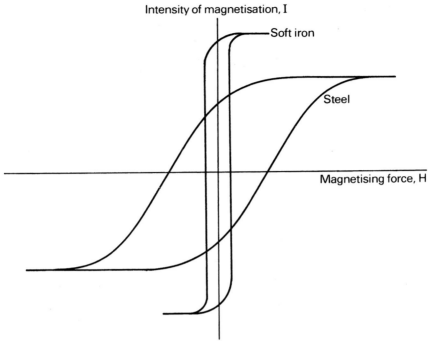

Figure 17.4   A comparison of the hysteresis loops for soft iron and steel.

where the induced magnetism may be switched off at will. *Note* that, although the remanence is greater for soft iron than for steel, the coercive force is so small that a slight agitation of the sample will cause it to demagnetise. Suitable applications for soft iron are electromagnetic relays (see Sect. 12.7) and transformer cores (used as an alloy—stalloy).

Steel is a more suitable material for permanent magnets since it has a higher coercive force than soft iron and is thus more difficult to demagnetise. The high coercive force and the large area of the hysteresis loop make it unsuitable for use in the transformer core.

Subsidiary hysteresis loops

It is not necessary to take a ferromagnetic sample around a *complete* hysteresis loop, i.e. from magnetic saturation one way to magnetic saturation the other. In such cases *subsidiary hysteresis loops* result as shown in Figure 17.5. This is the type of hysteresis loop produced in most transformers—the exception being the saturated core transformer which produces a complete hysteresis loop. The material with the hysteresis loop with the smallest area is still the most appropriate core material for a transformer.

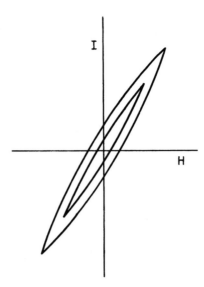

Figure 17.5 Subsidiary hysteresis loops where the ferromagnetic sample is not taken to full magnetic saturation.

The material usually selected for transformer cores is *stalloy* or *permalloy* as their small hysteresis loops limit the hysteresis 'loss'. The power loss due to hysteresis in the core increases the kinetic energy of the atoms of the core and so manifests itself in the form of heat.

17.6.3 Regulation

Regulation in a transformer is a consequence of the resistance of the windings. If the electrical load drawn from the secondary is *increased*—a higher current is made to flow in the secondary—it is found that the potential difference across the secondary is *decreased*. This effect is known as the transformer regulation.

Regulation occurs in any source of electricity which contains an internal resistance. In the case of the transformer, the internal resistance is taken as the resistance of the secondary winding. Figure 17.6 shows a graph of the voltage output from a given transformer for differing secondary currents. The output current is zero when the secondary is 'open circuit' and this corresponds to the open-circuit voltage (V_0 in the figure). In this condition the transformer has zero regulation—it behaves as an ideal transformer and so Equation 17.1 may be used to calculate the secondary voltage. When the secondary of the transformer is connected to a load, current will flow in the secondary winding and the output voltage falls linearly with the secondary current. The transformer regulation therefore varies with the

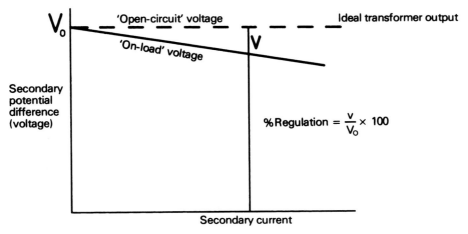

Figure 17.6 The greater the current drawn from the secondary winding of the transformer the smaller becomes the potential difference across it. This effect is caused by the resistance of the windings and is known as *transformer regulation*.

transformer load and so the output current is usually quoted with the regulation, e.g. *'a transformer has a regulation of 2% when the secondary current is 400 mA'*. The regulation is often expressed as a percentage and may be defined as follows:

Definition

The *percentage regulation* at a given load can be calculated by:

$$100 \times \frac{\text{(open-circuit voltage} - \text{on-load voltage)}}{\text{open-circuit voltage}}$$

In Figure 17.6:   percentage regulation $= 100 \times \dfrac{v}{V_0}$

Most transformers used in radiography have a low percentage regulation and so the on-load voltage is close to the open-circuit voltage. In the case of the high-tension transformer, however, there must be a correction for this regulation otherwise there would be a fall in the kV_p if the tube mA was increased. Such corrections are made by *compensating circuits* which are beyond the scope of this text.

Insight

The primary winding of a step-up transformer has such a low resistance that its effect on regulation may be ignored. If an EMF of V_0 is induced in the secondary and the secondary resistance is r, then a current I will produce a voltage drop of Ir (Ohm's Law:

$V = IR$) across the internal resistance r. This means that the potential difference which is available to the external circuit has been reduced by an amount Ir. Thus:

$$V = V_0 - Ir$$

This formula should explain why the regulation is linear with the current as shown in Figure 17.6. It should also be noted that when the secondary is 'open circuit' then the secondary current is zero and so the voltage drop because of the internal resistance is zero. In such a situation $V = V_0$.

17.7 THE AUTOTRANSFORMER

The autotransformer is a useful device for selecting a range of output voltages whose values are not very different from the input voltages (usually differing by a factor of between 0.5 and 2.0). It is constructed in such a way that the number of turns across which the primary voltage is applied can be varied (by moving S_1 in Fig. 17.7). It is also possible by moving the switch S_2 to alter the number of turns on the secondary or output side of the transformer—S_1 selects the number of primary turns, n_p, while S_2 selects the number of secondary turns, n_s.

The principle of operation of this transformer is illustrated in Figure 17.7. The transformer consists of a single winding (with a primary and a secondary side) around a soft iron core. This transformer therefore operates on the principle of *self-induction* (see Sect. 13.8). If we consider this as an 'ideal transformer', we can argue that the same magnetic flux links each turn of the winding and so the induced EMF in each turn is constant. Thus Equations 17.1 and 17.2 can also be applied to the autotransformer, the only difference being that the primary and secondary turns are selected

Figure 17.7 A circuit diagram for an autotransformer. This works on the principle of self-induction. The number of primary turns n_p can be varied at S_1 and the number of secondary turns n_s can be varied at S_2. Thus the output from the transformer can be varied.

from the same winding. As mentioned earlier, the differences between the input and output voltages at the autotransformer are restricted and so the ratio of n_s/n_p is usually between 0.5 and 2.0.

17.7.1 Losses and regulation

All the sources of power loss discussed in Section 17.6 also apply to the autotransformer. However, the less severe design constraints required for the autotransformer make it possible to use a thick winding of copper wire with a consequent reduction in winding resistance. Thus the copper losses and the regulation are lower for the autotransformer than for the conventional transformer as both these losses are dependent on the resistance of the windings. One practical consequence of this is that there is not a great deal of heat generated in the autotransformer and so it is air cooled.

17.7.2 Functions of the autotransformer

In the typical X-ray unit, the autotransformer is positioned between the mains supply and the input to the high-tension transformer. The autotransformer has a number of functions but only two of these are pertinent to this discussion. They are:

- mains voltage compensation
- kV selection.

Mains voltage compensation

In Figure 17.7 the mains voltage is connected to the autotransformer across n_p primary turns, selectable by switch S_1. To understand the workings of the mains voltage compensation at S_1 it is best to consider a numerical example. Let us assume that there are normally 200 turns across n_p and that the normal mains voltage to the transformer is 400 volts. If we assume that this is an ideal transformer, we have a normal volt-drop of 2 volts per turn in the transformer. To ensure the correct output from the transformer across n_s, this volt-drop must be maintained at this level irrespective of the mains voltage input to the transformer. If the mains voltage falls to 380 volts (because of increased demand), then the volt-drop per turn within the transformer will be less than 2 volts per turn (in fact it will be 1.9 V per turn). To get back to the 2 volts per turn and thus the correct operation of the transformer, the switch S_1 must be adjusted to spread this voltage across 190 turns. This gets the autotransformer back to its normal operating voltage of 2 volts per turn. For this reason the switch S_1 is usually referred to as the *mains voltage compensator*.

kV selection

Again this is probably easiest to understand if we consider a numerical example. As already mentioned, the output from the autotransformer forms the input to the high-tension transformer in the X-ray circuit. Suppose we have an ideal high-tension transformer with a turns ratio of 250:1. If we wish an output voltage from this transformer of 100 kV, then we need an input voltage of 400 V, and if we want an output voltage of 50 kV, then we need an input voltage of 200 V. The input voltages for the high-tension transformer are determined at the autotransformer. If we consider the autotransformer used in the previous example, it has a voltage difference of 2 volts per turn. Thus, if we wish to get 100 kV from the high-tension transformer, we move the switch S_2 until n_s is 200 turns. Similarly, if we wish to get 50 kV, S_2 is adjusted so that n_s is 100 turns. For this reason S_2 is referred to as the *kV selector*.

17.8 THE CONSTANT VOLTAGE TRANSFORMER

The constant voltage transformer is designed in such a way that there can be considerable variations in the input voltage to the transformer but the output voltage remains relatively constant. For reasons which will be discussed in Chapter 21, the output from the X-ray tube is sensitive to the temperature of the tube filament and so some units use a constant voltage transformer to ensure a well-stabilised voltage supply to the filament. Figure 17.8(a) gives a diagrammatic representation of the construction of such a transformer and Figure 17.8(b) shows a graph of the input and output voltages.

This transformer operates on the principle that the secondary limb of the core, B, is magnetically saturated during normal operation. The magnetic flux produced at the primary core, A, passes through two other magnetic circuits, the much thinner secondary core, B, and a central path of high magnetic resistance in core C—this high magnetic resistance is caused by the fact that there is an 'air gap' between one end of C and the rest of the core (remember air is less permeable than iron; see Table 11.1). The thinner core, B, is rapidly brought to magnetic saturation and the excess magnetic flux then passes through C. As can be seen from the graph, once B is saturated then an increase in input voltage does not produce any more magnetic flux in B and so the output voltage from the transformer remains fairly constant. Magnetic saturation occurs at an input voltage of X, and Y represents the normal operating input voltage of the transformer. *Note that a large fall in the input voltage (say to Z on the graph) can result in the limb B becoming unsaturated with a resultant fall in the output voltage.*

(a)

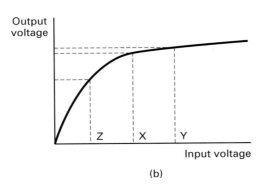

(b)

Figure 17.8   (a) shows the construction of a typical constant voltage transformer; (b) shows a graph of the input and the output voltage for such a transformer.

17.9 TRANSFORMER RATING

Transformer rating was already briefly discussed in Section 14.6. The term *rating* means the maximum combination of factors which a system can withstand without damage. If the rating is exceeded for a transformer, this may cause damage to the electrical insulation of the windings because of overheating or it may cause electrical breakdown.

The transformers in an X-ray unit are energised when the X-ray exposure is made. There are basically two types of exposure in radiography:

- fluoroscopy—this uses a low amount of power for a relatively long time
- radiographic exposures—these use a relatively large amount of power for a short time.

Each of the above produces heat in the high-tension transformer and this transformer thus requires oil cooling. In particular, a long exposure must be made at a relatively low current (and therefore low power), otherwise the heat generated in the transformer will not be convected away sufficiently quickly by the oil and overheating of the transformer results. Short exposures may use higher current values since the total energy deposited in the windings will still be low enough to cause no damage.

The detailed specification of the rating of any one transformer may be complicated, dealing with all the conceivable situations in which the transformer may be used. There are three main factors which must be considered:

- the maximum kV_p which the secondary winding may produce
- the maximum *continuous* current the transformer may supply—this would be used in fluoroscopy
- the maximum current supplied for *short* exposures—this would be used during radiographic exposures.

Summary

In this chapter you should have learnt:

- The concept of an ideal transformer and the equations for voltage and current produced from such a transformer (see Sect. 17.3)
- How Faraday's Laws and Lenz's Law apply to transformers (see Sect. 17.4)
- The types of losses which occur in a practical transformer and how these are minimised (see Sect. 17.6)
- Transformer regulation and its effect on the output voltage from a transformer (see Sect. 17.6.3)
- The operating principles and main functions of an autotransformer in an X-ray set (see Sect. 17.7)
- The operating principles of a constant voltage transformer (see Sect. 17.8)
- The factors to be considered for transformer rating in radiography (see Sect. 17.9).

SELF-TEST

a. If 110 V_{RMS} is applied to the primary of an ideal transformer with a turns ratio of 500:1, what is the RMS voltage output from the secondary? What is the peak voltage output from the secondary?

b. What is meant by the efficiency of a transformer? A transformer has a primary winding consisting of 500 turns and a secondary winding consisting of 50 000 turns. This transformer has an efficiency of 95%. The voltage applied to the primary is 240 V_{RMS} and the secondary current is 1.9 mA_{RMS}. What is the primary current?

c. Explain why the potential difference across the secondary of a high-tension transformer is reduced when the electric current drawn from it is increased.

d. A step-up transformer has a turns ratio of 500:1 and a regulation of 2% when the secondary output current is 400 mA. What is the secondary output voltage that accompanies this current if the primary input voltage is 200 V?

e. An ideal autotransformer normally has an input voltage of 200 V across a primary side consisting of 800 turns.
   (i) How many turns must be engaged on the secondary side to achieve an output voltage of 150 V?
   (ii) If the input voltage were now to fall to 160 V, what would be the secondary output voltage from the transformer assuming that the switches were in the same position as in (i)?
   (iii) How many turns should now be engaged at the input of the transformer to restore the output voltage to 150 V?

f. What is meant by the term *transformer rating*? Explain two ways in which damage may occur to a transformer if the rating is exceeded. Why is it necessary to contain some transformers (e.g. the high-tension transformer in the X-ray circuit) in an oil bath?

FURTHER READING

Ball J L, Moore A D 1986 Essential physics for radiographers, 2nd edn. Blackwell Scientific Publications, London, ch 10

Foster E 1985 Equipment for diagnostic radiography. MTP Press, Lancaster, ch 2

Gifford D 1984 A handbook of physics for radiologists and radiographers. John Wiley & Sons, Chichester, ch 6

Hay G A, Hughes D 1983 First year physics for radiographers. Baillière Tindall, London, chs 8, 13

Ohanian H C 1994 Principles of physics. W W Norton, London, ch 23

Stockley S M 1986 A manual of radiographic equipment. Churchill Livingstone, Edinburgh, chs 1, 3

Thompson M A 1994 Principles of imaging science and protection. W B Saunders, London, ch 5

18

Thermionic emission

18.1 AIM

The aim of this chapter is to introduce the reader to the physics of thermionic emission. Having explained the basic physics, the application of thermionic emission in the vacuum diode and the triode will be discussed. There is also an outline of the importance of thermionic emission to radiography.

18.2 THERMIONIC EMITTERS

A substance which readily releases electrons when heated is known as a *thermionic emitter* and the process responsible for the release of the electrons is called *thermionic emission*.

In the atoms which make up a body, the outer shell electrons are more loosely bound than the inner electrons because they are further away from the nucleus (remember $F \propto 1/d^2$). The application of heat to a body increases the kinetic energy of its atoms and so increases the violence of their collisions. As a result of these collisions the outer electrons may be dislodged from the atom. Electrons so released near the centre of a body travel only a relatively short distance but if they are released near the surface of the material they may have sufficient kinetic energy to leave the body. In thermionic emission this is the mechanism by which the electrons are emitted. It seems logical to assume that the higher the temperature of a body, the greater the kinetic energy of the atoms and so a greater number of electrons will have sufficient energy to break free from the influence of the surface atoms of the body. This is found to be true in practice.

We have also stated that the electrons which are released by thermionic emission are released from the surface atomic layers of the body. Any alteration to these outer layers will alter the ability of a body to perform as a thermionic emitter. This has two practical consequences in radiography:

- all the surfaces involved in thermionic emission (e.g. the tube filament) must be manufactured to a high degree of purity and must be kept scrupulously clean during assembly
- the thermionic emission characteristics of a body may be altered by the deliberate addition of 'impurities' either to the whole body or just to the body surface—thoriated tungsten has a different emission characteristic from pure tungsten (see Table 18.1).

The efficiency of thermionic emitters may be compared by comparing their *work function*, which is normally expressed in electron volts (eV) (see Sect. 6.5.3). The work function is the amount of work which must be performed by an electron in escaping from the body—alternatively it can be considered as the amount of work which must be performed on an electron to enable it to escape from the body. Substances which are good thermionic emitters have a lower work function than those which are poor thermionic emitters, since, in the former, less work is required to allow the electrons to escape. Table 18.1 shows the work function of three substances which are used in radiographic science as thermionic emitters.

From the discussion above it should be apparent that the amount of thermionic emission from a body is controlled by:

- the temperature of the body
- the material of the body
- the surface area of the body.

Table 18.1 Work functions for materials used as thermionic emitters in radiography

Substance	Work function	Comment
Tungsten	4.5 eV	Used as the filament of the X-ray tube to provide the electrons which form the tube current (mA). Its working temperature is around 2000°C
Thoriated tungsten	2.5 eV	Used as the filament in directly heated valves, e.g. switching triodes
Oxides of alkaline substances	1.0–1.3 eV	Used as electron source in indirectly heated devices, e.g. the electron gun in the television monitor

18.2.1 The space charge effect

If we assume that a body is electrically neutral before the application of heat, then each electron which leaves the body by thermionic emission will cause the body to have a net positive charge. After a very short period of time a state of equilibrium is set up where electrons leave the body and enter a 'cloud' of electrons near its surface and are then attracted back to the body, i.e. electrons are attracted back to the body as fast as they are emitted. The number of electrons in this cloud remains fairly constant since electrons are entering and leaving the cloud at equal rates. This cloud of electrons is known as the *space charge*. If the temperature of the body is increased, then the number of electrons in the space charge will also increase due to the increased electron emission from the body. If the body is left to cool, it will reduce the space charge to zero by attracting electrons from it back to the body. The relationship between the temperature of a tungsten filament and the number of electrons liberated in unit time is shown in Figure 18.1.

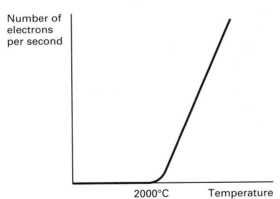

Figure 18.1 Graph of thermionic emission against temperature for a tungsten filament. Note that a small change in temperature produces a large change in emission.

> **Insight**
>
> If we take a normal tungsten filament light bulb and switch it on, then the filament of this bulb is producing significant numbers of electrons by thermionic emission. These electrons form a space charge around the filament and return to it in the process described above. If we bring a large positive charge close to this light bulb, we can cause these electrons to 'flash-over' to this positively charged body. If we switch off the power supply to the bulb, the filament cools down almost immediately, thermionic emission ceases and no further flash-over occurs until the bulb is switched on again.

If a positively charged body is placed close to the space charge, then some of the electrons within the space charge will be attracted towards that body and so an electrical current flows between the heated body and the positive body via the space charge. This is the principle of the thermionic vacuum diode of which the X-ray tube is a specialised type and will be further discussed in later sections of this chapter.

18.3 THERMIONIC EMISSION IN RADIOGRAPHY

Thermionic emission used to be significant in a number of devices used in radiography. However, many devices such as the thermionic rectifier valve and the thyratron valve have been replaced by solid-state equivalents which will be discussed in Chapter 19, and so discussion in this chapter will be limited to the diode valve, the X-ray tube and the triode valve.

18.4 THE VACUUM DIODE

The vacuum diode is a device which will allow a current to flow in one direction only and is thus often referred to as a diode *valve*. Vacuum diodes were of two types: the directly heated and the indirectly heated cathode. As only the principle of the device is considered here, details of the difference between the construction of the two types will not be considered.

Figure 18.2 shows the principal components of such a vacuum diode. The filament is heated to produce electrons by thermionic emission and these are attracted to the positive anode to produce a current flow through the diode. To allow us to control the current through the diode, the anode and cathode are enclosed in an evacuated glass envelope.

Suppose the diode is connected as shown in Figure 18.3. The battery B1 supplies the current which heats the filament allowing it to produce electrons by thermionic emission. The battery B2 is connected across the

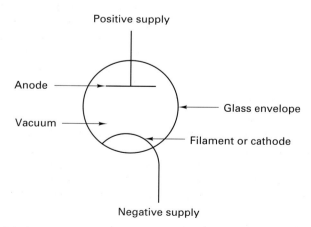

Figure 18.2 Principal components of a vacuum diode illustrated by means of its circuit symbol.

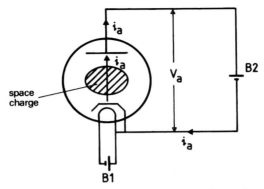

Figure 18.3 Flow of electric current through a vacuum diode. For explanation of its function, see text.

diode so that the anode has a positive potential V_a with respect to the cathode. The effect of the positive anode is to move the position of the space charge from the immediate vicinity of the cathode to a position somewhere between the cathode and the anode. Under these circumstances some of the electrons produced at the filament will gain sufficient kinetic energy to pass through the space charge and reach the anode. Other electrons will be repelled by the space charge and return to the filament. Thus, the space charge has a limiting effect on the flow of current across the diode and the diode is said to be *space-charge limited*. If we make the anode more positive, then the space charge will move further away from the cathode and more electrons will flow across the diode—there is an increase in the diode current i_a.

At a particular value of anode potential all the space charge is collected by the anode as soon as it is produced by the filament. This represents the maximum flow of electrons through the diode at that filament temperature, as electrons will travel across the diode as soon as they are produced by the filament. The diode is then said to be *saturated* or *temperature limited*.

If the temperature of the filament is increased, then it will produce more electrons by thermionic emission and so the saturation current of the diode will have a higher value.

If the polarity of the battery is reversed, only a very small current will flow through the diode due to limited thermionic emission at the anode. If, however, the reverse bias is very large, there can be a breakdown in insulation either inside or outside the diode and a large current can flow in the reverse direction. If we wish to use the diode as a one-way electrical valve (a rectifier; see Ch. 20) then it makes sense to use it at a value below its breakdown voltage—thermionic diodes are seldom used as rectifiers in modern radiographic apparatus but their solid-state equivalent, the *PN* junction diode, must also be used below its breakdown voltage (see Ch. 19).

Figure 18.4 Current and voltage characteristics for a vacuum diode at two values of filament temperature.

These points can be seen in the graph (often referred to as a *diode characteristic curve*) shown in Figure 18.4. As can be seen, there is no increase in the current through the diode once the diode has saturated despite the fact that the potential difference across the device is increased. However, the current can be increased by increasing the temperature of the filament. X-ray tubes are designed to operate in the saturated region as this allows the radiographer to have independent control of the tube current (mA) and the potential across the tube (kV_p)—the radiographer can select *either* a high kV_p and a low mA *or* a low kV_p and a high mA.

If we consider applying an alternating voltage across the X-ray tube, this means that the current through the tube will rise rapidly and then reach a plateau due to the fact that the tube is saturated. During the inverse half-cycle no significant current will flow through the tube as the anode will be negative with respect to the cathode—this will be further discussed in Chapter 20. A graph of the current and voltage for such a tube is shown in Figure 18.5.

18.5 THE TRIODE

The triode valve is similar to a vacuum diode valve except that a third electrode, *the grid*, is inserted between the anode and the cathode (see

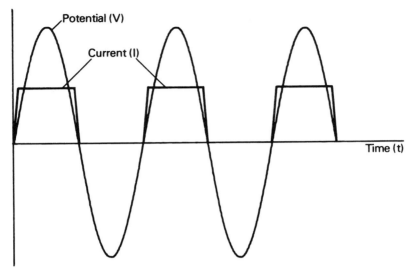

Figure 18.5 The current and voltage waveforms for an X-ray tube which also operates as its own rectifier. The current waveforms are flat topped because the tube is operated in the saturated region.

Fig. 18.6(a)). Electrons flow from the cathode (or filament) to the anode by passing through the grid. The potential difference between the anode and the cathode would allow a *diode* of similar design to operate in the saturated region. The current through the triode is controlled by the negative bias on the grid. If the grid is very negative, then it will repel electrons from the cathode so that none pass through it. Thus there is no current through the triode. If the grid is made less negative (or more positive!), then current will flow through the triode, the amount of current

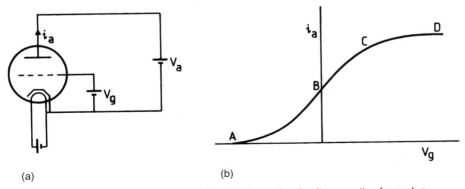

(a)   (b)

Figure 18.6 The thermionic vacuum triode: (a) shows the circuit connection for such a device and (b) shows its characteristic curve.

being controlled by the bias on the grid. Like the diode, the triode will eventually saturate as shown in section CD of the triode characteristic curve (see Fig. 18.6(b)). This ability to switch the triode on and off by altering the potential on the grid allows us to use such devices for switching the X-ray exposure on and off in the constant potential unit (see Ch. 20).

The solid-state equivalent of the triode is the *transistor*.

Summary

In this chapter you should have learnt:

- When certain substances are heated they can be made to liberate electrons by thermionic emission (see Sect. 18.2).
- The amount of energy required to liberate an electron by thermionic emission is known as the thermionic work function of the material (see Sect. 18.2).
- Electrons liberated by thermionic emission form a cloud called the space charge in close proximity to the emitter. An equilibrium exists between the rate of thermionic emission of electrons and the rate of return of electrons form the space charge to the material (see Sect. 18.2.1).
- In a vacuum diode, electrons produced by the filament can be attracted to the anode through the space charge. Depending on the potential difference across the diode, it can be space-charge limited or saturated (see Sect. 18.4).
- The value of the saturation current through a diode depends on the temperature of the filament (see Sect. 18.4).
- X-ray tubes are used in saturated mode so that there is independent control of the tube voltage and the current through the tube (see Sect. 18.4).
- A triode is similar to a diode but it has a grid situated between the cathode and the anode. The current through the triode can be controlled by altering the bias on the grid—the more negative the grid, the less current flows (see Sect. 18.5).

SELF-TEST

a. Describe the process of thermionic emission and discuss how this is affected by the temperature of the body.

b. Discuss the space charge effect in the thermionic diode. How is it affected by the temperature of the filament?

c. List devices in radiography which utilise thermionic emission.

d. What is meant by the terms:
   - space-charge limited
   - temperature limited?

e. Describe the operation of a vacuum triode valve.

FURTHER READING

Ball J L, Moore A D 1986 Essential physics for radiographers, 2nd edn. Blackwell Scientific Publications, London, ch 11

Curry T S et al 1990 Christensen's Physics of diagnostic radiology. Lea & Febinger, London, ch 2

Hay G A, Hughes D 1983 First year physics for radiographers. Baillière Tindall, London, ch 11

Hendee W, Ritenour R 1992 Medical imaging physics, 3rd edn. Mosby Year Book, London, ch 5

Johns H E, Cunningham J R 1983 The physics of radiology, 4th edn. Charles C Thomas, Illinois, USA, ch 2

Thompson M A 1994 Principles of imaging science and protection. W B Saunders, London, ch 6

Semiconductor materials

19.1 AIM

The aim of this chapter is to introduce the reader to semiconductors and semiconducting devices which are important to radiography. While this is a very large field, the chapter concentrates on the barrier layer rectifier, the transistor and the thyristor, all of which have made a major impact on radiographic science. Finally, there is an overview of the uses of semiconductor devices in radiography.

19.2 INTRODUCTION

The use of semiconductor materials and the associated technology play an increasingly important part in our everyday lives as well as in radiographic science. It is possible to produce many thousands of electronic circuits on a small *silicon chip* using large-scale integration (LSI) techniques. This enables the production of microprocessors which are capable of being programmed to perform specific tasks. Such devices are cheap, easy to programme, can perform a wide range of functions and are very reliable. Because of this, microprocessors are found in devices from wrist watches to aircraft flying systems and it is not surprising to learn that they are used in many devices in diagnostic imaging and radiotherapy departments.

However, the microprocessor is a complicated solid-state device and a detailed description of its operation is beyond the scope of this text. Other, simpler, solid-state devices are widely used in X-ray circuitry and hence are suitable for inclusion in this chapter after a general description of the properties of semiconductor materials.

19.3 INTRINSIC SEMICONDUCTORS

An *intrinsic semiconductor* is a chemically pure semiconductor which is also assumed to have perfect regularity of atoms within its crystal lattice. The concept of semiconducting materials was briefly introduced in Section 10.3.2 where the properties of conductors, insulators and semiconductors were compared in terms of the energy band model for the orbiting electrons. This was illustrated in Figure 10.3 and this diagram is again reproduced here as Figure 19.1. As shown in Figure 19.1(b), one of the characteristics of semiconductors is that there is a small energy gap (up to a few eV) between the top of the valence band and the bottom of the conduction band. At very low temperatures all the outer electrons have energies near the bottom of the valence band. Thus no electrons are able to take part in electrical conduction as there are no free electrons in the

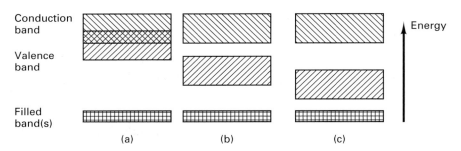

Figure 19.1 Energy level bands for (a) a conductor, (b) a semiconductor and (c) an insulator.

conduction band. As mentioned in Chapter 10, increasing the temperature of a semiconductor increases its conductivity. Thus at normal room temperatures many electrons are able to gain sufficient energy (because of the increased kinetic energy of the atoms) to jump up to the conduction band and so take part in electrical conduction.

19.3.1 Positive holes

Associated with each electron which is able to jump up to the conduction band is a 'vacancy' in the valence band, referred to as a *positive hole* or just *hole*. This hole may be filled by an electron from the *valence* band of a neighbouring atom, but in doing so the electron leaves a hole in the valence band of that atom. In this way a hole may appear to move around the crystal lattice of a semiconductor (behaving like a positive charge) until eventually an electron drops down from the *conduction* band to fill the hole and remove it from the valence band. This process is referred to as *recombination*. At any one moment all three of the above processes are occurring:

- electrons are being excited into the conduction band creating holes in the valence band
- there is movement of electrons in the conduction band and holes in the valence band
- there is a recombination of electrons in the conduction band with holes in the valence band.

The overall conductivity of such an intrinsic semiconductor is the sum of the effects of the movements of the electrons in the conduction band and the holes in the valence band.

Insight

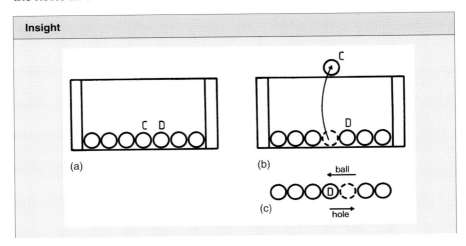

Consider the situation depicted in part (a) of the diagram, where there is a row of ball bearings at the base of a box, with no available space between them for sideways movement to take place. If we now lift ball bearing C on to the lid of the box, it is possible for ball bearing D to move to the left to fill the space once occupied by C. In doing so, D has now created a space to its right, i.e. the hole may be considered as moving in the opposite direction to the ball.

Now consider the above situation as it refers to the valence and conduction bands of a semiconductor. No net movement is initially possible in the valence band because it is full of electrons. When an electron is raised to the conduction band, movement within the valence band is possible. Thus if an electron moves from right to left within the band, it leaves a hole in its starting position, i.e. the hole appears to move from left to right. If an electron is removed from the valence band of an atom, then the atom is positively charged since the protons in the nucleus now outnumber the orbiting electrons; the hole is referred to as a *positive hole*. Thus if a semiconductor is passing current such that the electron flow in the conduction band is from left to right, there will also be an effective flow of positive charge associated with the movement of positive holes in the valence band in the opposite direction.

19.3.2 Silicon

Silicon is currently the most widely used general semiconductor material. Silicon has an atomic number of 14 and hence has 14 protons in its nucleus and 14 electrons orbiting that nucleus (see Ch. 26). This means that the two inner shells (K- and L-shells) are completely full and contain 2 and 8 electrons respectively. The next shell out from the nucleus is the M-shell and this exhibits a stable configuration when it contains either 8 or 18 electrons (see Ch. 26). In this case, it contains 4 electrons and so may be regarded as an incomplete shell in the solitary silicon atom. However, in the silicon crystal there is a regular arrangement of atoms in which each silicon atom shares its outer electrons with 4 neighbouring atoms so that each atom appears to have 8 electrons in its M-shell and thus stability (see Fig. 19.2). Such electron bonds are known as *covalent bonds* and the electrons are termed *valence electrons* and inhabit the valence energy band of the atom. The covalent bonds give the crystal its regularity by inhibiting the movement of any particular atom. At room temperature, these bonds are being continuously broken and re-formed as some of the valence electrons are gaining sufficient energy to reach the conduction band (bond broken) and electrons from the conduction band fall back into the valence band (bond re-formed). The 8-electron configuration of the M-shell behaves like a full shell and so the valence band is effectively full until an electron moves up to the conduction band. As previously explained, when this happens, electron flow in the conduction band and positive-hole flow in the valence band are both possible.

Intrinsic semiconductors, such as the silicon we have just considered, have very limited practical use. If small amounts of specific impurities are added to them (this process is called *doping*), then they exhibit properties which allow us to use them as rectifiers, transistors, thyristors and

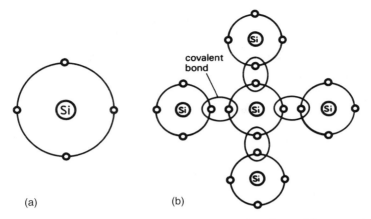

Figure 19.2 Pure silicon as an example of an intrinsic semiconductor: (a) represents a silicon atom showing the 4 electrons in its valence shell; (b) demonstrates the covalent bonds formed in a pure silicon crystal by each silicon atom sharing electrons with 4 neighbouring silicon atoms.

integrated circuits, all of which are found in most X-ray generators. Intrinsic semiconductors which have impurities added to them in this way are known as *extrinsic semiconductors* and will now be discussed.

19.4 EXTRINSIC SEMICONDUCTORS

The addition of small amounts of specific impurities to silicon or germanium is the basis on which most extrinsic semiconductors are produced. The doping may be heavy or light depending on the component being produced. A typical concentration is 1 part of impurity to 10 million parts of pure silicon. The electrical conductivity of the extrinsic semiconductor is much greater than that of an intrinsic semiconductor and the level of conductivity can be controlled by altering the ratio of doping material to pure material. The impurity atoms within the silicon crystal lattice are therefore the source of this greatly increased electrical conductivity. This is because the type of impurity is chosen either to enhance electron flow in the conduction band (this gives an *N-type* semiconductor) or to enhance the flow of positive holes in the valence band (this gives a *P-type* semiconductor). These two types of extrinsic semiconductor will now be considered.

19.4.1 *N*-type semiconductors

As we have already seen, single atoms of intrinsic semiconductors have 4 valence electrons. To produce an *N*-type extrinsic semiconductor, a *pentavalent impurity* (one with 5 valence electrons) is used as the doping

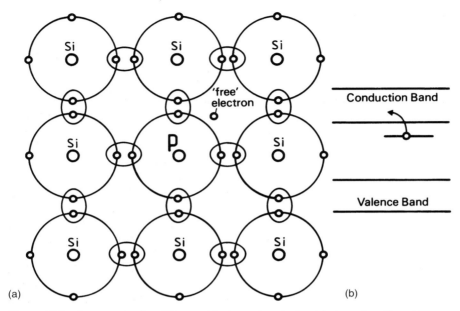

(a)   (b)

Figure 19.3   An example of an *N*-type extrinsic semiconductor: (a) shows how the addition of a pentavalent impurity produces a 'free' electron which does not take part in the covalent bond formation; (b) shows how the energy of such free electrons is close to the conduction band so that they can readily be enabled to take part in electrical conduction.

material. Arsenic, antimony and phosphorus are examples of pentavalent elements which are suitable. Figure 19.3 illustrates the effect of introducing an atom of phosphorus, for example, into the crystalline structure of silicon. Four of the valence electrons in the phosphorus form covalent bonds and the fifth electron is unbonded. This electron has an energy level which is just below the bottom of the conduction band (see Fig. 19.3(b)). At normal room temperatures it is therefore virtually a *free* electron since it is easily lifted into the conduction band and can therefore take part in electrical conduction if a potential difference is applied across the crystal.

Since such pentavalent atoms provide a 'spare' electron, they are known as *donor impurities*.

However, it must be remembered that some electrons from the valence band will also be able to jump into the conduction band due to the normal vibrational energy within the atom at room temperature (this is similar to the intrinsic semiconductor; see Sect. 19.3). Positive holes will also be produced in the valence band and add to the conductivity. At normal room temperatures, this effect is much less than the effect produced by the donor atoms. Thus, in the case of an *N*-type semiconductor, the *majority carriers* are the electrons in the conduction band and the *minority carriers* are the holes in the valence band.

19.4.2 *P*-type semiconductors

As we discussed in the previous section, the *N*-type semiconductor has enhanced conductivity because of the movement of electrons (negative hence the *N*) and so it seems logical to assume that the *P*-type semiconductor functions because of the movement of positive holes. In the case of intrinsic semiconductors, we saw that holes were in the valence band and that this allowed the movement of electrons within this band thus giving the appearance of positive-hole movement (see previous 'Insight'). In the *P*-type semiconductor the movement of electrons within the valence band is encouraged by the creation of more positive holes within this band.

Figure 19.4 illustrates the result of introducing a trivalent material (one with 3 valence electrons) into a silicon crystal lattice. The material used in this case is aluminium, and it results in a broken covalent bond between it and the silicon atoms as there are not sufficient electrons in its outer shell to form the four covalent bonds. The energy level of this broken bond is only just above the valence band (see Fig. 19.4(b)) and so, at normal room temperatures, electrons have sufficient energy to leap this small gap. Thus the electrons which have left the valence band of the silicon leave positive holes behind them and so there is an increase in the number of positive holes in the valence band because of the trivalent impurity. This type of impurity is known as an *acceptor impurity* since it accepts electrons from the silicon atoms, thus creating holes in the valence band.

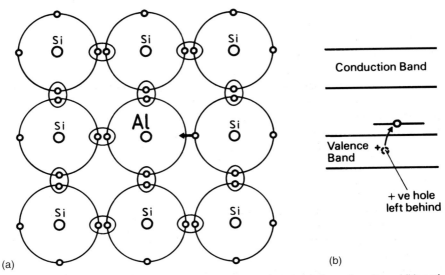

Figure 19.4 An example of a *P*-type extrinsic semiconductor: (a) shows how the addition of a trivalent impurity produces a 'hole' in the outside electron shell; (b) shows how such acceptor atoms take an electron from the valence band leaving a positive hole capable of flowing through this band.

Table 19.1 Summary of the properties of semiconductors

	Intrinsic semiconductor	Extrinsic semiconductor	
		N-type	P-type
Typical material	Pure silicon or germanium	Silicon or germanium with added impurities	
Type of impurity	None	Pentavalent	Trivalent
Term for impurity	—	Donor	Acceptor
Conductivity	Low	High	High
Majority carrier	Electrons and positive holes in equal numbers	Electrons in conduction band	Positive holes in valence band
Minority carrier		Positive holes in valence band	Electrons in conduction band
Effect of temperature	Increases both the number of electrons and the number of positive holes	Increases number of minority carriers (+ve holes) only	Increases number of minority carriers (electrons) only

The *majority carriers* in the *P*-type material are positive holes in the valence band and the *minority carriers* are electrons which have sufficient energy to rise to the conduction band at room temperature as in pure silicon (see Sect. 19.3.2).

Table 19.1 summarises the main points we have considered so far regarding intrinsic semiconductors and the *N*-type and *P*-type of extrinsic semiconductor. *Note* that an increase of temperature does not affect the conductivity due to the majority carriers, but only that due to minority carriers. This is due to the increased number of electrons able to reach the conduction band from the valence band as the temperature increases.

19.4.3 Diagrammatic representation of *N*- and *P*-types

When we discuss the *PN* junction in the next section we need to form a mental picture of what occurs when an *N*-type and a *P*-type semiconductor are fused together. This is made easier if we have a simple symbolic representation of each as shown in Figure 19.5. In the *N*-type the majority carriers are the free donor electrons represented by the minus (–) sign. Each nucleus of the donor impurity has an excess positive charge because of the loss of its outer electron. These fixed positive charges are represented by the symbol $\oplus$. In the *P*-type, the positive holes are free and so are shown as a plus (+) sign while the electrons captured by acceptor atoms give these an overall negative charge. Since these atoms form part of the crystal lattice they are not free to move and so the minus sign is shown

N-Type   P-Type

Figure 19.5 A diagrammatic representation of *N*- and *P*-type semiconductors. In both illustrations the ringed charges represent the fixed charges while the unringed charges represent the free charges which form the majority carriers (electrons for the *N*-type and positive holes for the *P*-type).

ringed ($\ominus$). Thus in both the diagrams the ringed charges are fixed and the unringed charges are free or mobile.

Note that in both the diagrams there are minority carriers caused by the elevation of electrons from the valence band to the conduction band. Since these play little part in the electrical properties of the material they have been omitted from the diagrams for simplicity.

19.5 THE *PN* JUNCTION

When *P*- and *N*-types are heat fused together to form *PN junctions*, interesting effects appear. Examples of the *PN* junction include the *PN* junction diode, the transistor and the thyristor, which have one, two and three *PN* junctions respectively.

If we use the diagrammatic representation which we have just discussed, then the *PN* junction may be shown as in Figure 19.6. When *P*- and *N*-types are brought together and heat fused in intimate contact, then free electrons from the *N*-type and free positive holes from the *P*-type are able to penetrate across the boundary between them. This diffusion of charge across the barrier results in recombination of the positive holes and the free electrons (the free electrons drop into the positive holes so that their charges are cancelled; see Sect. 19.3.1). Thus for a short distance on either side of the *PN* junction (about 0.5×10^{-6} m) no free carriers exist—this is therefore known as a *depletion layer*. However, a net charge exists on either side of the junction because the *N*-type has lost electrons and the *P*-type has lost positive holes (see Fig. 19.6(b)). Thus there is a negatively charged area just within the *P*-type region and a positively charged area just within the *N*-type region. The two peaks of charge shown in Figure 19.6(b) increase in size until no further net flow of majority carriers takes place. For example a free electron from the *N*-type will only be able to pass over to the *P*-type if it has sufficient energy to overcome the repulsion of the negative peak at the *PN* junction.

The charge distribution produces its own potential difference as depicted in Figure 19.6(c). The height of CD is known as the *potential barrier* since it acts in opposition to the flow of majority carriers from either side of the barrier. For a silicon *PN* junction this potential barrier is about

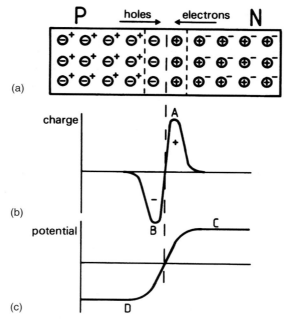

(a)

(b)

(c)

Figure 19.6 The *PN* junction. The diffusion of electrons across the *PN* junction in one direction and positive holes in the other forms a charge barrier which prevents further flow: (b) shows the gain in charge across the junction and (c) shows the potential difference established across the barrier.

0.4 volt so that free carriers of energy lower than 0.4 eV cannot overcome this barrier.

19.5.1 Minority carriers at the *PN* junction

The above discussion concerned only the effect of the *PN* junction on the majority carriers. For majority carriers a potential barrier is formed which prevents any further flow.

However, this barrier actually aids the transport of *minority* carriers between the materials. Consider the potential gradient between D and C (Fig. 19.6(c)). If a free electron (the minority carrier in a *P*-type material) is in position D it is strongly attracted by the positive potential of the *N*-type material and rapidly moves to C. At equilibrium of course there are equal numbers of minority carriers moving in both directions.

Minority carriers are dependent on temperature, since an increase in temperature increases the number of electrons which can jump from the valence to the conduction band. Thus the flow of minority carriers across a *PN* junction increases with temperature. This affects the behaviour of the *PN* junction under conditions of *reverse bias* as will be explained later in this chapter.

19.5.2 Forward bias

If a source of potential difference (e.g. a battery) is connected across a *PN* junction as shown in Figure 19.7(a), then a current will flow across the junction because the potential barrier is lowered. This is shown graphically in Figure 19.7(b). The negative side of the battery reduces the positive potential of the *N*-type and the positive side of the battery reduces the negative potential of the *P*-type. Thus the original height of the barrier is lowered and energetic free carriers from either side are able to surmount the barrier. A steady electrical current is therefore set up as long as the battery is connected. This type of connection, which produces current flow across the *PN* junction, is called *forward bias*. The removal of the battery results in the full height of the barrier being re-established and so no further current can flow.

(a)

(b)

Figure 19.7   The *PN* junction connected in forward bias. The potential from the battery lowers the potential barrier and allows current to flow across the junction: (b) shows the position of the barrier before connection into the circuit and after the device is connected as shown in (a).

19.5.3 Reverse bias

If the source of potential difference is now connected in the opposite orientation as shown in Figure 19.8(a), then this is known as *reverse bias*. No current flows through this circuit due to the increase in the potential

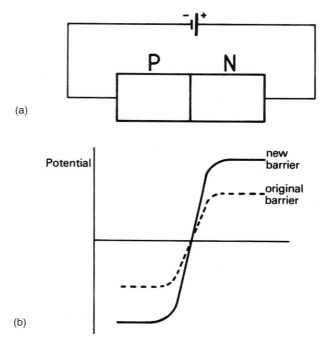

(a)

(b)

Figure 19.8 The *PN* junction connected in reverse bias. The potential from the battery raises the potential barrier as shown in (b) and further prevents electrical conduction.

barrier at the *PN* junction. The graph in Figure 19.8(b) shows that the negative side of the battery increases the negative potential of the *P*-type and the positive side of the battery increases the positive potential of the *N*-type. Thus no current flows, as none of the majority carriers have sufficient energy to surmount this higher barrier. In fact when a *PN* junction is connected in reverse bias, the depletion layer extends further into each semiconductor on either side of the *PN* junction.

The discussion so far has been regarding majority carriers. However, as discussed earlier, a small electrical current due to the thermally generated minority carriers is able to flow.

19.5.4 The *PN* junction as a diode

In our discussion in the last two sections we have shown that current will readily flow through a *PN* junction when it is forward biased, but very little current will flow through the junction when it is reverse bias. Thus the *PN* junction can act as a one-way valve (a diode) which allows current only to flow in one direction. For this reason *PN* junctions are used to create *solid-state rectifiers* or *PN junction diodes*. The symbol for such a device is shown below.

Note that electrons may only flow through the diode *against* the direction of the arrow of the symbol. Such devices have largely replaced thermionic diodes (see Ch. 21) for the following reasons:

- they contain no filament and thus have a longer life, consume less power and produce less heat
- they are smaller in size than thermionic diodes thus enabling the production of a more compact X-ray unit
- they have a smaller forward voltage drop thus enabling a higher kV_p to be applied to the X-ray tube (see Ch. 19)
- the reverse current is less than a vacuum diode and so they are more efficient rectifiers.

19.5.5 *PN* junction characteristic

If the current flowing through a *PN* junction is plotted against the potential difference across it, then the graph produced is referred to as the *characteristic curve* for the device. Such a graph is shown in Figure 19.9.

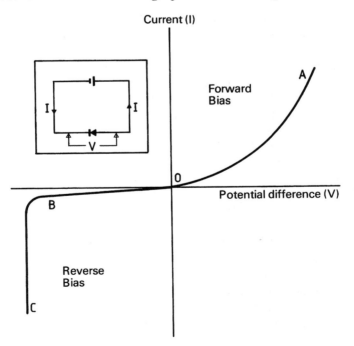

Figure 19.9 The *PN* junction characteristic. For explanation see text.

As the potential difference across the diode is increased in a forward direction, so the current through it increases as shown by OA on the figure. If we compare this with the forward bias characteristic for the vacuum diode (Sect. 18.4) we can note that, in this case, there is no saturation current. However, passing too high a current through a *PN* junction diode can cause irreparable damage.

A normal reverse bias produces only a very low reverse current due to the flow of minority carriers which happen to move into the vicinity of the *PN* junction and so get swept across it. As we have already discussed, this reverse current is very sensitive to temperature as this alters the production of minority carriers due to thermal excitation. If the reverse bias is further increased, then the reverse current increases dramatically (see BC in the graph). This is called the *zener voltage* or *breakdown voltage* and at this value of reverse bias the diode ceases to act effectively as a rectifier. At this negative bias the minority carriers which cross the potential barrier gain enough energy to ionise atoms with which they collide. This results in the liberation of additional electrons and hence the large current. This phenomenon is also referred to as *solid-state multiplication* or *electron avalanching*.

19.6 THE TRANSISTOR

The transistor has replaced the triode valve in most electronic circuits. The transistor itself as a single item has been replaced by large numbers of transistors and other components produced in a silicon chip. Large-scale integration of this sort was mentioned in the introduction to this chapter and the silicon chip so produced is referred to as an *integrated circuit* (IC). The transistors in such an IC are the *field effect* type and will be discussed later in this chapter. First, however, the *junction* transistor is considered.

19.6.1 The *NPN* junction transistor

The junction transistor is composed of three alternating layers of semiconductor materials so both *NPN* junction transistors and *PNP* junction transistors exist, although only the *NPN* transistor is considered in this section. An *NPN* transistor is shown in Figure 19.10(a) together with its electrical symbol (Fig. 19.10(b))—the symbol for a *PNP* transistor is shown in Figure 19.10(c). The central *P*-type semiconductor is known as the *base* and the *N*-types on either side of it are known as the *emitter* and the *collector. Note* that the direction of the arrow on the emitter in the transistor symbol indicates the direction of positive-hole flow—electron flow will be in the opposite direction.

The factors which determine which is the emitter and which is the collector are the geometry of the device and the amount of doping in each. Typically the emitter contains 1000 times more doping than the

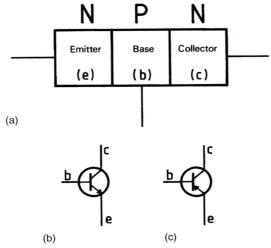

(a)

(b)   (c)

Figure 19.10 The *NPN* junction transistor (a) and its symbol (b). The symbol for the *PNP* transistor is shown in (c).

collector and 100 times more than the base. The emitter thus contains a ready supply of free electrons (from the *N*-type doping) which are available to flow through the transistor as a whole.

Figure 19.11 shows the separate actions of the transistor in terms of its two *PN* junctions. In Figure 19.11(a) the base and the collector are connected to a battery in reverse bias conditions. Thus only the very small current, due to the thermally generated minority carriers, flows. Figure 19.11(b) shows the junction between the emitter and the base connected in forward bias. This time a larger current than in the previous section is able to flow. However, if these two circuits are connected simultaneously (see Fig. 19.11(c)), it is found that almost the same current flows through the

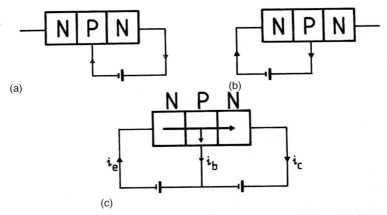

(a)

(b)

(c)

Figure 19.11 The principle of operation of the *NPN* junction transistor (see text for explanation).

emitter and the collector, while the current through the base is much smaller. At first sight this suggests that the base to collector *PN* junction has been destroyed thus allowing a larger current to flow than was previously possible. *This is, in fact, not the case.* It should be remembered that reverse bias applies to *majority carriers*—positive holes in the base. Thus, when electrons are injected into the base from the emitter, they become *minority carriers* within the base and so readily cross the collector-to-base *PN* junction. This process is so efficient that approximately 98% of the electrons injected into the base from the emitter are able to diffuse across the base and form the collector current. The remaining 2% form the base current. This ratio of approximately 50 : 1 for the collector current and the base current remains constant for a particular transistor. Thus the base current may be used to control the collector current, as an increase in the base current will allow a subsequent increase in the collector current. A small signal to the base will produce an amplified signal (amplification 50 : 1) between the emitter and the collector.

19.6.2 The field-effect transistor

The field-effect transistor (FET) varies the current flowing through the semiconductor by varying the electrical field. In this way it can be used to rapidly alter the current in a circuit in a similar way to the function of the triode valve, which it has largely replaced. A simple cross-sectional diagram of the FET is shown in Figure 19.12 where a central rod of *N*-type material has a collar of *P*-type material around it. When the transistor is in a circuit, current flows along the central rod (from left to right in the diagram) one end of which is referred to as the *source* and the other as the *drain*—electrons flow from source to drain. If a negative potential is put on the *P*-type collar (the *gate*), then the *PN* junction is under reverse bias and this extends the depletion layer further into the *N*-type material as shown by the dotted line in Figure 19.12. This means that the majority carriers have been removed from this area and so the electrical conductivity of the

Figure 19.12 A section through a field-effect transistor (FET). The connection of a reverse bias between *P*- and *N*-type semiconductors extends the depletion layer and inhibits electron flow.

area is reduced with a consequent reduction in the current flowing through the N-type. Hence the current through the FET can be reduced by increasing the negative bias on the gate. At a particular *pinch-off potential* no current is able to flow.

The FET has a high input impedance compared to a junction transistor and that means that a lower current is needed to control the device. A typical value of input impedance for such a device is $10^8 \, \Omega$ compared to $10^5 \, \Omega$ for a junction transistor. This is an important consideration when trying to amplify very low signals. However, the FET is a more delicate device and is easily damaged by voltage surges or by static electricity (e.g. touching it may supply sufficient static to cause damage).

19.7 THE THYRISTOR

The thyristor is a silicon-controlled rectifier (SCR) and can be made to act as an *electronic switch*. Its behaviour is similar to that of the thyratron valve which it has largely replaced. Its structure is shown in Figure 19.13(a) showing that it is composed of four alternating N and P semiconductor layers (both NPNP and PNPN thyristors are available but in this case only the operation of the NPNP type is described). Junctions J1 and J3 are forward biased but junction J2 is reverse biased. Consequently, if the thyristor is connected into a circuit, only a small leakage current flows through it—it behaves as an open switch. If a positive pulse is applied to the P-type layer (the gate) at junction J1, then positive holes are injected into the P-type material and flow across the junction J1 so that the potential barrier at that junction is greatly reduced. The reduced potential difference across J1 means that a higher reverse potential difference than before exists across J2 and, if high enough, will cause electrical breakdown to occur at

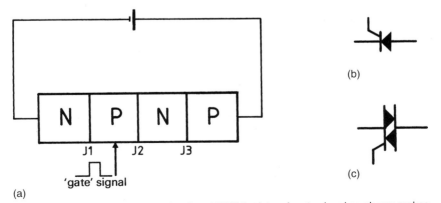

(a)

Figure 19.13 (a) shows an example of an NPNP thyristor. A gate signal as shown makes the thyristor conduct until the potential across the device is reduced to zero; (b) and (c) show the symbols for the thyristor and the triac respectively.

this junction due to the avalanche effect (see Sect. 19.5.5). Once this breakdown occurs, a large current may flow through the thyristor—it behaves as a closed switch. It is not possible to switch the thyristor off by applying a negative pulse to the gate but it will switch off when the potential difference across it is zero—the avalanching effect can no longer be maintained under such conditions. This makes the thyristor very suitable for switching alternating currents as the potential difference across it drops to zero every 0.01 seconds.

The thyristor does have a slight disadvantage when used with alternating currents in that it will only allow current to flow when the N end is negative and the P end is positive. This is overcome by connecting two thyristors in parallel but facing in opposite directions—this is known as a *flip-flop circuit*. A *triac* is, however, able to switch alternating currents. The symbol for this is shown as Figure 19.13(c). It behaves in the same way as the two thyristors connected in parallel but facing in opposite directions. Triacs or flip-flop circuits are often used to switch the X-ray exposure on and off.

19.8 SEMICONDUCTOR DEVICES IN RADIOGRAPHY

Semiconductor devices are used extensively in radiography. This final section gives only a brief overview, mainly of the types of semiconductor devices considered in this chapter. Electromechanical circuits employing semiconductor *logic* components are increasingly used instead of relays because they are more dependable and are inertia free. Microprocessors

Table 19.2 Applications of semiconductor devices

Semiconductor device	Applications
Solid-state diode	Rectification of the HT supply to the X-ray tube using multiple PN junctions connected in series to form stick rectifiers Rectification of the supply to devices which require a unidirectional supply, e.g. certain types of meter
Transistors	Electronic timing circuits Safety interlocks which avoid exceeding the rating of the X-ray tube Amplifying circuits, e.g. in the closed-circuit television chain
Thyristors/triacs	Primary switching of the X-ray exposure, i.e. the triac switches the exposure on and off—following the signal from the timer
Logic circuits	These can check that a number of functions have taken place in sequence, e.g. they can check that the anode is rotating at the correct speed before an exposure is made
Microprocessors	These have many applications in more sophisticated measurement and controls, e.g. microprocessors can check a certain set of exposure factors to ensure that they are not outwith the rating of the selected tube focus

are used in many parts of the X-ray generator circuitry and also in film processors. Unfortunately, the description of the function of such circuits is the subject of a book in its own right and is beyond the scope of this text. Table 19.2 gives an indication of some of the areas where semiconductor devices are used.

Summary

In this chapter you should have learnt:

- A semiconductor has a conductivity between that of an insulator and a conductor, reflecting the small energy gap between the conduction and the valence bands (see Sect. 19.3).
- An intrinsic semiconductor, such as silicon, is a chemically pure semiconductor with a regular arrangement of atoms within its crystal lattice (see Sects 19.3 and 19.3.2).
- Extrinsic semiconductors have carefully measured quantities of impurity added to the intrinsic semiconductor by a process known as doping (see Sect. 19.4).
- An N-type semiconductor is produced when a pentavalent or donor impurity is added to the silicon. This gives a supply of free electrons in the semiconductor (see Sect. 19.4.1).
- A P-type semiconductor is produced when a trivalent or acceptor impurity is added to the silicon. This gives a supply of positive holes within the semiconductor (see Sect. 19.4.2).
- The majority carrier in the N-type material is the free electron and the majority carrier in the P-type is the free positive hole (see Sects 19.4.1 and 19.4.2).
- Minority carriers are thermally produced and are present in all types of semiconductor at room temperature. Minority carriers in the N-type are positive holes and in the P-type are free electrons (see Sects 19.4.1 and 19.4.2).
- A PN junction produces a potential barrier to the flow of electrons and holes. The height of this barrier grows when the junction is reverse biased and diminishes when the junction is forward biased. Thus the PN junction will allow current to flow in one direction only—electrons can flow from N to P (see Sects 19.5 to 19.5.5).
- A transistor is a solid-state device consisting of two PN junctions. A small base current is used to control a larger collector current so that signal amplification using a transistor is possible (see Sects 19.6 to 19.6.2).
- A thyristor is a solid-state device which acts as an electronic switch. A gate signal switches the device on and it can be switched off by allowing the potential difference across the thyristor to drop to zero. Triacs are similar to thyristors but will switch alternating current (see Sect. 19.7).
- Semiconductor devices have many uses in radiography including rectification, signal amplification, switching and microprocessor control (see Sect. 19.8).

SELF-TEST

a. What is meant by the term *intrinsic semiconductor*?

b. How is the conductivity of an intrinsic semiconductor altered by the addition of trivalent or pentavalent impurities? What is meant by the terms:
   (i) extrinsic semiconductor
   (ii) *P*-type semiconductor
   (iii) *N*-type semiconductor?

c. What are the majority carriers and the minority carriers in the *P*-type and the *N*-type semiconductors?

d. What is meant by the term *PN* junction? Explain the meaning of the terms:
   (i) depletion layer
   (ii) potential barrier
   as applied to a *PN* junction. Explain why the *PN* junction conducts current when it is forward biased but will not normally conduct current when it is reverse biased.

e. What are the advantages of a solid-state rectifier over a diode valve?

f. Describe the action of a junction *NPN* transistor.

g. Describe the action of a thyristor.

FURTHER READING

Ball J L, Moore A D 1986 Essential physics for radiographers, 2nd edn. Blackwell Scientific Publications, London, ch 13

Foster E 1985 Equipment for diagnostic radiography. MTP Press, Lancaster, ch 3

Hay G A, Hughes D 1983 First year physics for radiographers. Baillière Tindall, London, ch 11

Ohanian H C 1994 Principles of physics. W W Norton, London, ch 30

Stockley S M 1986 A manual of radiographic equipment. Churchill Livingstone, Edinburgh, chs 5, 7

20

Rectification

20.1 AIM

The aim of this chapter is to consider the various aspects of rectification as it applies to the X-ray generator. There is some initial discussion regarding the need for rectification and the ideal voltage waveform to apply to the X-ray tube. There is then a description of types of rectification of increasing complexity which move towards this ideal voltage.

20.2 INTRODUCTION

In Chapters 13 and 17 we saw that it is convenient to use an AC supply for an X-ray set because of the ease with which the potential can be stepped up or stepped down. The X-ray tube requires a high potential difference across it in order to produce X-rays of the required energy (usually between $40\,\text{kV}_\text{p}$ and $150\,\text{kV}_\text{p}$ for diagnostic radiography but considerably higher than this for therapy radiography). The voltage across the tube is thus stepped up using the high-tension transformer. On the other hand, the filament of the X-ray tube only requires about 10 volt and a few amperes to heat it to a temperature sufficient for thermionic emission (see Sect. 18.2) and so the filament transformer is a step-down transformer. As we will see in Chapters 22 and 28, the X-ray tube is designed to emit X-rays when the anode is positive and the cathode is negative. This means that ideally we would like to change the alternating voltage supplied by the high-tension transformer to a *constant unidirectional voltage*. It is not always possible to achieve this and the best we may be able to get is a *pulsating unidirectional voltage*. The process of converting an alternating voltage to a unidirectional voltage is called *rectification*. As outlined below, the more closely the voltage across the tube resembles the ideal voltage pattern, the more efficient the production of X-rays from the tube. We will now consider different types of rectification.

20.3 Half-wave rectification

As the name suggests, half-wave rectification only utilises half of the available cycles during a given exposure—one-half of each cycle is used and the other half-cycle suppressed. Thus there is X-ray production during the 'used' half-cycle but no X-rays are produced during the suppressed half-cycle. The two basic circuits which used this type of rectification are now seldom encountered in medical radiography (due to the advantages of solid-state rectification) but will be covered in this chapter to show the logical development to more sophisticated types of rectification.

20.3.1 Self-rectification

Figure 20.1 shows a simplified self-rectified circuit. Here the X-ray tube acts both as a rectifier and as a producer of X-rays. The filament of the tube is supplied with power from the filament transformer (FT) and the potential difference across the tube is supplied by the high-tension transformer (HTT). Electrons can only flow through the tube and strike the anode (this is necessary for the production of X-rays; see Ch. 28) when the anode is positive and the cathode is negative. The voltage across the tube is an alternating voltage as shown by V_AB in Figure 20.1(b). The current through the tube is also shown in the diagram and is flat-topped due to the fact that the tube is operating under saturation conditions (see Sect. 18.4).

Note that no current flows through the tube when the anode is negative and the cathode is positive. Thus during this inverse half-cycle the transformer is *off load* and so has zero regulation (see Sect. 17.6.3). This means that the voltage generated in the inverse half-cycle is greater than the vol-

Figure 20.1 (a) shows a self-rectified circuit and (b) shows its current and voltage waveforms.

tage in the forward half-cycle, the difference being the 'on load' regulation of the transformer.

The *advantages* of the self-rectified circuit are:

- the circuit is simple and thus little can go wrong
- the unit is relatively inexpensive
- because of the absence of rectifiers it is possible to incorporate the circuit in a single tank and thus eliminate the need for external high-tension cables.

Note that most of the above advantages are minimal if we are using solid-state rectifiers, which are small and reliable (see Sect. 19.5.4).

The *disadvantages* of the self-rectified circuit are:

- because the temperature of the anode cannot be allowed to rise to the level where there is significant thermionic emission from the anode, the unit is suitable only for low-power work—most dental units used to be of this type
- only half of the available voltage waveform is used during the production of X-rays
- the inverse voltage is larger than the forward voltage and this may restrict the maximum kV_p which can be applied to the tube during X-ray production
- because of the above, the rating of this tube (see Ch. 23) is low: if this rating is exceeded, then damage to the tube may occur.

The restriction on the rating of the tube when in a self-rectified circuit is probably its most significant disadvantage. The remaining circuits in this chapter overcome this disadvantage by the insertion of rectifiers.

Insight

The target of the X-ray tube is made of tungsten and so readily emits electrons by thermionic emission (see Sect. 18.2). If the anode is allowed to rise to a temperature where significant thermionic emission occurs (about 1500°C), then electrons will travel from anode to cathode in the X-ray tube during the inverse half-cycle. This will cause irreparable damage to the cathode assembly of the tube. Thus the target temperature must be kept below the value where significant thermionic emission occurs, so restricting the load which can be applied to the X-ray tube.

20.3.2 Two-diode half-wave rectification

The insertion of two diodes into the secondary circuit of the high-tension transformer overcomes some of the rating problems of the self-rectified circuit. Figure 20.2(a) shows two solid-state rectifiers inserted in the appropriate orientation in the high-tension circuit. Figure 20.2(b) shows the current and voltage waveforms which are applied to the X-ray tube. *Note* that the inverse voltage half-cycle is no longer applied to the tube—it is 'stopped' by the rectifiers and so thermionic emission at the target is no longer a problem. This means that the temperature of the target can be allowed to rise to near the melting point of tungsten (the target working temperature is usually about 2500–3000°C) thus allowing an increase in the applied load of about 50%.

The main reasons for production of this type of unit as opposed to a full-wave rectified unit were that it was significantly cheaper and significantly smaller. Both of these advantages have been eroded by the production of solid-state rectifiers, and this type of unit is no longer in production.

Figure 20.2 (a) shows a two-diode rectified circuit and (b) shows its current and voltage waveforms. Note the absence of the inverse voltage shown in Figure 20.1.

Insight

Two diodes are used to ensure that there is electrical symmetry in the high-tension circuit. This means that the mid-point of the high-tension transformer is at earth potential and that an equal but opposite potential is applied to each end of the X-ray tube, e.g. if 100 kV$_p$ is applied to the X-ray tube then +50 kV$_p$ is applied to the anode end and −50 kV$_p$ is applied to the cathode end. Also, the use of two diodes means that if one should fail, there will not be damage to the X-ray tube as the other diode will continue to function.

20.4 FOUR-DIODE FULL-WAVE RECTIFICATION

The two circuits described in the previous section for half-wave rectification have the disadvantage that only alternate half-cycles are used to produce X-rays. Thus we can consider the X-ray tube as being 'switched off' for half of any exposure time. In order to utilise both halves of the AC cycle, four diodes are used in the secondary circuit of the high-tension transformer (see Fig. 20.3). Figure 20.3(a) and Figure 20.3(b) may at first sight look different but they are, in fact, just two different ways of drawing the same circuit. Figure 20.3(a) is similar to Figure 20.2 in that diodes D1 and D2 are the same in both figures. These diodes rectify one half-cycle

Figure 20.3 (a) and (b) are two different circuits which represent full-wave rectification. Diodes D1 and D2 conduct in one half-cycle and diodes D3 and D4 conduct in the next half-cycle. (c) shows the current and voltage waveforms.

while diodes D3 and D4 rectify the other half-cycle. The direction of electron flow in the circuit is shown by the arrows and it can be seen that the electron flow through the tube for both half-cycles is in the same direction.

Figure 20.3(b) is known as a *Gratz bridge circuit,* which serves the same function as the circuit shown in Figure 20.3(a). A useful tip in drawing this diagram is that, if the tube is in the same orientation as it is in the figure, the arrows on the diode symbols will always point away from G.

Figure 20.3(c) shows the voltage and current waveforms for the full-wave rectified circuit. The voltage across the transformer secondary is still alternating but the voltage across the X-ray tube (V_{AB}) has been fully rectified so that the anode is always positive with respect to the cathode. A current therefore flows during each half-cycle as shown in the lower graph.

Note that in both (a) and (b) of Figure 20.3, the mA meter is also full-wave rectified. The reason for this is that the current through the HT transformer is an alternating current flowing in both half-cycles. The mA meter can only read a unidirectional current and so the current is rectified before it passes through the meter.

20.4.1 Comparison of X-ray tube current for half-wave and full-wave rectification

Figure 20.4(a) and (b) shows the current waveforms for half-wave and full-wave rectification *for the same mA selector setting.* The current waveforms for the half-wave rectified set are twice the height of those for full-wave rectification. The reason for this is that the mA which the radiographer

Figure 20.4 The current and mA (average current) for (a) half-wave rectification and (b) full-wave rectification for the same mA selection.

selects is the *average value* of the mA through the X-ray tube (see Sect. 14.4.2). Since, in the half-wave rectified circuit, every other current waveform is missing the height of each of the remaining waveforms must be doubled to achieve the same average current. This is an important consideration for short exposure times as the half-wave rectified circuit inevitably deposits twice as much energy at the anode during the 'on' half-cycles. Thus, at the same mA in the half-wave rectified circuit, the anode reaches a higher temperature than it would in the full-wave rectified circuit, so restricting the loading. For longer exposure times the effect of individual half-cycles on the anode temperature is less important and so both units have similar ratings. These differences in ratings will be further discussed in Chapter 23.

20.5 CONSTANT POTENTIAL CIRCUITS

None of the circuits described so far conforms to the ideal situation described in the introduction to this chapter where a *constant potential* (or *voltage*) is applied to the X-ray tube. In all of the circuits described so far the voltage has been *pulsating* and not constant. This has three practical disadvantages:

- the anode of the X-ray tube receives rapidly varying amounts of energy
- the intensity of the X-ray beam varies over each half-cycle—the beam intensity is related to the voltage as will be explained in Chapter 28
- the effective energy of the X-ray beam varies over each half-cycle—again, as will be explained in Chapter 28, the effective energy (or quality) of an X-ray beam is related to the voltage across the X-ray tube.

The anode of the X-ray tube is better able to cope with the considerable energy deposited on it if the energy is at a steady level over the period of the exposure. This means that there are no periods when the thermal stress is higher than others. The variation in the output of the X-ray tube over each half-cycle means that the shortest practical exposure time is one half-cycle (0.01 s in the UK) and this can have implications if rapid sequential radiographs are required. As noted above, the effective energy of the X-ray beam is related to the voltage across the X-ray tube. This means that, during any exposure, low-energy X-rays are produced, which add to the absorbed dose in the patient without contributing to the diagnostic information on the radiograph (remember that the voltage across the X-ray tube ranges from zero to the peak value of the kV during any exposure). While it is possible to remove much of this low-energy radiation using filters (see Ch. 29), the best way of solving all of the above problems is to have a constant potential across the X-ray tube during the whole length of the exposure. The four circuits discussed in the remainder of this chapter attempt to apply a less pulsating voltage to the X-ray tube.

20.5.1 Capacitor smoothing of the full-wave rectified voltage

Capacitor smoothing of a pulsating unidirectional voltage has already been discussed in Section 16.11.3. A full-wave rectified circuit with capacitor smoothing is shown in Figure 20.5(a) and the resultant waveform is shown in Figure 20.5(b). (The similarities between this graph and

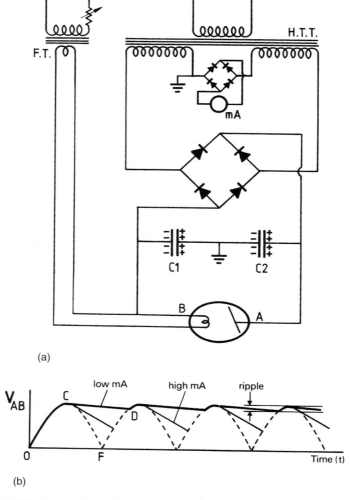

(a)

(b)

Figure 20.5 (a) shows a circuit diagram for a capacitor-smoothed circuit. Capacitors C1 and C2 store charge and discharge it slowly through the X-ray tube as represented by CD on graph (b).

Fig. 16.9(b) should be noted.) The capacitors charge up quickly when the exposure starts (OC on the graph) but discharge more slowly through the X-ray tube (CD on the graph). There is therefore a reduction in the voltage ripple across the X-ray tube compared to a full-wave circuit.

Note that the depth of the voltage ripple depends on the value of mA selected as, if the current through the X-ray tube is large, the capacitor will be able to discharge more quickly and thus its potential will fall more rapidly.

The high-tension cables used to connect the HT transformer to the X-ray tube also possess capacitance but this is quite small so only has a significant smoothing effect when the current is very small, e.g. during fluoroscopy.

Although this voltage is smoother—it has less ripple—it is still not a constant potential. A constant potential can be produced if this voltage is now *triode smoothed* as in the case of the *constant potential generator*.

20.5.2 Triode smoothing—the constant potential generator

The circuit shown in Figure 20.6 shows both *triode smoothing to produce a constant potential* and *secondary switching* of the exposure. It uses triode valves to switch the X-ray tube on and off as well as to absorb the residual voltage ripple after capacitor smoothing.

Before the exposure is made, the X-ray tube is in the *off* condition because the grids of each triode (see Sect. 18.5) are strongly negative, and so no current will flow through them and no potential is applied to the X-ray tube. To start the exposure, the timer sends a signal which makes the triode grids strongly positive thus allowing them to conduct, and so the X-ray exposure starts. The timer terminates the exposure after the pre-selected time by restoring the strong negative bias on the triode grids.

However, *during the exposure* small signals are applied to the grids of the triodes by circuits Y1 and Y2. When the potential from the capacitors is at a high value the grids of the triodes are made more negative, thus effectively resulting in an increase in the resistance of the triodes. This means that there is a greater volt-drop across the triodes and so there is less kV 'left' to apply to the X-ray tube. When the voltage is at its trough, the triode grids are less negative, the resistance of the triodes is less and so they have a smaller volt-drop. By altering the grid bias to correspond to the voltage ripple from the capacitors, this ripple can be totally absorbed allowing us to apply a *constant potential* to the X-ray tube. This has now achieved the ideal situation set out in the introduction to this chapter.

20.6 THREE-PHASE RECTIFICATION

In Chapter 14 we considered three-phase electrical supplies. If all three

(a)

(b)

Figure 20.6 (a) shows a circuit diagram for a constant potential generator; (b) shows the effect of triode smoothing on the output from the capacitors before it is applied to the X-ray tube. For a fuller explanation see the text.

phases are used to supply an X-ray generator, the resultant voltage across the X-ray tube is not a constant potential but the ripple is very small. There are two types of three-phase generator:

- the six-pulse generator
- the twelve-pulse generator.

The circuits in these generators may or may not have capacitor smoothing as described for the single-phase generators. In this case, to allow greater clarity in the diagrams, capacitor smoothing has not been considered. Each generator will now be considered in turn.

20.6.1 The six-pulse generator

A diagram of this generator is shown in Figure 20.7. The movement of electrons through this circuit is slightly more complicated because of the three phases. Figure 20.7(b) shows the voltage waveforms from the three secondaries of the high-tension transformers. Consider the point in time when phase 1 is at peak negative and phases 2 and 3 are at half their positive peaks (this point is shown by a heavy line through the graph). At this stage all the electrons flow through rectifier D1 which is forward biased. They then flow through the X-ray tube from cathode to anode. After this, half of the electrons will flow through D4 and the other half will flow through D6 to transformers 2 and 3 respectively. Thus no electrons are gained or lost in the circuit. (You may wish to test your understanding of the circuit by checking that you can identify the electron flow at some other stage of the voltage cycle shown in Fig. 20.7(b).)

Note: The primary of the high-tension transformer is delta wound and the secondary is star wound (see Sect. 14.8.1). The delta winding of the primary allows a higher primary current to flow. The star winding of the secondary means that the centre of the star is at earth potential, thus giving electrical symmetry around the X-ray tube.

20.6.2 The twelve-pulse generator

The twelve-pulse generator uses three phases but this time the secondary side of the high-tension transformer is split into two sets of secondary windings. One set of windings is in a star winding formation and the other set is in delta winding formation. The point midway between each set of windings is at earth potential so that there is electrical symmetry around the X-ray tube. Each set has six rectifiers associated with it as shown in Figure 20.8(a). The voltage from the star winding is 90° out of phase with the voltage from the delta winding. The generator thus behaves like two three-phase generators which are producing voltages which are 90° out of

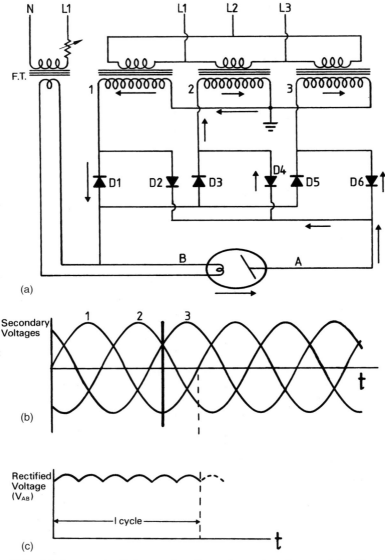

Figure 20.7 (a) shows a circuit diagram for a three-phase, six-pulse generator. Electron flow through the diodes in (a) is shown for a moment in time indicated by the thick line in diagram (b). The rectified voltage results in a waveform across the X-ray tube as shown in (c).

phase with each other. This combined voltage (see Fig. 20.8(b)) is now applied to the X-ray tube. Thus the tube is operating at almost constant potential.

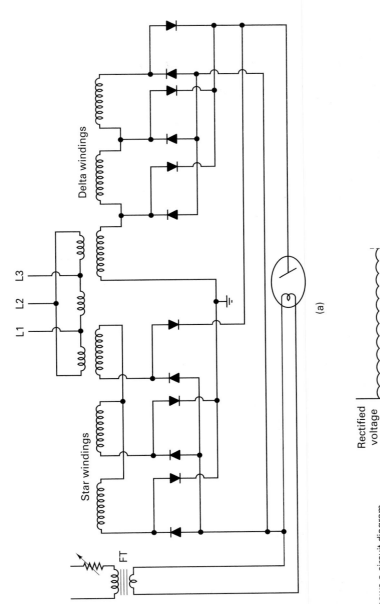

Figure 20.8 (a) shows a circuit diagram for a three-phase twelve-pulse generator. Note that the secondary of the high-tension transformer is in two halves, one half being star wound and the other delta wound. The rectified voltage from each half is applied to the X-ray tube resulting in 12 pulses per 0.02 s as shown in (b).

20.7 RECTIFICATION IN THE PRIMARY CIRCUIT OF AN X-RAY GENERATOR

In all the units we have considered so far, rectification occurs in the secondary circuit—between the high-tension transformer and the X-ray tube. In the *medium-frequency generator* there is also rectification in the primary circuit—between the mains and the primary side of the high-tension transformer. Figure 20.9 shows a box diagram of such a unit. The mains supply is rectified and capacitor smoothed to produce an almost constant potential. This is then passed through a frequency invertor to produce an alternating voltage of frequency 5000 Hz. This high-frequency AC is now passed through the high-tension transformer and the resultant voltage is again rectified and capacitor smoothed before being applied to the X-ray tube—this is equivalent to a 200 pulse unit! The voltage thus applied to the tube is almost a constant potential. The unit has the additional advantage of improved transformer efficiency because of the increased frequency.

Figure 20.9   A box diagram of a medium-frequency generator. Note that this unit has rectification both in the low-tension and in the high-tension circuits.

Summary

In this chapter you should have learnt:

- The reasons why an AC supply is required for the X-ray set and why this needs to be rectified before it is applied to the X-ray tube (see Sect. 20.2)
- The operation, advantages and disadvantages of a self-rectified X-ray unit (see Sect. 20.3.1)
- The mode of operation of a two-diode half-wave rectified unit (see Sect. 20.3.2)
- The mode of operation of a four-diode full-wave rectified unit (see Sect. 20.4)
- A comparison of the current waveforms for a two-pulse unit and a four-pulse unit (see Sect. 20.4.1)
- How the voltage waveform from full-wave rectification can be smoothed using capacitors (see Sect. 20.5.1)
- How a constant potential can be applied across the X-ray tube as a result of capacitor smoothing and triode smoothing in the constant potential generator (see Sect. 20.5.2)
- The mode of operation of a six-pulse generator (see Sect. 20.6.1)
- The mode of operation of a twelve-pulse generator (see Sect. 20.6.2)
- The role of rectification in the primary and secondary circuits of the medium-frequency generator (see Sect. 20.7).

SELF-TEST

a. Why is an AC supply desirable for the operation of an X-ray unit but a unidirectional supply desirable for the operation of the X-ray tube? How are these contradictory requirements achieved?

b. What are the advantages of the self-rectified unit over a full-wave rectified unit and why are these not so relevant in the modern X-ray unit?

c. With the aid of a diagram describe the operation of a four-diode full-wave rectified unit.

d. Describe the mode of operation of the constant potential generator.

e. Discuss the function of the main components of a medium-frequency X-ray generator.

FURTHER READING

Ball J L, Moore A D 1986 Essential physics for radiographers, 2nd edn. Blackwell Scientific Publications, London, ch 13
Curry T S et al 1990 Christensen's Physics of diagnostic radiology. Lea & Febinger, London, ch 3
Foster E 1985 Equipment for diagnostic radiography. MTP Press, Lancaster, chs 2, 9
Hay G A, Hughes D 1983 First year physics for radiographers. Baillière Tindall, London, ch 12
Hendee W, Ritenour R 1992 Medical imaging physics, 3rd edn. Mosby Year Book, London, ch 5

Johns H E, Cunningham J R 1983 The physics of radiology, 4th edn. Charles C Thomas, Illinois, USA, ch 2

Ohanian H C 1994 Principles of physics. W W Norton, London, ch 30

Stockley S M 1986 A manual of radiographic equipment. Churchill Livingstone, Edinburgh, ch 5

Thompson M A 1994 Principles of imaging science and protection. W B Saunders, London, ch 7

21

Exposure and timing circuits

21.1 AIM

The aim of this chapter is to introduce the reader to the principles involved in switching the X-ray exposure on and off. The chapter will also consider the physics involved in timing the X-ray exposure.

21.2 PREPARATION FOR EXPOSURE

Before the X-ray tube can deliver an exposure for a predetermined time interval, it must first be 'prepared' for exposure. This is done during the 'prep' stage of the exposure sequence and during this time two major things happen:

- The appropriate filament of the X-ray tube is raised to its working temperature so that it emits the required number of electrons by thermionic emission (see Sect. 18.2) to allow the tube current (mA) to flow during the exposure.
- If it is a rotating anode X-ray tube (see Ch. 22), the anode is made to rotate at the required speed prior to the exposure being made.

At the end of the prep sequence, the tube is now ready for the exposure. There are two circuit sections responsible for this event:

- the switching section
- the timing section.

21.3 THE SWITCHING SECTION

The function of the switching section is to connect the high voltage (kV_p) to the X-ray tube during the exposure and to disconnect this supply from the tube at the end of the exposure. Such switching commonly occurs between the autotransformer and the high-tension transformer where it is known as *primary switching* or between the high-tension transformer and the X-ray tube where it is known as *secondary switching*.

21.3.1 Primary switching

In a number of older X-ray units this may be in the form of a mechanical switching system. This involves a heavy duty electronic relay switch (see Sect. 12.7) which closes to start the exposure and a second relay which is opened by the timing circuit at the end of the predetermined time to terminate the exposure. Such a system has some in-built inertia and so is not capable of the rapid exposure switching demanded by many modern X-ray generators. For this (and a number of other reasons) it is now replaced by *electronic* or *solid-state switching*.

A simple diagram of a circuit containing a solid-state switching system is shown in Figure 21.1. This type of switching has no moving parts and utilises two thyristors connected as a flip-flop circuit to perform the switching sequence. As you may remember from Chapter 19.7, two thyristors are required to switch an alternating current as each conducts the

Figure 21.1 Simplified circuit diagram of primary switching using two thyristors. The timer produces voltage pulses for the set exposure time, so ensuring that the thyristors are switched on for alternate half-cycles. (For a more detailed description see text.)

half-cycle when that thyristor is forward biased. At the end of each half-cycle each thyristor will cease to conduct as the potential difference across it drops to zero and so a voltage pulse must be applied to its gate if it is required to conduct during the next half-cycle. Thus, during the exposure the timer is simply required to apply a sequence of synchronised pulses to the gates of the thyristors at a time slightly later than the mains zero to switch them back on and ensure their continued conduction. At the end of the exposure these pulses stop and the thyristors cease to conduct at the end of the next half-cycle. This system is inertia free and allows an accuracy of one voltage pulse (i.e. an exposure time of 0.01 second in the case of a two-pulse unit; see Sect. 20.4).

21.3.2 Secondary switching

Secondary switching of the X-ray exposure may be in one of two forms:

- secondary switching using triode valves
- secondary switching using a grid-controlled X-ray tube.

Secondary switching using triode valves

The use of triode valves for secondary switching of the X-ray exposure has already been discussed in the previous chapter (see Sect. 20.5.2). The triode valves are placed between the high-tension generator and the X-ray tube. Electrons from the cathode of the valve must pass through a grid to reach the anode and thus allow a current flow through the valve and in the rest of the high-tension circuit during the exposure. If the grid is sufficiently negative, then electrons will be repelled by it and so no current flows through the valve. Because of this, no potential is applied to the X-ray tube and therefore no exposure is made. As can be seen in Figure 20.6, two triodes are used to give electrical symmetry around the X-ray tube.

Secondary switching using a grid-controlled X-ray tube

As will be seen in Chapters 22 and 28, X-rays are produced when electrons flow from the cathode to the anode of the X-ray tube. These electrons are normally focused on to the target of the tube by a focusing cup, which is at a negative potential equal to that of the filament. If a separate bias is applied to the focusing cup, then it is possible to make it more negative than the filament. Tubes which offer this facility are known as grid-controlled tubes. If the focusing cup is made about 3 kV more negative than the filament, it will produce a sufficiently large electrostatic field to prevent any electrons from crossing the X-ray tube and therefore no exposure is made. When the bias is reduced to make it equal that of the filament, electrons will flow across the tube and X-rays will be produced. At the end of the exposure the high negative bias is re-established on the focusing cup, thus stopping electron flow. The grid-controlled tube is therefore acting as an electronic exposure switch as well as a producer of X-rays. This arrangement is used in cine-radiography where the system is capable of giving up to 500 exposures per second. It is also used in capacitor discharge units where the charge from the capacitor is allowed to pass through the X-ray tube during the exposure time. In such cases the switch shown in Figure 16.7 does not exist as the X-ray tube will act as the high-tension switch.

Insight

A similar form of grid-controlled switching is now used in a number of dental units. In such units the current through the tube is switched off when the voltage falls below a certain percentage of the peak kV. The principles of the process are shown in Figure 21.2.

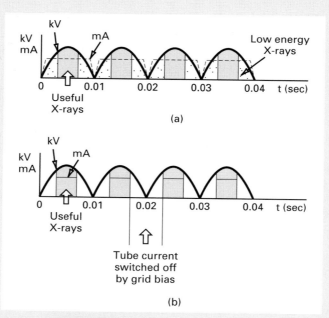

Figure 21.2 The use of a grid-biased X-ray tube to limit patient dose. In (a), low-energy X-rays are produced which contribute to the patient radiation dose but do not contribute to the image. In (b), by applying the necessary bias to the tube, current is prevented from flowing when the tube voltage is below a predetermined limit, thus preventing the production of much of the low-energy X-rays.

As we can see from Figure 21.2(a), in a conventional X-ray unit, X-rays are produced during each of the voltage pulses but only the X-rays produced at the centre of each pulse (near the peak kV) are of diagnostic value. X-rays produced when the tube voltage is significantly lower than the peak kV have very low photon energies and so will be absorbed by the patient and contribute nothing to the diagnostic image. If we can prevent production of these low-energy X-rays, we can limit the patient radiation dose and also help to prolong the life of the X-ray tube. This is achieved by applying a strong negative bias to the focusing cup if the tube voltage is below a certain value and so no current will flow through the tube and no X-rays are produced. This is shown in Figure 21.2(b).

21.4 THE TIMING SECTION

The function of the timing section is to ensure that the appropriate signals are passed to the switching section to allow X-ray production to be switched on and switched off at the appropriate times. The principles of a capacitor/resistor timer were discussed in Chapter 16 and Figure 16.8 is reproduced in this chapter as Figure 21.3. As we can see from this diagram, the time taken to charge a capacitor so that there is a predetermined potential across its plates, is determined by the resistance in the line. When this trigger voltage is achieved, a signal is sent to the switching system which terminates the X-ray exposure by stopping current flow through the X-ray tube. If we consider the situation for thyristor switching (see Sect. 21.3.1), then it can be seen that the exposure can be terminated by simply removing the triggering voltage pulses from the gates of the

Figure 21.3   Simplified circuit diagram (a) and output graph (b) for a capacitor-controlled timer. *Note* that when the switch (S) is in position B the timer is switched off. To switch the timer 'on' the switch should be moved to position A. This will allow the capacitor (C) to receive charge through the variable resistor (R).

thyristors. Thus, at the end of the next half-cycle, the thyristors will cease to conduct and the exposure will terminate.

21.4.1 Time-based timers

If the circuit in Figure 21.3 is arranged in such a way that the capacitor receives charge from a fixed single source (e.g. a rectified supply from the autotransformer), then the time it takes to charge the capacitor will be influenced only by the resistor selected by the radiographer. This is the basis of a *time-based timer*, i.e. a timer where the radiographer selects the exposure time (along with the kV_p and the mA). The X-ray output at a given value of kV_p is a function of the tube current (mA) and the exposure time (see Ch. 28). As the time-based timer controls only the exposure time, it cannot compensate for any fluctuations in the tube current which would influence the X-ray output from the tube. This problem is overcome by the *mAs timer* which will be discussed in the next section.

21.4.2 The mAs timer

A simplified diagram to show the operating principles of an mAs timer is shown in Figure 21.4. Note that on this occasion the capacitor is charged from two sources V_1 and V_2. V_1 is a stable source of voltage (e.g. a rectified supply from the autotransformer). The amount of charge which the capacitor receives from V_1 is controlled by the variable resistor R. This supply is connected to the capacitor (C) when the switch S moves from position B to position A at the start of the exposure. V_2 is a rectified supply from the mid-point of the high-tension transformer so that the amount of charge from this source is directly related to the amount of charge passing through the X-ray tube (the mAs). This supply is again switched on with the exposure. (In the discussion below it is assumed, for simplicity, that the charge from V_2 is the same as the charge through the X-ray tube. This is not always the case but the principle of operation of the timer is still the same.)

Figure 21.4 Simplified diagram showing the operating principles of an mAs timer. When the timer is switched on, the capacitor (C) receives charge from V_1 and V_2. For further explanation of the operating principles, see text.

Suppose the capacitor requires 500 milicoulomb of charge to raise its potential (V_C) to the trigger voltage of the electronic switch. Consider the situation where the variable resistor, R, is set in such a position that the capacitor will receive 400 milicoulomb from V_1. Then the capacitor must receive 100 milicoulomb (or 100 mAs) from V_2 to reach its trigger voltage and terminate the exposure. If we assume that the charge to the capacitor from V_2 is the same as the charge passing through the X-ray tube, then the exposure will be terminated when 100 mAs has passed through the tube.

From the above discussion it can be seen that the radiographer will position the variable resistor, R, to determine the charge from V_2 and hence the charge passing through the X-ray tube during the exposure—the radiographer therefore selects the required mAs.

This has the advantage over the time-based timer that fluctuations in the tube current (mA) will be accommodated by the timer so as to achieve the selected mAs. As the output from the tube at a given kV is proportional to the mAs, the above timer will give a more stable output than the time-based timer in situations where the mA is prone to fluctuations.

In both the time-based timer and the mAs timer we have the fundamental problem that they control the output from the X-ray tube according to a judgement made by the radiographer of the amount of radiation which will be absorbed by the patient. The density (or blackening) on a piece of film is related to the amount of radiation striking the imaging device. In the situations described so far the radiographer judges how much radiation should leave the tube so that when this beam passes through the patient the correct amount will strike the imaging device. The principles of this process are shown in Figure 21.5. If R units of radiation leave the X-ray tube and A units are absorbed by the patient then $(R - A)$ units will strike the imaging device. Thus, ensuring the correct exposure to the film depends on the radiographer's skill in judging how much radiation the patient will absorb. The *autotimer*, which we will now consider, actually measures the amount of radiation to a small sample of the film and terminates the exposure when this radiation has reached the required value.

21.4.3 The autotimer

The principles of the autotimer can be explained using Figure 21.6. As in the case of the mAs timer, the capacitor is charged from two sources. V_1 is a stable source of voltage (e.g. a rectified supply from the autotransformer). The amount of charge which the capacitor receives from V_1 is controlled by the variable resistor R. V_2 is an amplified supply from an ionisation chamber or a photocell, either of which can measure the amount of radiation which has passed through the patient. If we assume that the amount of charge from V_1 is determined by the position of the variable resistor, R, then the remainder of the charge required to raise the potential of the

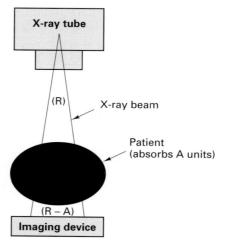

Figure 21.5 Diagram showing the X-ray absorption involved in image production. If R units of radiation leave the X-ray tube and the patient absorbs A units, then $(R - A)$ units of radiation will reach the imaging device.

capacitor to the trigger voltage of the switching device must be from the source V_2. As this is directly related to the amount of radiation passing through the patient on to the imaging device, this will be constant irrespective of the amount of radiation absorbed by the patient. The timer, in this case, terminates the exposure when the correct amount of radiation has passed through the ionisation chamber or photocell. Thus, if the ionisation chamber or photocell is positioned over the correct part of the patient, the radiograph should always receive the correct exposure. If we vary the position of the variable resistor, R, we can vary the amount of charge required from V_2 thus allowing imaging devices of differing sensitivities (speeds) to be used.

Figure 21.6 Simplifed diagram to show the operating principles of an autotimer. When the timer is switched on, switch (S) is in position A and so the capacitor (C) receives charge from two sources. V_1 is a stable voltage supply and the charge from V_2 is from the ionisation chamber or the photocell. Further explanation is in the text.

An autotimer is usually used in conjunction with a guard timer. This is a time-based timer (see Sect. 21.4.1) which will terminate the X-ray exposure should the autotimer fail.

Summary

In this chapter you should have learnt:

- The role of the circuits which prepare the X-ray unit for exposure (see Sect. 21.2)
- The role of the switching section in the X-ray generator (see Sect. 21.3)
- The function and operation of primary exposure switching (see Sect. 21.3.1)
- The function and operation of secondary exposure switching using triode valves or using a grid-controlled X-ray tube (see Sect. 21.3.2)
- The principles of the timing section of the X-ray generator (see Sect. 21.4)
- The principles and mode of operation of time-based timers (see Sect. 21.4.1)
- The principles and mode of operation of the mAs-based timer (see Sect. 21.4.2)
- The principles and mode of operation of autotimers utilising either an ionisation chamber or a photocell (see Sect. 21.4.3).

SELF-TEST

a. Discuss the role of the 'prep' circuits in preparing a rotating anode X-ray tube for exposure.

b. Describe the role of primary exposure switching using thyristors in the X-ray circuit.

c. Describe how the X-ray exposure can be switched on and off using a grid-controlled X-ray tube. Give two uses of such an arrangement.

d. Describe the operation of a time-based timer in an X-ray circuit.

e. Describe the operation of an mAs-based timer in an X-ray circuit.

f. Describe the operation of an autotimer in an X-ray circuit.

FURTHER READING

Carter P H 1994 Chesneys' Equipment for student radiographers. Blackwell Scientific Publications, London, ch 4
Foster E 1985 Equipment for diagnostic radiography. MTP Press, Lancaster, ch 4
Gifford D 1984 A handbook of physics for radiologists and radiographers. John Wiley & Sons, Chichester, ch 23
Hay G A, Hughes D 1983 First year physics for radiographers. Baillière Tindall, London, ch 13
Stockley S M 1986 A manual of radiographic equipment. Churchill Livingstone, Edinburgh, ch 7
Webb S (ed) 1988 The physics of medical imaging. Institute of Physics Publishing, Bristol, ch 3

The construction and operation of X-ray tubes

22

Diagnostic X-ray tubes

22.1 AIM

The aim of this chapter is to discuss the factors involved in the construction of diagnostic X-ray tubes.

22.2 INTRODUCTION

The stationary anode tube has a very limited application in a modern diagnostic imaging department. It has a very low rating (see Ch. 23) and so the amount of electrical power which can be applied to it without causing thermal damage is severely limited. Its main areas of use are in dental or portable X-ray units. In such cases, the unit is connected to a 13 amp main and this restricts the power to the unit, making a tube with high rating irrelevant. Stationary anode tubes—often with heat exchangers—are used in radiotherapy, as the longer exposure time allows sufficient time for cooling by conduction.

In the case of the rotating anode tube there is improved anode rating by more efficient cooling of the focal spot and so such tubes are used extensively in the modern department. The two types of tube are considered in turn in this chapter.

Figure 22.1   A simplified diagram of a stationary anode X-ray tube shield and diaphragm assembly. *Key:* L—lead lining; P—tube support; I—electrical insulator; C—bellows; S—microswitch; O—oil; A—tube aperture or port; F—aluminium filter; B—light bulb; M—mirror; D—movable diaphragms (only one pair shown); R—plastic diaphragm front.

22.3 CONSTRUCTION OF X-RAY TUBES

The X-ray tube consists of two main components:

- *the insert* (shown in detail in Fig. 22.2) which is usually bolted inside the second component
- *the shield* which forms the external casing of the X-ray tube.

These components and the light beam diaphragm—we will discuss its role later in this chapter—are shown in Figure 22.1. We will consider the inserts for the stationary anode tube and the rotating anode tube separately as these differ substantively but the shields for both types of tube are very similar and so will be considered together.

22.4 CONSTRUCTION OF THE STATIONARY ANODE TUBE INSERT

The construction of the stationary anode tube insert is shown diagrammatically in Figure 22.2 and is discussed in the following sections.

22.4.1 Glass envelope

X-ray production is at its most efficient when a vacuum exists between the cathode and the anode of the X-ray tube, and so the glass envelope must be sufficiently strong to preserve this vacuum. The envelope is joined to the anode stem at one end and to the nickel cathode support at the other end by *re-entrant seals*, so called because the glass is shaped to point inwards at the area of contact. Slightly different glass seals are used at each end so that the thermal expansion of the glass is similar to the nickel at the cathode end and is similar to the copper at the anode end. This reduces the stress on the glass when the insert is hot and so limits the chance of cracking.

Figure 22.2 A stationary anode X-ray tube insert. *Key:* T—tungsten target; A—copper anode; S—re-entrant seal; G—glass envelope; V—vacuum; F—tungsten filament; C—focusing cup; K—cathode support.

The glass must be a good electrical insulator or a substantial current will flow through it when the high potential difference is applied between the anode and the cathode. However, electrical charges are built up on the inside of the glass during operation and so the glass must have sufficient electrical conductivity to allow these to leak away—usually between exposures—avoiding the build-up of high amounts of static charge. The glass is gently rounded so that there are no sharp corners which would allow the build-up of high amounts of static charge (see Sect. 9.9).

During operation of the X-ray tube, a thin film of tungsten will be deposited on the inside of the glass as a result of the release of tungsten vapour from the filament and the target. This may eventually cause electrical breakdown within the tube as it can act as an electrical conductor around the inside wall of the glass envelope. If this happens, the tube is classed as 'gassy' and is of no further use. The rate of tungsten deposition can be reduced by not keeping the tube in the 'prep' mode (see Sect. 21.2) any longer than is required and by keeping exposures well within the rating of the tube (see Ch. 23).

22.4.2 Cathode and filament(s)

The terms 'cathode' and 'filament' are often interchanged when discussing the X-ray tube. However, the correct usage of the term 'cathode' implies the whole cathode assembly including the filament, focusing cup, supporting wires and cathode support. The filament is therefore part of the cathode but not vice versa.

The focusing cup is made of either nickel or stainless steel, each of which has a high melting point and is a relatively poor thermionic emitter—each has a high thermionic work function (see Sect. 18.2). In addition, the thermal expansion of these materials is close to that of certain types of glass, thus reducing the stress on the seals during operation of the tube. When the filaments produce electrons by thermionic emission these would repel each other by electrostatic repulsion—like charges repel—and so would strike a large area of focal spot. The area of the focal spot is reduced by the negative bias on the focusing cup which 'squeezes the electrons together' (see Sect. 22.7.2).

The filament is made of a thin tungsten wire for the following reasons:

- Tungsten has a low thermionic work function (see Sect. 18.2) and so will readily emit electrons by thermionic emission.
- Tungsten has a low vapour pressure and so does not easily evaporate. This helps prolong the life of the filament as evaporation would cause the wire to become thin. It also prolongs the life of the tube as it prevents the formation of a tungsten film on the inner wall of the glass envelope.

• Tungsten is a strong metal which can be drawn into a thin wire which will not easily distort. This helps to maintain the shape of the filament helix over a period of time.

An X-ray tube may have two filaments side by side as shown in Figure 22.3. This is known as a dual-focus X-ray tube. The differing sizes of filament result in differing sizes of electron foci on the anode. The larger is known as the *broad focus* and would be used in situations where a high radiation output was required from the tube, while the smaller—the *fine focus*—would be used in situations where it is desirable to keep geometric unsharpness (see Sect. 2.6) to a minimum.

One side of each filament is connected to the focusing cup while the other is insulated from it (see Fig. 22.3(c)). This connection between both

(a)

(b)

(c)

(d)

Figure 22.3 Details of a dual-filament cathode assembly: (a) 'face-on' view; (b) from above; (c) from the side; (d) showing electrical connections.

filaments also forms the common connection between the filament circuit and the high-tension circuit. This is represented by point P in Figure 22.3(d). From this diagram it can be seen that three conductors are required in the high-tension cable coming to the cathode end of the X-ray tube.

The secondary side of the filament transformer is also connected to one side of the high-tension circuit and so this transformer could be a source of electrical hazard to the operator of the X-ray unit. For this reason and for reasons of ensuring good electrical insulation and heat dissipation, the filament transformer is contained in the same oil-filled tank as the high-tension transformer.

Insight

All high-tension cables for X-ray units contain at least three conducting wires even though only one is required at the anode end of the tube. This means that manufacturers only need to make (and X-ray departments only need to stock) one type of cable. Only one of the three wires at the anode end is used to make an electrical connection to the tube.

22.4.3 The anode

The anode of the stationary anode tube (see Fig. 22.4) is constructed of two materials, copper and tungsten, and so is known as a *compound anode*. The main part of the anode assembly is made of copper because of its good thermal conductivity. (Note that the cooling of the target of the stationary anode tube is discussed in detail in Sect. 8.7.1.) The inclined face of the anode block has an inset of a thin (about 2–3 mm) tungsten plate known as the *target* on which the electrons are focused. The target is made of tungsten for the following reasons:

- Tungsten has a high atomic number ($Z = 74$) and so is an efficient producer of X-rays (see Ch. 28).
- Tungsten has a high melting point (3387°C) so it can withstand the heat generated during the X-ray exposure without melting.
- Tungsten has a low vapour pressure so it does not readily vaporise at its normal working temperature.
- Tungsten can be readily machined to give the smooth surface required for X-ray production.

The face of the anode is set at an angle to the central axis of the X-ray beam. This has already been considered in Section 2.3 and gives rise to the *line focus principle*. As already discussed in Section 2.3, this results in an effective focus which is smaller than the real focus. The advantages of the line focus principle are:

- The real focus can be longer than the effective focus. Thus the filament may be relatively long without giving rise to excessive geometric

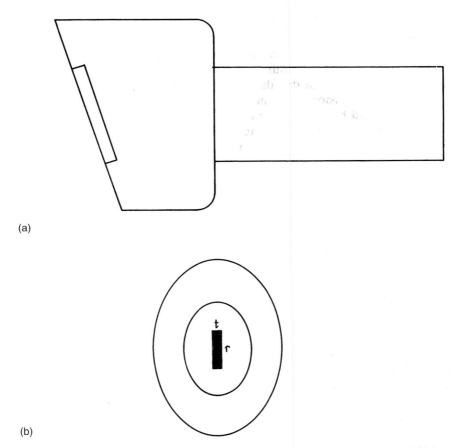

(a)

(b)

Figure 22.4 The line focus principle: (a) shows the anode viewed from the side and (b) is a view of the front surface of the anode. The electrons are focused on a small rectangle of breadth *t* and length *r*—the line focus.

unsharpness. Thermionic emission from the filament is proportional to its surface area and so a long filament will provide the high values of mA required by many exposures.

● The area over which the heat is deposited is the larger area of the real focus. The temperature rise experienced by a large area for a given amount of heat is less than that experienced by a small area since more atoms are able to take part in the heat dissipation processes. The line focus principle enables the anode to be designed so that the area of the real focus is about three times the area of the apparent focus. This enables a reasonable compromise between the need to minimise the temperature rise at the target (thus requiring a large focal area) and the need for minimising the geometric unsharpness (thus requiring a small focal area).

The anode face is usually set at an angle between 15° and 20° to the central axis of the X-ray beam. This is called the *target angle*.

22.4.4 The anode heel effect

Consider Figure 22.5. X-rays are produced slightly below the surface of the target material. X-rays passing along path 1 will therefore pass through a smaller section of the target than those passing along path 2. There is absorption of the X-rays as they pass through the target and so the rays which pass through the greatest thickness of target are the more heavily absorbed—there will be a lower intensity of X-rays along path 2 than along path 1. This means that the X-ray intensity at the anode end of the beam will be less than at the central axis while the intensity at the cathode end will be greater than at the central axis. This is known as the *anode heel effect*. The effect increases as the target angle is reduced and also increases with the age of the X-ray tube. This latter increase is caused by the fact that the target becomes pitted with use.

Insight

Some of the electrons which strike the target cause secondary electrons to be emitted from the target surface. Many of these electrons strike other points on the anode outside the focal area while others strike the glass and produce a static charge on it. X-rays are therefore produced at points on the anode outside the area of the original electron beam to the focus. This is called *extra-focal radiation* and, if it occurs in significant amounts, can contribute to image unsharpness. The electrons which strike the surface of the glass prevent further electrons from doing the same by mutual repulsion and leak away between exposures because of the small but finite conductivity of the glass.

Figure 22.5 The anode heel effect: ray 2 is more attenuated than ray 1 owing to its longer pathway through the tungsten target.

22.5 CONSTRUCTION OF THE ROTATING ANODE TUBE INSERT

(Note that the heat loss from the target of the rotating anode tube to the air of the X-ray room was discussed in detail in Sect. 8.7.2.)

The rotating anode X-ray tube is the most common type of X-ray tube found in diagnostic imaging departments. The reason for this is that it is able to produce higher intensities of X-rays than the stationary anode tube. This is due to two factors:

• The heat deposited in the anode during an X-ray exposure is spread over a larger area and so there is a smaller temperature rise at the anode surface.

• The cooling characteristics of the rotating anode are superior to those of the stationary anode and this effective dissipation of heat means that larger loads can be applied without causing thermal damage to the target.

The construction of the insert and the stator coils is shown in a simplified form in Figure 22.6. The components of this tube will now be individually discussed.

22.5.1 The cathode assembly

The cathode assembly is essentially the same as for the stationary anode tube in that it consists of two filaments in focusing cups held in position by

Figure 22.6 A rotating anode tube insert and shield (housing). *Key:* A—anode disk; F—focal track; S—anode stem; R—rotor assembly; T—rotor support; W—stator windings; E—glass envelope; K—cathode assembly; O—oil; L—lead lining; N—neoprene expansion diaphragm; M—microswitch; HT—high-tension cable receptacle; P—tube port.

a cathode support. The filaments are offset from the central axis of the tube so that the electrons emitted are aligned with the bevelled edge of the anode disk. In some tubes the filaments are positioned end to end instead of side by side. This means that the electron beams fall on different parts of the bevelled surface of the disk and that these can be set at differing angles. This is referred to as a *bi-angular tube*.

In the most common type of rotating anode X-ray tube the filaments are connected as previously described in Figure 22.3(d).

22.5.2 The anode assembly

The simplest anode configuration is shown in Figure 22.6 where the anode consists of a molybdenum disk with an accurately bevelled edge on which is deposited a tungsten/rhenium focal track. Electrons from the filament strike this track and dissipate some of their kinetic energy as X-ray photons. The disk has a central hole in it through which it is connected to a molybdenum anode stem and hence to the rotor of the induction motor. The rotor, stem and anode disk are accurately balanced so that no appreciable wobble occurs when the whole assembly rotates. The rotor is made to spin by the rotating fields produced by the stator coils—this is a similar process to the AC induction motor described in Section 15.7. The rotor moves smoothly on steel ball bearings coated in a soft metal, such as tin or silver, which acts as a lubricant but does not destroy the vacuum inside the envelope—a lubricant such as oil would evaporate and compromise the vacuum. The positive terminal from the high-tension supply is connected to the rotor support and through this there is a continuous electrical connection to the anode disk.

The conduction of heat from the anode disk to the ball bearings is inhibited by the fact that the anode stem is made of molybdenum (a relatively poor thermal conductor) and the fact that the stem has a small cross-sectional area (see Sect. 8.4.1). However, some heat will inevitably reach the ball bearings and could cause sufficient expansion to produce a risk of seizure. This risk is reduced by applying a black coating to the outer surface of the rotor so that it loses heat efficiently by black body radiation (see Sect. 8.4.4). Many modern X-ray tubes also have a graphite backing on the anode disk. This draws heat from the anode and then dissipates it by black body radiation. This results in the possibility of greater loads being applied to the anode and also in a reduced heat dissipation to the ball bearings.

The materials used in the disk design of the modern rotating anode tube are given in Table 22.1.

A rotating field is produced by the stator coils and thus the rotor (and the anode disk) rotate at the same frequency as the applied voltage.

Table 22.1 Materials used in the design of the modern rotating anode disk

Material	Use	Reason for use
Molybdenum	Disk	Half the density and twice the specific heat capacity of tungsten
Tungsten	Focal track (90%)	High atomic number; high melting point; low vapour pressure; suitable mechanical properties
Rhenium	Focal track (10%)	High atomic number. More elastic than tungsten therefore less pitting of the focal track
Graphite	Disk backing	Low density. Acts as 'heat sink'. Radiates heat by black body radiation

22.6 CONSTRUCTION OF THE TUBE SHIELD (HOUSING)

It is necessary to protect the patient and the radiographer from the electrical and radiation hazards posed by the X-ray tube insert while in operation. The insert is therefore incorporated within a suitable container, the shield, which must satisfy the following criteria:

- There must be no danger of electrical shock if the shield is touched during operation of the X-ray tube.
- No significant amounts of radiation should escape from the shield other than the radiation necessary for taking the radiograph.
- The shield must give secure support to the X-ray tube, the high-tension cables and the connector cables within the shield.
- Adequate insulation must be provided between the insert and the tube shield to avoid electrical breakdown.
- There must be adequate cooling of the insert and facilities to allow expansion of the cooling oil.
- There must be facilities at the tube port to allow adequate filtration of the emergent beam so that low-energy radiations may be removed from the beam.

As can be seen from this list, the shield must satisfy many requirements. Schematic diagrams of shields for stationary anode and rotating anode X-ray tubes are shown in Figures 22.1 and 22.6 respectively. Note that in both cases the insert is held in position by a support at the anode end.

The metal casing surrounding the insert is made either of aluminium or steel and is lined with about 3 mm of lead to provide sufficient radiation protection. This housing is filled with pure oil which acts as an insulator and as a coolant. A metal bellows or neoprene diaphragm at one end of the shield allows for expansion of the oil when the oil is heated. This assembly may be fitted with a microswitch which will prevent further exposures if the oil is very hot. Within the casing there is a radiolucent window—the tube port—which will allow the useful beam of radiation to leave the tube via the light beam diaphragm.

22.6.1 Electrical safety

Electrical safety is designed around three basic principles:

- insulation of live components
- earthing of component housings
- restricted access to live components.

All of the above are utilised in the design of the X-ray tube. Insulation exists between the live components and the housing in the form of the oil in the housing. As we saw in Section 10.3.3, the resistance of an insulator (and so its insulating properties) diminishes as the temperature of the insulator increases and so the role of the oil in heat dissipation is also important from the point of view of electrical safety.

The tube shield is connected to earth via the outer braiding of the high-tension cables (see Fig. 22.7) and so the casing will always remain at earth potential. If a live wire within the casing becomes disconnected and touches the shield, then the current will readily flow to earth and the casing will present minimal electrical hazard to someone touching it at the time.

The live components in the X-ray tube are secured inside the tube shield and the ends and the high-tension cable connectors are securely fixed. This means that, under normal circumstances, the operator has no easy access to the live components.

In addition to this, the circuits may be isolated from the mains by switches, fuses or circuit breakers.

Figure 22.7 (a) Structure of a high-tension cable. (b) The X-ray tube shield is made electrically safe by connecting the copper braiding of the high-tension cables to both the shield and the high-tension transformer casing. The latter is securely earthed.

22.6.2 Radiation safety

Radiation safety is important for the operators of X-ray equipment and for patients and others who may be in the vicinity at the time of making an X-ray exposure. The lead lining of the tube housing (see Fig. 22.6) limits the radiation leakage from the tube and so provides protection to both the operator and the patient. It should be borne in mind that X-rays are emitted *in all directions* from the focus on the anode but only those which pass through the tube port are allowed to leave the housing. The anode itself has a high absorption and so the lead lining at the anode end of the shield is often thinner than at the cathode end. The radiation leakage rate from the tube is normally measured at a distance of 1 metre from the housing and should not exceed an air kerma of 1.00 mGy per hour measured at a distance of 1 metre from the focus (for definitions of the kerma and the gray, see Ch. 33). Any break in the lead lining will result in radiation leakage from the tube, so the leakage levels should be checked at regular intervals as part of the quality checks on the X-ray unit.

Radiation safety means exposing the patient only to the minimum dose necessary to produce a radiograph of acceptable quality. As we will see in Chapter 28, the spectrum of X-rays produced at the target is a continuous spectrum containing a mix of low-energy, medium-energy and high-energy photons. Some of the photons have very low energy and will not be able to pass through the patient to reach the imaging device. These photons would contribute to the patient dose but not to the image production. Some of these are removed by the glass envelope of the insert and the oil as the beam passes to the tube port. This is known as the *inherent filtration* of the tube. Further filtration takes place through the aluminium filters (see Fig. 22.1). Thus the *total filtration* of the beam is determined by the *inherent filtration* plus the *added filtration*.

Scattered radiation contributes to the patient dose and the operator dose and causes a degradation in the radiographic image quality. As we will see in Chapter 30, the amount of scatter produced at a given set of exposure factors, is dependant on the volume of tissue irradiated. The volume can be reduced by reducing the area irradiated using a *light beam diaphragm* (see Fig. 22.1). This also means that parts of the body not required on the radiograph can be protected from the radiation. In this way, adequate collimation using a light beam diaphragm (or cones) will reduce the patient dose and the operator dose and produce an improvement in the image quality.

22.7 PRINCIPLES OF OPERATION OF THE X-RAY TUBE

As we will see in Chapter 28, X-rays are produced when electrons are accelerated from the cathode to the anode of the X-ray tube. The number of electrons crossing the tube is controlled at the mA selector and the kinetic energy of the electrons—and thus the photon energy of the X-ray beam—at the kV selector.

22.7.1 Tube current (mA) and filament current

Figure 22.8 shows a circuit diagram of the X-ray tube and high-tension circuit which has been greatly simplified to illustrate the difference between the tube current (mA) and the filament current (I_f). The relationship between the temperature of the tungsten filament and the number of electrons released by thermionic emission has already been discussed in Section 18.2.1 and this section will look at the application of this information to the X-ray tube. In Figure 22.8, B1 represents the power supply across the X-ray tube and B2 represents the power supply across the filament. Suppose B2 causes a current I_f to flow through the filament circuit. The passage of this current through the filament causes heating of the filament and the subsequent temperature rise will cause electrons to be emitted by thermionic emission. Because of the potential difference placed across the tube during the exposure, these electrons will flow across from the cathode to the anode and thus a current, mA, will flow through the tube and circuit B1. If the radiographer increases the value of I_f, then the temperature of the filament will increase and so will the number of electrons emitted by thermionic emission. As these electrons constitute the tube current—assuming the tube is operating under saturation conditions (see Sect. 18.4)—we can say that *as a result of an increase in the filament heating current, there will be an increase in the tube current.* Thus the radiographer actually selects, at the mA selector, the filament heating current which will produce the required tube current. A typical set of figures for an X-ray tube are shown in Table 22.2.

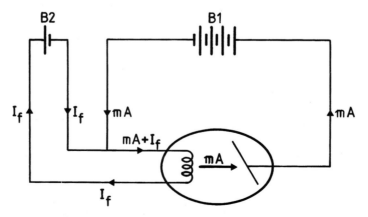

Figure 22.8 The difference between tube current (mA) and filament heating current (I_f). For explanation of the difference see text.

Table 22.2 Filament heating currents for different tube currents for a typical X-ray tube

Filament heating current	Tube current
5 A	200 mA
7.5 A	400 mA
9 A	800 mA

22.7.2 Electron focusing

During the X-ray exposure, the anode of the X-ray tube is positively charged and the cathode is negatively charged. As a result of this, the electron space charge emitted from the filament (see Sect. 18.2.1) is repelled from the negative cathode and attracted to the positive anode. The situation which would arise if both the cathode and the anode were flat plates is shown in Figure 22.9(a). The electric force field (see Sect. 9.4) consists of parallel lines starting at the anode and finishing at the cathode. Electrons are emitted from the filament, F, and are attracted to the positive anode. However, the electrons repel each other so the plume of electrons will increase in size as it travels across the X-ray tube. The area W on the anode represents an unacceptably large focal area as this would produce a large geometric unsharpness (see Sect. 2.6) on the resultant radiograph. This problem is overcome by the use of a focusing cup (see Sect. 22.4.2) as shown in Figure 22.9(b). The thermionic electrons from F now experience two forces, one towards the anode and the other towards the central axis of the beam. The force towards the central axis of the beam is greater than the

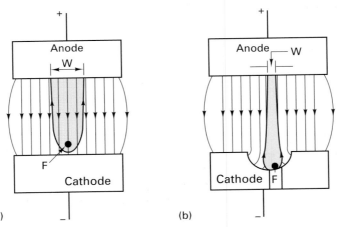

Figure 22.9 Simplified explanation of the focusing of electrons in the X-ray tube: (a) shows the result of no focusing cup on the cathode; in (b), the concave focusing cup directs the electrons from the thermionic emitter F towards the central axis, so that they strike a smaller area (W) on the anode.

force of electrostatic repulsion between the electrons and so the plume of electrons is focused on to a small area of the anode—W in Figure 22.9(b).

22.7.3 Tube voltage (kV$_p$)

The kV$_p$ selected by the radiographer controls the peak potential difference across the X-ray tube. The higher the kV$_p$, the higher the peak potential difference and so the greater the force of attraction between the anode and the cathode. Because of this, the electrons will strike the anode with greater kinetic energies and so will produce more energetic X-ray photons. This will be discussed in more detail in Chapter 28 when we consider X-ray production in detail. In this chapter we will finish with a brief synopsis of the process so that the construction of various parts of the X-ray tube may be more clearly understood.

22.7.4 X-ray production

In the X-ray tube, electrons are produced at the cathode by thermionic emission. These electrons are then accelerated towards the anode and are made to give up their energy when they collide with the atoms of the target material. The main mechanism of X-ray production is when the electron is made to lose kinetic energy because of the pull of the positive nucleus of the target atoms. This is known as *Bremsstrahlung radiation*. The intensity (I) of the Bremsstrahlung radiation varies with both the energy (E) of the electrons striking the target and with the atomic number (Z) of the target material as shown in the equations below:

$$I \propto Z \times E$$

Equation 22.1

or $\quad I \propto Z \times kV_p^2$

Equation 22.2

The process of X-ray production is very inefficient and up to 99% of the energy of the electrons may be converted into heat which must rapidly be transferred from the focal area to avoid damage to the target of the tube (see Sect. 8.7.2).

22.8 MODERN TRENDS IN X-RAY TUBE DESIGN

There are a number of modern trends in the design of specialist X-ray tubes which are not within the scope of this text. The reader should either consult more specialist texts on tube design or should consult manufacturers' literature. Specialist designs include:

- the metal/ceramic X-ray tube insert
- grid-biased X-ray tubes

- high-speed anode X-ray tubes
- stress-relieved anodes in rotating anode X-ray tubes
- X-ray tubes which allow automatic measurement of anode temperature
- alteration of the shape of the anode disk to allow improved loading (e.g. discus-shaped discs).

Summary

In this chapter you should have learnt:

- The reasons why the stationary anode X-ray tube is of limited use in the modern X-ray department and why it has largely been replaced by the rotating anode X-ray tube (see Sect. 22.2)
- The fact that X-ray tubes consist of two major components, the insert and the shield (see Sect. 22.3)
- The construction of the glass envelope of the stationary anode X-ray tube (see Sect. 22.4.1)
- The construction of the cathode and filaments of the stationary anode X-ray tube (see Sect. 22.4.2)
- The construction of the anode of the stationary anode X-ray tube (see Sect. 22.4.3)
- The reason for and the result of the anode heel effect (see Sect. 22.4.4)
- The construction of the rotating anode tube insert (see Sect. 22.5)
- The construction of the cathode assembly of the rotating anode X-ray tube (see Sect. 22.5.1)
- The construction of the anode assembly of the rotating anode X-ray tube (see Sect. 22.5.2)
- The construction of the X-ray tube shield (see Sect. 22.6)
- The methods of ensuring the electrical safety of the X-ray tube shield (see Sect. 22.6.1)
- The methods of ensuring the radiation safety of the X-ray tube shield (see Sect. 22.6.2)
- The principles of operation of the X-ray tube (see Sect. 22.7)
- The interrelationships between the filament heating current and the X-ray tube current (mA) (see Sect. 22.7.1)
- The requirement for and the method of achieving focusing of the electron beam across the X-ray tube (see Sect. 22.7.2)
- The effect of the tube voltage (kV_p) on the emergent X-ray beam (see Sect. 22.7.3)
- A basic description of X-ray production (see Sect. 22.7.4).

SELF-TEST

a. Draw a sketch diagram of a stationary anode X-ray tube to show the insert and housing. Indicate the function(s) of each of the major components.

b. Draw a sketch diagram of a rotating anode X-ray tube to show the insert and housing. Indicate the function(s) of each of the major components.

c. List the reasons why tungsten is used in the construction of the filament and the reasons why tungsten is used in the construction of the target of the X-ray tube.

d. Tabulate the materials used in the construction of a modern rotating anode X-ray tube disk, indicating where each is used and the reasons for its use.

e. Discuss why a change in the filament heating current produces a change in the X-ray tube current (mA).

f. Why is it possible to have a filament heating current without a tube current but it is not normally possible to have a tube current without a filament heating current?

FURTHER READING

You will find further information on the rating of X-ray tubes in Chapter 23 of this text and more information on the factors affecting the X-ray spectrum produced in Chapter 28. In addition you may find sections from the following texts provide useful further reading:

Ball J L, Moore A D 1986 Essential physics for radiographers, 2nd edn. Blackwell Scientific Publications, London, ch 12

Carter P H 1994 Chesneys' Equipment for student radiographers. Blackwell Scientific Publications, London, ch 1

Curry T S et al 1990 Christensen's Physics of diagnostic radiology. Lea & Febinger, London, ch 2

Foster E 1985 Equipment for diagnostic radiography. MTP Press, Lancaster, ch 5

Gifford D 1984 A handbook of physics for radiologists and radiographers. John Wiley & Sons, Chichester, chs 19, 20

Hay G A, Hughes D 1983 First year physics for radiographers. Baillière Tindall, London, ch 11

Hendee W, Ritenour R 1992 Medical imaging physics, 3rd edn. Mosby Year Book, London, ch 5

Johns H E, Cunningham J R 1983 The physics of radiology, 4th edn. Charles C Thomas, Illinois, USA, ch 2

Stockley S M 1986 A manual of radiographic equipment. Churchill Livingstone, Edinburgh, ch 6

Thompson M A 1994 Principles of imaging science and protection. W B Saunders, London, ch 6

Webb S (ed) 1988 The physics of medical imaging. Institute of Physics Publishing, Bristol, ch 2

Rating of X-ray tubes

23.1 AIM

The aim of this chapter is to enable the reader to understand the concept of the rating of X-ray tubes. This will allow the use of rating charts to ensure that exposures are within safe limits. The chapter will also consider the limitations of rating charts in certain circumstances.

23.2 DEFINITION OF RATING

The general term *rating* is used to describe the practical limits which are inherent in any device. An example of this is that a fuse rated at 5 amp will tolerate currents up to 5 amp. If a current above 5 amp passes through the fuse then the fuse will melt causing a break in the circuit. A high-tension transformer is a more complicated device than a fuse and so has a more complicated set of rating conditions (see Sect. 17.9). Similarly the rating of an X-ray unit—the X-ray tube and the associated equipment—depends both on how it is constructed and how it is being used. The rating may be defined as follows:

Definition

The *rating* of an X-ray unit is the combination of exposure settings which the unit can withstand without incurring unacceptable damage.

Any radiographic exposure causes slight wear and tear on the X-ray tube, since the anode becomes slightly pitted and the filament becomes slightly thinner as a result of any exposure. However, in this context 'unacceptable damage' means damage which would seriously impair the performance of the unit for further exposures or might indeed make it inoperative. In this context, a single short exposure where the mA was out-with the rating of the tube, might damage the anode by melting the focal track. Alternatively, a long exposure at low mA may again damage the anode if the total amount of heat generated in the anode caused a sufficient temperature rise to melt the tungsten. It is also true that multiple expo-sures, each of which is individually within the tube rating, might damage the tube because of the total heat accumulated in the anode by the expo-sure series. As the anode takes a finite time to cool after an exposure, the closer the exposures follow each other, the more likely the anode is to suffer thermal damage. For this reason the rating for single and multiple exposures will be considered separately in this chapter.

23.3 SINGLE EXPOSURES AND RATING CHARTS

Some of the exposure factors are under the control of the operator while others are not, as shown in Table 23.1.

In any particular unit, the non-selectable factors are fixed and so a rating chart must be used which is applicable to that set of circumstances, e.g. a rating chart might be appropriate to an X-ray tube connected to a two-pulse unit. This chart shows the effect on the rating of varying the quantities in the selectable group. A simplified form of such a chart is shown in Figure 23.1 where the rating curve corresponds to a 1.2 mm focus

Table 23.1 Selectable and non-selectable factors which affect the single-exposure rating of a particular X-ray unit

Selectable factors	kV_p, mA, exposure time, focal spot size, radiography/fluoroscopy
Non-selectable factors for stationary anode tube	Rectification, thermal capacity of anode, thermal capacity of tube shield, efficiency of heat loss from anode and tube shield, anode angle, rating of high-tension cables and transformers
Non-selectable factors for rotating anode tube	Rectification, thermal capacity of anode, diameter of the anode, rate of anode rotation, thermal capacity of tube shield, efficiency of heat loss from anode and tube shield, anode angle, rating of high-tension cables and transformers

Figure 23.1   A simplified rating chart. All points below the curve are permissible for radiographic exposure.

selection and a kV_p selection of 80 kV_p. The curve indicates the upper limit for all combinations of mA and time for this value of kV_p. Thus, points *below* the line are safe whereas points *above* the line are unsafe in that they would result in unacceptable damage to the X-ray tube. If we consider an exposure of 80 kV_p, 100 mA and 0.2 s, then we can see that this exposure may be safely made, as the point P is below the 80 kV_p line. *Note* that because of the wide range of exposure times possible it is usual to use a logarithmic scale on the X-axis.

It can also be seen from the graph that higher values of mA will be tolerated for short exposure times—150 mA at a time of 0.1 s is within the rating—whereas, at long exposure times, only lower values of mA are within the rating—for an exposure time of 2 s the maximum mA permissible within the rating is 50 mA. In each case the limiting factor is the anode temperature. For longer exposure times there can be significant cooling of the anode during the exposure. This is shown by the flattening off of the curve at longer exposure times.

In practice, rating charts are produced for a variety of kV_p values which might be applied to the X-ray tube and there are separate rating charts for *broad focus* and for *fine focus*. Examples of such charts are shown in Figure 23.2 where (a) is the rating chart for the broad focus and (b) for the fine focus. As can be seen from these charts, the rating of the tube is lower for the fine focus than for the broad focus. This is caused by the fact that for a fine focus the electron beam is concentrated on to a smaller area, thus producing a higher temperature rise for the same value of mA.

Figure 23.2 Comparison of rating charts for broad and fine focus.

Figure 23.2 also shows that larger values of mA are permitted as the kV_p is reduced, the difference between the curves being most marked for the shorter exposure times. As was discussed in the last chapter, electrons are produced at the filament of the X-ray tube and are accelerated towards the anode. The higher the kV_p across the tube, the more kinetic energy each electron possesses when it interacts with the anode target. Thus, the same number of electrons per second (mA) will deliver more energy per second to the target and so will increase the possibility of thermal damage. The rating chart shows this inverse relationship between the kV_p and the mA.

Insight

Consider a situation where for a given exposure time (t) the anode may be given a total energy E without causing thermal damage. The energy of a single electron crossing the X-ray tube is proportional to the kV_p across the tube. The total number of electrons is related to the current (mA) and the exposure time (t).

$$\therefore E \propto kV_p \times mA \times t$$

Thus for a given exposure time, halving the kV_p should double the permissible mA. Reference to an exposure chart for an X-ray tube should confirm that this is the case.

Finally, different rating charts are required for different types of rectification when using the same X-ray tube. Figure 23.3 summarises this effect for four different types of rectification, where the same focal spot and the same kV_p have been selected. As can be seen from the graphs, the self-rectified circuit has the poorest rating, while the constant potential circuit has the best rating. Also note that the differences in rating are most marked at short exposure times. This is because the heating effect of individual pulses is most apparent in this situation. The more constant the heat production the less likelihood of thermal damage to the target—hence the best rating for constant potential. For longer exposure times, the thermal

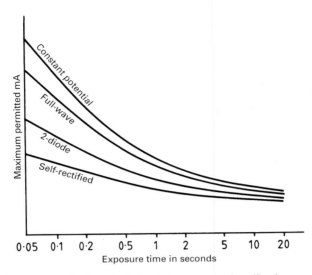

Figure 23.3 Comparison of rating charts for different types of rectification.

capacity (see Sect. 8.3.2) of the anode disk is the dominating factor. This is independent of the type of rectification and so the curves all tend to come closer together as the exposure time increases. Also note that for longer exposure times the cooling of the tube shield and the heat dissipation within the high-tension transformer are significant factors in determining the rating of the tube and X-ray unit.

23.4 RATING OF STATIONARY ANODE AND ROTATING ANODE X-RAY TUBES

The rating of the stationary anode X-ray tube is significantly less than the rating of the rotating anode tube. The limitations of the stationary anode tube are caused by its anode construction and its method of cooling. The anode consists of a small target of tungsten embedded in a block of copper. Copper is used because of its high thermal conductivity but it has a relatively low melting point (1083°C), which limits the temperature rise that the anode will tolerate. Heat loss by conduction (see Sect. 8.4.1) is a relatively sluggish process and so both of the above factors limit the heat which can be produced at (and therefore the power applied to) the target.

In the rotating anode X-ray tube, heat loss by conduction is discouraged by the design of the anode stem (see Sect. 22.5.2) and the main method of heat loss is by radiation. Efficient heat loss by radiation is achieved by designing the anode disk so that it can tolerate high temperature rises (remember that the rate of heat loss by radiation is proportional to the fourth power of the Kelvin temperature). During large exposures the anode disk often becomes incandescent and at such temperatures can lose heat effectively by radiation—hence the higher rating of the rotating anode tube.

23.5 EFFECTS OF ANODE DIAMETER AND SPEED OF ANODE ROTATION ON TUBE RATING

When we consider the rating of the rotating anode tube we must consider all the factors discussed so far plus the effect of the *anode diameter* and the *rate of anode rotation*. In the rotating anode tube the electrons land on the focal track around the bevelled circumference of the disk. This means that the heat is deposited around the whole disk instead of in the same area, as in the case of the stationary anode tube. Because this heat energy is now deposited over a larger area, there is a smaller temperature rise and so improved rating.

If we increase the anode diameter we will also increase its circumference. This means that the heat energy is now deposited over a larger area and, as more atoms are involved in cooling, leads to more efficient cooling, improving the rating. Doubling the diameter of the disk will increase its rating by 40–50% but this has practical limitations because of the extra mechanical stress this imposes on the bearings. A simplified graph showing the improvement in rating is shown in Figure 23.4(a).

If we double the speed of rotation of the anode, this means that only half the heat energy is deposited on to the anode for each rotation although it makes twice as many rotations during a given exposure time. If there was no cooling between successive heatings of the same point, there would be no advantage of increasing the rotational speed. The temperature changes at the anode because of the heating and cooling are shown graphically in

Figure 23.4   Effect on rating of (a) anode diameter and (b) rate of anode rotation.

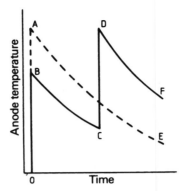

Figure 23.5 The advantage of a high-speed anode is due to anode cooling. The dotted line represents the rating for an anode rotating at half the speed of the full line. Cooling of the anode allows a higher anode loading (OB + CD compared to OA).

Figure 23.5. Points A and D represent the maximum permissible temperature of the anode but it should be noted that the high-speed anode will tolerate two applications of heat before it reaches this temperature whereas the disk which is rotating more slowly reaches this temperature after one application of heat. For the high-speed anode, cooling—represented by the curve BC—takes place between the applications of heat.

The effect of increased anode rotation on the tube rating is shown in Figure 23.4(b). Doubling the speed of rotation will again increase the rating by about 40–50%. It should also be noticed that the difference in rating diminishes with longer exposure times, since it is the overall thermal capacity of the anode that is the dominant factor.

23.6 MULTIPLE EXPOSURES

If multiple exposures are to be made, where there is insufficient time for the anode disk to cool between exposures, then the rating charts discussed so far must be used with extreme caution. While a single exposure may be within the rating of the tube, the heating effect of subsequent exposures may raise the temperature of the tungsten above the permitted level, resulting in thermal damage to the focal track. In such cases it is necessary to use the rating charts in conjunction with the anode cooling curves to predict the safety of any combination of exposures.

23.6.1 Anode cooling curves

An example of a cooling curve is shown in Figure 23.6 where Heat Units (see Sect. 6.4.4) are plotted against time. Note that a number of manufacturers now present this graph for joules plotted against time but the principles are still the same. The anode disk has a given mass and thermal

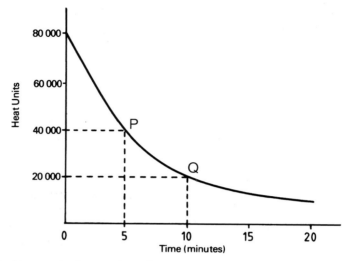

Figure 23.6 An example of an anode cooling curve.

capacity and so there is a given quantity of heat which will raise the whole anode disk to its maximum desirable operating temperature. This is known as the heat storage capacity of the anode and is expressed in Heat Units or joules—in the example chosen this is 80 000 Heat Units. The cooling curve in the figure shows the number of Heat Units left after a given time, assuming that the anode has received its maximum permitted number of Heat Units at $t = 0$. Suppose an exposure of 80 kV$_p$, 250 mA and 2 s has just been made. The heat produced in Heat Units is $80 \times 250 \times 2 = 40\ 000$ HU. This is shown by the point P on the graph. The anode loses heat as given by the curve below P such that it stores only 20 000 HU 5 minutes later (see point Q on the graph). An example of the use of such a graph is given below.

Example

An exposure of 100 kV$_p$, 400 mA and 1.5 s is made on the X-ray tube for which Figure 23.6 is the cooling curve. The exposure requires to be repeated as soon as possible. How long must we wait between exposures to ensure that the anode does not exceed its maximum heat storage capacity?

HU produced by the exposure = 100 × 400 × 1.5
= 60 000 HU

The maximum heat storage capacity of the anode is 80 000 HU and so it must cool down till it stores only 20 000 HU before the exposure is repeated. By consulting the graph, it can be seen that this takes approximately $10 - 3 = 7$ minutes.

In the cases discussed so far using cooling curves, it is assumed that *no significant cooling of the anode takes place during the exposure*. If this is not the case, e.g. during fluoroscopy, then anode heating curves are used as described below.

23.6.2 Anode heating curves

For long exposures such as fluoroscopy, the cooling which occurs during the actual exposure becomes important in calculating tube ratings. The anode initially heats up fairly quickly but then tends towards a *thermal equilibrium* which occurs when the rate of heat generated in the anode by the electron beam is exactly balanced by the rate of heat loss from the anode. Examples of anode heating curves for a particular tube are shown in Figure 23.7 where the number of Heat Units stored by the anode at any moment is plotted against time. The maximum heat storage capacity of this anode is 100 000 HU. Three different exposure rates are shown:

- The rate of 1000 HU per second fairly rapidly exceeds the heat storage capacity of the anode and further exposure beyond this time would result in thermal damage.
- The rate of 500 HU per second establishes thermal equilibrium at the maximum heat storage capacity of the anode.
- The exposure at 100 HU per second—this would be the rate of heat production for a fluoroscopic kV of 100 kV$_p$ and a fluoroscopic current

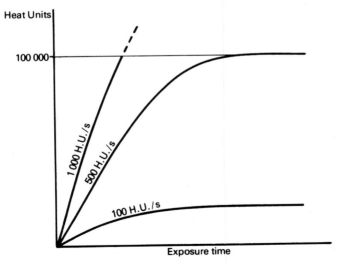

Figure 23.7 An example of a series of anode heating curves. The maximum thermal capacity of the anode is 100 000 Heat Units and this may be exceeded if the rate of heat production is sufficiently high.

of 1 mA—produces thermal equilibrium with the anode at a fairly low temperature.

Note that in many cases it is convenient to show the heating and cooling curves on the same graphs.

23.6.3 Angiographic rating charts

In the case of rapid sequential imaging, as in angiography, it is necessary to consult the heating and cooling curves and the rating charts to determine whether a proposed series is within the rating of the particular tube. Such calculations may be time consuming and prone to arithmetical error if performed under specific time constraints. This problem is overcome by the use of *angiographic rating charts*. Table 23.2 is an example of such a rating chart supplied with an X-ray tube where the maximum tube loading for an exposure is 40 kW. Similar rating charts are usually provided for different exposure loadings.

Let us consider an exposure series of 4 exposures per second for a time of 5 seconds where each exposure has the following exposure factors 80 kV$_p$, 500 mA, 0.05 s. (For the purpose of the following calculation it is assumed that the generator is a constant potential unit so that the peak value and the RMS value of the kV are the same.) First the single exposure should be checked against a single exposure rating chart to ensure that it is within the rating—for the purpose of the discussion which follows we will assume that it is within the rating of the tube for a single exposure. The loading produced by each exposure will be:

$$80 \times 10^3 \times 500 \times 10^{-3} = 40\,000 \text{ W}$$

Thus the 40 kW rating chart is the one we require to consult.

If we now consider the line for 4 exposures per second and an exposure time of 50 ms, we find that a series of 35 exposures is permissible. The

Table 23.2 Angiographic rating chart for a tube loading of 40 kW per exposure. For this tube the interval to be observed *before* and *between* series must not be shorter than 20 minutes (for details of how to use the chart, see accompanying text)

Tube load	Exposure rate (exposures/s)	Exposure time for each radiograph in ms												
		3	6	10	20	25	32	40	50	63	80	100	120	160
	12	100	100	100	82	60	42	30	22	16	—	—	—	—
	10	100	100	100	88	64	45	33	24	17	12	—	—	—
	8	100	100	100	97	71	50	36	26	19	13	10	—	—
40 kW	6	100	100	100	100	80	56	41	30	21	15	11	4	—
	4	100	100	100	100	95	67	49	35	25	18	13	10	7
	3	100	100	100	100	100	75	55	40	29	20	15	11	8
	2	100	100	100	100	100	90	66	48	34	24	18	14	9
	1	100	100	100	100	100	100	88	64	46	33	24	18	12

proposed series consisted of 20 exposures and so is within the rating of the tube.

Insight

Many modern units are fitted with devices which can measure the amount of heat stored in the anode disk and then calculate whether the proposed exposure is within the rating of the tube. Also, for serial radiography, many units have angiographic rating computers which can work out the heat generated by an exposure series and check if this is within the rating of the tube, taking into account any heat already stored by the anode disk. As microprocessors have ever more applications it may well be the case that the rating chart is simply used by the engineer during the tube installation and will require no further consultation by the radiographer.

Summary

In this chapter you should have learnt:

- The definition of rating when applied to the X-ray tube and its associated equipment (see Sect. 23.2)
- How to interpret and use single exposure rating charts (see Sect. 23.3)
- A comparison of the rating of stationary anode and rotating anode X-ray tubes (see Sect. 23.4)
- The effects of the anode diameter and the speed of rotation on the rating of the rotating anode tube (see Sect. 23.5)
- The use of anode cooling curves in checking rating for multiple exposures (see Sect. 23.6.1)
- The use of anode heating curves to check the rating during fluoroscopy (see Sect. 23.6.2)
- The use of angiographic rating charts in checking that a proposed angiographic series is within the rating of the X-ray tube (see Sect. 23.6.3).

SELF-TEST

a. What is meant by the rating of an X-ray tube?

b. How does the rating of the X-ray tube depend on:
   (i) the focal spot size
   (ii) the kV_p
   (iii) the exposure time
   (iv) the rectification
   (v) the diameter of the anode disk
   (vi) the rate of anode rotation?

c. Why are the curves in a typical rating chart further apart for short exposure times than they are for long exposure times?

d. Under what circumstances can a single exposure which is within the rating of the X-ray tube nevertheless cause thermal damage to the anode? How can the radiographer avoid such damage?

e. Referring to the rating charts below, indicate whether the following single exposures or series of exposures are within the rating of the X-ray tube when used with a constant potential generator:

(i) a single exposure on the 0.6 × 0.6 mm focus of 80 kV$_p$, 200 mA at a time of 0.5 s

(ii) a single exposure on the 1.2 × 1.2 mm focus of 80 kV$_p$, 1250 mA at a time of 0.5 s

(iii) cine-fluoroscopy performed at 100 kV$_p$ and 5 mA for a time of 4 minutes

(iv) an angiographic series of 4 exposures per second for a time of 6 seconds where the exposure factors are 80 kV$_p$, 500 mA and 0.08 s on the 1.2 × 1.2 mm focus (assume that the anode is not storing any significant amount of heat at the start of the exposure series).

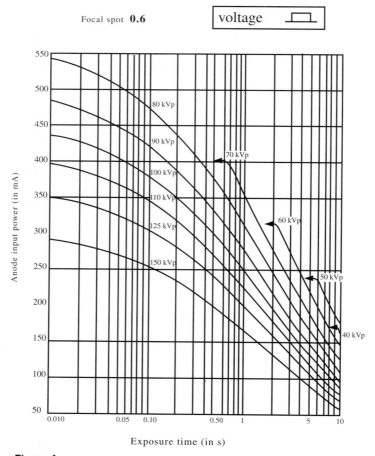

Figure A

Figures A, B and D are reproduced by kind permission of General Electric.

Focal spot **1.2**

voltage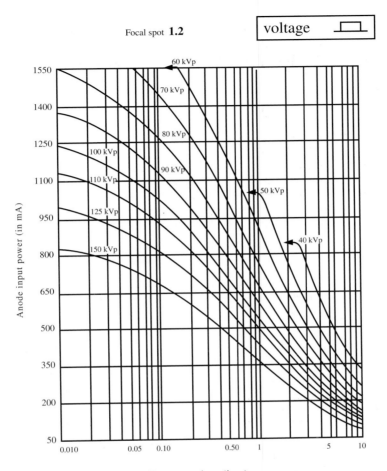

Figure B

Tube load	Exposure rate (exposures/s)	Exposure time for each radiograph in ms											
		3	6	10	20	25	32	40	50	63	80	100	120	160
	12	100	100	100	82	60	42	30	22	16	—	—	—	—
	10	100	100	100	88	64	45	33	24	17	12	—	—	—
	8	100	100	100	97	71	50	36	26	19	13	10	—	—
40 kW	6	100	100	100	100	80	56	41	30	21	15	11	4	—
	4	100	100	100	100	95	67	49	35	25	18	13	10	7
	3	100	100	100	100	100	75	55	40	29	20	15	11	8
	2	100	100	100	100	100	90	66	48	34	24	18	14	9
	1	100	100	100	100	100	100	88	64	46	33	24	18	12

Figure C Angiographic rating chart.

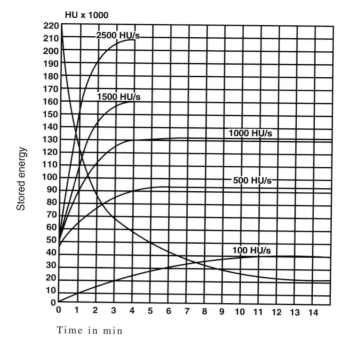

Figure D

FURTHER READING

Carter P H 1994 Chesneys' Equipment for student radiographers. Blackwell Scientific Publications, London, ch 1

Foster E 1985 Equipment for diagnostic radiography. MTP Press, Lancaster, ch 6

Gifford D 1984 A handbook of physics for radiologists and radiographers. John Wiley & Sons, Chichester, ch 22

Hendee W, Ritenour R 1992 Medical imaging physics, 3rd edn. Mosby Year Book, London, ch 5

Johns H E, Cunningham J R 1983 The physics of radiology, 4th edn. Charles C Thomas, Illinois, USA, ch 2

Stockley S M 1986 A manual of radiographic equipment. Churchill Livingstone, Edinburgh, ch 6

PART 4

Atomic physics

PART CONTENTS

24

Laws of modern physics

24.1 AIM

The aim of this chapter is to introduce the reader to the laws of modern physics. In many cases these are refinements or extensions to the laws of classical physics which were discussed in Chapter 5 and reference will be made to the laws outlined in Chapter 5 in this chapter. In other areas there is disagreement between the classical and the modern laws and these will be identified and discussed.

24.2 INTRODUCTION

The laws of classical physics were discussed in Chapter 5 and these have been sufficient to explain the phenomena outlined in previous chapters of this text. However, in the following chapters on atomic and radiation physics, some important aspects of modern physics must be introduced in order to explain many of the phenomena discussed. The purpose of this chapter is to describe the laws of modern physics which are relevant to our need in the rest of the text.

24.3 CLASSICAL VERSUS MODERN LAWS

Modern physics started at the turn of the twentieth century with *Planck's quantum hypothesis* in 1900 in which he conjectured that radiation energy could only be absorbed or emitted by a body at discrete values of energy. Other dates of interest to the rest of this text include the *mass–energy relationship* postulated by Einstein in 1905, the *Bohr model of the atom* which was suggested in 1913 and the *de Broglie wavelength of particles* which was introduced in 1924. Since these dates there have been major technical and theoretical strides, but these form part of the firm experimental foundation upon which modern physics is built.

One of the essential differences between classical and modern physics is the way in which matter is regarded. In classical physics matter and energy are completely separate entities and so we have the *Law of Conservation of Matter* (see Sect. 5.2) and the *Law of Conservation of Energy* (see Sect. 5.3) with no interconnection being produced between the two laws. Also, in classical physics, *matter* is supposed to behave in one way—like matter!—and *waves* are supposed to behave like waves, and one cannot behave like the other; classical physics does not allow for the existence of a particle with a wavelength. However, there are no such rigid boundaries in modern physics. In particular, the work of Einstein showed that matter can be thought of as being interchangeable with energy if the conditions are right. This principle is known as *mass–energy equivalence* and will be discussed in more detail later in this chapter (see Sect. 24.4.1). In addition, it is found in modern physics that particles of matter do behave like waves and vice versa and this is known as the *wave–particle duality principle* (see Sect. 24.6).

With these concepts in mind, we will now consider the laws of modern physics in more detail in the remainder of this chapter.

24.4 LAW OF CONSERVATION OF ENERGY

This law now states that *the amount of energy in a system is constant*. In the context of modern physics this can be thought of as the sum of all the energies (rest energies + kinetic energies + potential energies) being a constant for any given system. The phrase '*a system*' can be used to define either a very small or a very large area, provided the influence of other bodies outside the system is negligibly small. In the context of modern physics, the use of the term *energy* in the above law embraces the contribution of matter to the total energy of a system under consideration. This concept of *mass–energy equivalence* will now be discussed.

24.4.1 Mass–energy equivalence

Einstein showed that the mass of a body, m, and its energy, E (excluding potential energy), are related by the formula:

$$E = mc^2$$

Equation 24.1

where c is the velocity of electromagnetic radiation (often referred to as the velocity of light, as light is probably the best-known form of electromagnetic radiation). Thus the energy of a body is proportional to its mass (and vice versa) since c is a constant. If we consider a stationary body with a rest mass, m_0, then the rest energy of this body is given by $E_0 = m_0c^2$. If we now consider this body travelling with a velocity, V, then its energy is now E_V and Einstein's equation is $E_V = m_Vc^2$. Since the energy of the body when moving, E_V, is greater than the energy of the body when at rest, E_0, and since c is a constant then m_V must be greater than m_0—*a body increases in mass as its velocity increases.* The above statement seems to contradict our common experiences (because of the small values of velocity which we can normally produce) but if we take particles and accelerate them until they travel with a velocity close to the velocity of light (3×10^8 m·s^{-1}) then there is a measurable increase in the mass of the particles. The mass which they then possess is known as the *relativistic mass* of the particles.

The Law of Conservation of Energy stated earlier is sometimes referred to as the Law of Conservation of *Mass–Energy* because of the concept of equivalence between mass and energy. It is also not uncommon to quote the *rest mass* of subatomic particles, either in units of mass or in units of energy—the rest mass of the electron can be stated as 9.1×10^{-31} kg (mass) or 0.511 MeV (energy).

As we can see from the above discussion, energy and mass can be considered as two manifestations of the same thing, and may be changed from one form to the other in appropriate circumstances, as the following examples show:

● The forces which hold the atomic nucleus together are obtained because some of the mass of the nuclear particles is converted into energy. Because of this the mass of the nucleus is less than the sum of the masses of the individual nuclear particles.

● If a gamma ray has an energy greater than 1.02 MeV and passes close to the nucleus of an atom, the ray may spontaneously disappear and create two particles of matter—an electron and a positron. This process is known as *pair production* and will be described in more detail in Chapter 30. The positron created in this interaction will interact with an electron and their mass will be converted into two photons of radiation, each photon having an energy of 0.51 MeV. The positron and the electron will now cease to exist and the radiation is referred to as *annihilation radiation*. This interaction shows that energy can be converted into mass and that mass can be converted into energy.

24.5 THE LAW OF CONSERVATION OF MOMENTUM

This law may be stated as *the total linear momentum in a system is constant.* The word '*system*' is used in the same context as for the Law of Conservation of Energy. As we discussed in the section dealing with the laws of classical physics, the momentum of a body is the product of its mass and its velocity. Thus we can say:

sum of all (mass × velocity) = constant for a system.

Here, the mass referred to in the equation is the relativistic mass of the body, i.e. its mass when it is moving with the velocity, V. An example of the Law of Conservation of Momentum being applied to modern physics is in Compton scattering (see Ch. 30) when some of the momentum of the incoming photon is given to an electron—the combined momentum of the scattered photon and the ejected electron is the same as the momentum of the incident photon.

24.6 WAVE–PARTICLE DUALITY

As we have just seen, modern physics regards mass and energy as being two manifestations of the same phenomenon. Similarly, modern physics blurs the distinction which exists in classical physics between a particle and a wave.

24.6.1 Waves as particles

Classical physics was very successful in explaining many of the phenomena associated with electromagnetic radiation (e.g. diffraction and interference) by assuming that such radiation was made up of waves travelling at the velocity of light, c. In this case $c = v\lambda$, where v is the frequency of vibration of the radiation and λ is its wavelength. However phenomena like the Compton effect and photoelectric absorption (both will be discussed in detail in Ch. 30) are not easy to explain using the wave theory. These effects are explained by considering that sometimes electromagnetic radiation behaves as 'packets' of energy which have an associated momentum. Such a packet of energy is called a *photon* or a *quantum* and the *quantum theory* predicts that:

- the quantum will have an energy, E, given by:

$$E = hv \hspace{4cm} \text{Equation 24.2}$$

where h is a constant known as *Planck's constant* and v is the frequency of vibration of the associated wave. We will frequently use this formula in the chapters which follow on atomic physics!
- the quantum will have a momentum, p, given by:

$$p = \frac{hv}{c}$$
Equation 24.3

Thus, the electromagnetic wave may also behave like a particle, possessing energy and momentum.

24.6.2 Particles as waves

Moving particles of matter, whether these are large or very small, have both kinetic energy and momentum. Are there then occasions when they behave as waves? Perhaps the most dramatic example of particles behaving like waves is in the operation of the electron microscope. Here high-energy electrons are passed through or are scattered by a sample. A very highly magnified image of the sample is obtained so that individual large molecules may be seen in materials. The reason for the high degree of magnification is due to the very small wavelength of the electrons. Whether we consider an optical microscope or an electron microscope, the smaller the wavelength of the radiation used the finer the detail it is possible to see.

De Broglie proposed the following relationship to exist between the momentum, p, of the particle and its associated wavelength, λ:

$$p = \frac{h}{\lambda}$$
Equation 24.4

In such cases λ is called the *de Broglie* wavelength and the existence of particles behaving like waves can be verified by a number of experiments.

Note the *inverse* relationship between the momentum of the particle and its associated wavelength. Thus the wavelength decreases as the momentum increases and vice versa. For example the de Broglie wavelength associated with an electron moving at half the velocity of light is about 4×10^{-12} m which is less than the diameter of the hydrogen atom (100×10^{-12} m). When the velocity of the electron is one-hundredth of that of light then the de Broglie wavelength is at the larger value of 240×10^{-12} m, which is now in the X-ray range of wavelengths (see Ch. 25) and so such electrons can be used for X-ray crystallography.

Within the context of radiographic science, it is more common to consider waves behaving as quanta rather than quanta behaving as waves. This is particularly true when we consider the production of X-rays (see Ch. 28) and the interactions of X-rays with matter (see Ch. 30).

24.7 HEISENBERG'S UNCERTAINTY PRINCIPLE

In classical physics it is possible *in principle* to measure exactly a number of quantities concerning the state of a body, e.g. the body's energy, position and momentum. Furthermore, if it were possible to build measuring apparatus which was infinitely precise, it would be possible to make *simultaneous exact measurements* of several of these quantities.

According to modern physics, it is not possible to treat quantities like mass and energy or matter and waves as being totally independent of each other. *Heisenberg's uncertainty principle* is an extension of the principle of wave–particle duality and concerns the maximum possible precision which may be obtained in ideal circumstances when measuring two quantities simultaneously. The central point of the principle is that *measuring one quantity affects another quantity* so that it is never possible to measure both quantities simultaneously with complete accuracy—if we try to measure the momentum of a particle this will automatically affect the position of the particle so that it is never possible to measure momentum and position *simultaneously* with complete accuracy. Effects due to this principle are too small to be observed in everyday life and concern atomic and nuclear systems. This principle is yet another difference between modern and classical physics—in classical physics it is assumed that perfect instruments produce perfect results.

If we now apply Heisenberg's uncertainty principle to the duality theory we can say that, although we can demonstrate that waves can behave like particles and that particles can behave like waves, it is not possible to set up a situation where both properties are demonstrated *simultaneously*.

Summary

In this chapter you should have learnt:

- The differences which exist between the laws of classical physics and the laws of modern physics (see Sect. 24.3)
- The Law of Conservation of Energy as applied to modern physics (see Sect. 24.4)
- The concept of mass–energy equivalence (see Sect. 24.4.1)
- The Law of Conservation of Momentum as applied to modern physics (see Sect. 24.5)
- The concept of wave–particle duality (see Sect. 24.6)
- The concept that waves may behave as particles and that particles may behave as waves with examples of each situation (see Sects 24.6.1 and 24.6.2)
- A brief outline of Heisenberg's uncertainty principle (see Sect. 24.7).

SELF-TEST

a. Discuss the concept of *mass–energy equivalence* and define the terms:
   (i) rest mass
   (ii) relativistic mass.

b. Discuss the concept of wave–particle duality and identify a situation where a wave behaves as a particle and a situation where a particle behaves as a wave.

c. Outline Heisenberg's uncertainty principle.

FURTHER READING

You may find Chapter 25 of this text and chapters from the following texts provide useful further reading:

Johns H E, Cunningham J R 1983 The physics of radiology, 4th edn. Charles C Thomas, Illinois, USA, ch 1

Ohanian H C 1994 Principles of physics. W W Norton, London, ch 27

Wheeler J, Wojciech Z 1983 Quantum theory and measurement. Princetown University Press, USA

25

Electromagnetic radiation

25.1 AIM

The aim of this chapter is to discuss the properties of electromagnetic radiations. The wave–particle duality of such radiations will be further discussed. Having identified the contents of the electromagnetic spectrum we will finally consider some parts of this spectrum in more detail as these are of particular relevance to radiography.

25.2 INTRODUCTION

As we will see from Figure 25.3, the electromagnetic spectrum encompasses a wide range of radiation types and we are only sensitive to a small section of these radiations. We can see the world around us because the retinae of our eyes are sensitive to a section of the electromagnetic spectrum which we know as *light*. Similarly we can feel heat from the sun because our skin responds to the infra-red part of the electromagnetic spectrum. However, we can accidentally walk through a beam of X-rays or we may handle an isotope which is producing gamma (γ) radiation but we cannot feel the presence of these radiations as none of our sense organs are able to detect them. It is important to remember, when we consider radiation protection, that although our sense organs are not immediately able to detect the presence of ionising radiations (X or γ) they may still be damaged by them.

25.3 PROPERTIES OF ELECTROMAGNETIC RADIATIONS

All electromagnetic radiations exhibit a set of general properties which are listed below:

- The waves are composed of transverse vibrations of electric and magnetic fields.
- The vibrations have a wide range of wavelengths and frequencies.
- All electromagnetic radiations travel through a vacuum with the same velocity—3×10^8 m·s^{-1}.
- All electromagnetic radiations travel in straight lines.
- The radiations are unaffected by electric or magnetic fields.
- The radiations may be polarised so that they vibrate in one plane only.
- The radiations are able to produce constructive or destructive interference.
- All the radiations obey the duality principle (see Sect. 24.6) and so can either be considered as waves or as quanta with energy and momentum.

From the above list it is obvious that all electromagnetic radiations have a lot in common, so how can they be used for such widely differing purposes? The answer to this lies in the differences which they exhibit in their interactions with matter. These are outlined in Table 25.1.

Table 25.1 Interactions of different electromagnetic radiations with matter

Interaction	Notes
Emission	All bodies will emit electromagnetic radiation in certain circumstances but the most efficient emission is from a 'black body' (see Sect. 8.4.4)
Reflection	Reflection of electromagnetic radiation is not possible for the higher-energy radiations (X- and γ-radiation)
Refraction	Refraction of electromagnetic radiation is not possible for the higher-energy radiations (X- and γ-radiation)
Transmission	Different materials are transparent to different wavelengths or photon energies
Attenuation	Different attenuation processes are possible depending on the photon energy of the radiation but, if the photons all have the same energy, the attenuation is always exponential *Photoelectric absorption* can occur from UV to γ-radiations *Compton scattering* is produced by X- and γ-radiations *Pair production* is an absorption process possible if the photon energies are higher than 1.02 MeV
Luminescence —fluorescence and phosphorescence	Electron transitions within the material being irradiated cause the emission of photons which have less energy than the incident radiation. A single photon of incident radiation can produce many fluorescent photons

As discussed in the previous chapter, there is a wave–particle duality which exists when electromagnetic radiation interacts with matter. This will now be discussed further in the following sections.

25.3.1 Wave-like properties of electromagnetic radiation

As the term *electromagnetic* suggests, electromagnetic radiation consists of both *electric* and *magnetic* fields. These fields are at right angles to each other and to the direction of propagation and are shown diagrammatically in Figure 25.1. As shown in E and B of the figure, both the electric and the magnetic vectors (see Sect. 6.3) vibrate *transversely* to the direction of propagation of the wave. In addition, the vectors vary in a sinusoidal manner as shown in the figure. Thus, if we draw the variations of the electric vector (for example), a sine wave results, as shown in Figure 25.2. These periodic variations of the vectors are the reason why electromagnetic radiations are often referred to as *electromagnetic waves* and this was the sole method of explaining the behaviour of such radiations adopted by classical physics (see Sect. 24.6). The same parameters can be used to describe this type of wave formation as can be used for any sinusoidal waves. These are:

- the *cycle*—one complete waveform (this can start from any point on the wave and end at the corresponding point on another wave)

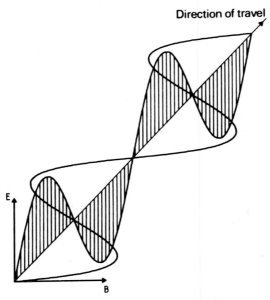

Figure 25.1 Electromagnetic radiation depicted as a wave consisting of alternating electrical and magnetic vectors vibrating at right angles to each other and to the direction of motion of the wave.

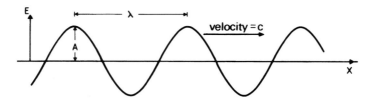

Figure 25.2 An electromagnetic sine wave produced by plotting energy (E) against distance (X). The wave has an amplitude of A and a wavelength λ and travels at the velocity of light, c (3×10^8 m·s^{-1}).

- the *wavelength*—the distance travelled in completing one cycle (λ)
- the *frequency*—the number of cycles per second (Hz)
- the *amplitude*—the magnitude of the peak of the wave above the X axis (A).

If we consider Figure 25.2, it should be apparent that we can calculate the distance travelled by the radiation in 1 second by multiplying the wavelength (λ) by the frequency (v). However, the distance travelled in 1 second is simply the velocity of the radiation (c in a vacuum) and so we have:

$$c = v\lambda \qquad\qquad \text{Equation 25.1}$$

in a vacuum.

As we mentioned earlier, one of the features of electromagnetic radiations is that they all travel with the same velocity (3×10^8 m·s^{-1}) in a vacuum. One ray is distinguished from another by the difference in wavelength and frequency—*blue light* has a wavelength of about 400 nm and a frequency of 7.5×10^{14} Hz while *red light* has a wavelength of about 800 nm and a frequency of 3.75×10^{14} Hz. From this it can be seen that *the greater the frequency, the smaller the wavelength* and vice versa.

In a transparent medium the waves travel at a velocity V given by the equation $c = nV$, where n is a constant for a given medium and a given incident wavelength and is known as the *refractive index*. The frequency of the radiation is unaltered as it passes through a transparent medium but the wavelength is reduced due to the reduction in the velocity of the wave. If the wavelength in the medium is λ', then Equation 25.1 becomes:

$$V = v\lambda'$$

Substituting the value of V for $c = nV$ we obtain:

$$c = nV\lambda' \qquad\qquad \text{Equation 25.2}$$

in a medium of refractive index, n.

> **Insight**
>
> Chapters 12 and 13 showed that it is possible to produce both a magnetic field from moving electrical charges (electromagnetism) and an electric field from a changing magnetic flux (electromagnetic induction). It can be shown mathematically that a changing electric field can sustain a changing magnetic field and vice versa, if they both travel at the velocity of light. This is the basis both for the linear propagation of electromagnetic radiations and for the fact that the wave does not gradually diminish in amplitude with time. Electromagnetic radiation can therefore be described as *a self-sustaining interaction of electric and magnetic fields travelling with the velocity of light.*

Two further properties of electromagnetic radiation which are a consequence of its wave-like nature are *polarisation* and *interference.*

Polarisation

A beam of light, from a bulb for instance, consists of many millions of waves whose electric vectors are pointing in random directions with respect to each other. If this light beam is passed through a polarising lens (similar to the one found in polarising sunglasses), then there is optimum transmission of the waves whose electric vectors are pointing in one direction and complete absorption of those at right angles to this direction (this is the mechanism by which polarising sunglasses limit the glare due to light reflection from water). The emergent light is said to be *plane polarised*—all its vibrations are in the one plane.

Interference

Further evidence of the wave-like properties of electromagnetic radiations comes from the phenomenon of interference where the amplitudes of two coherent beams (beams which are in phase with each other) can be added together. If the peaks of the waves coincide, then we get *constructive interference* and this produces bright areas. If the peak of the wave from one source coincides with the trough of the wave from the other source, then we get *destructive interference* and this produces a dark area. Such interference patterns are used in radiographic science to produce *holograms* but further discussion on this topic is well outside the scope of this text.

25.3.2 Particle-like properties

In Chapter 24 we discussed how consideration of electromagnetic radiations as quanta or photons having energy and momentum, enabled us to explain a number of properties which are not explained by the wave theory. The energy of such a quantum, E, is proportional to the frequency of the associated wave such that:

$$E = h\nu \qquad\qquad \text{Equation 25.3}$$

where h is a constant known as *Planck's constant* and ν is the frequency of vibration of the associated wave. The momentum, p, of the quantum is also proportional to the frequency, and is given by:

$$p = \frac{h\nu}{c} \qquad\qquad \text{Equation 25.4}$$

where c is the velocity of electromagnetic radiation in a vacuum.

The photon energy and its wavelength can now be related. If we take Equation 25.3 and substitute $\nu = c/\lambda$ from Equation 25.1 we get:

$$E = \frac{hc}{\lambda} \qquad\qquad \text{Equation 25.5}$$

In this equation h is Planck's constant (6.62×10^{-34} J·s), c is the velocity of electromagnetic radiation in a vacuum (3×10^8 m·s^{-1}), λ is the wavelength measured in metres and E is the photon energy measured in joule. For practical purposes in radiography it is more convenient to measure the photon energy in keV (1 keV = 1.16×10^{-16} J) and the wavelength in nanometres (1 nm = 10^{-9} m). Because h and c are constants, Equation 25.5 can now be rewritten:

$$E = \frac{1.24}{\lambda} \qquad\qquad \text{Equation 25.6}$$

This equation gives us an easy link between the energy of the photon in keV and the wavelength of the radiation in nanometres.

Example

If the energy of the X-ray photon is 100 keV, what will be its wavelength in nanometres?

Using Equation 25.6:

$$E = \frac{1.24}{\lambda}$$

$$\therefore \lambda = \frac{1.24}{E}$$

$$= \frac{1.24}{100} \text{ nm}$$

$$= 0.0124 \text{ nm}$$

Lengths as small as 0.0124 nm or 1.24×10^{-11} m are difficult to imagine. This is less than the diameter of an atom of body tissue (about 10^{-10} m) but is greater than the diameter of the atomic nucleus (about 10^{-14} m).

25.4 THE ELECTROMAGNETIC SPECTRUM

The previous sections of this chapter have shown that electromagnetic radiation may have a very large range of wavelengths, i.e. a *spectrum* of wavelengths (and frequencies). It is convenient to split up such an electromagnetic spectrum into bands which are broadly categorised by their interaction with matter and hence the use to which the bands of radiation may be put. This is illustrated in Figure 25.3, which also shows the wavelengths, frequencies and energies corresponding to the approximate boundaries between the various bands. As we have previously discussed, the table of the electromagnetic spectrum shows that the smaller the wavelength of the radiation the higher the frequency and the energy.

The common factor which links the interactions between different types of electromagnetic radiations is that *the value of the wavelength determines the size of object with which the radiation will directly interact*. This is illustrated in Table 25.2.

Insight

At the beginning of this chapter (see Table 25.1) are the types of interactions which are possible between electromagnetic radiations and matter with brief comments. From this table you will note that refraction is associated with electromagnetic radiations which have wavelengths larger than X-rays. Refraction is a phenomenon associated with an interaction between a photon and the outer electron orbitals of atoms. It is therefore associated with wavelengths which are able to interact with these electrons—ultra-violet and longer wavelengths. Smaller wavelengths become progressively less affected by the outer electron orbitals and so it is just possible to demonstrate refraction with very large wavelength X-rays but it is not possible to refract X-rays which have shorter wavelengths.

Table 25.2   Common electromagnetic radiations and the type of body with which they will directly interact

Type of radiation	Body with which radiation directly interacts
Radio waves	Transmitted and received by large metallic conductors—aerials
Infra-red radiation	Interacts with whole molecules or atoms giving them an increase in their kinetic energy in the form of heat
Visible light and ultra-violet radiation	Interact with the outer electrons (more loosely bound) of an atom
X-rays and γ-rays	Interact with the inner electron shells or, if they have very high energy, will interact with the tiny nucleus of the atom

Figure 25.3 The electromagnetic spectrum (not drawn to scale). Typical values for wavelengths, frequencies and photon energies for different bands of the spectrum are shown together with some of the methods used for their detection. (*Note:* 1 Hz = 1 cycle per second; 1 pm = 10^{-12} m, etc.)

The interactions between X-rays and matter, which are of great relevance to radiographic science, are discussed in detail in Chapter 30 of this book.

25.5 ELECTROMAGNETIC RADIATIONS AND RADIOGRAPHY

The process of taking a radiograph results in the emission of radiations whose wavelengths and energies are from three different parts of the

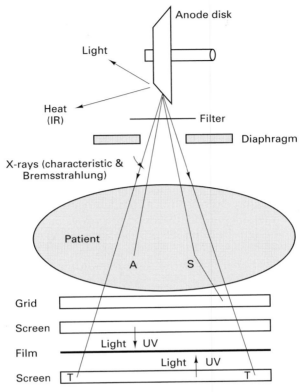

Figure 25.4 The production of radiation from different parts of the electromagnetic spectrum when a radiograph is taken.

electromagnetic spectrum described in the previous section. These are summarised in Figure 25.4.

When the anode is bombarded by electrons it emits both *heat* and *light* as well as X-rays. The X-ray spectrum is composed of a continuous or Bremsstrahlung spectrum upon which is superimposed a characteristic or line spectrum from the tungsten target. The absorption processes within the aluminium filter and the lead collimators also produce characteristic radiation from these elements, although these are of fairly low intensity. When the radiation beam passes through the patient, some of the photons are absorbed (A in the diagram) and some are scattered (S in the diagram). The above processes produce a minute amount of heat and other characteristic radiations from the elements which make up the body tissues. Some of the scattered radiation is absorbed by the grid. When the transmitted X-ray beam (T) strikes the intensifying screens in the cassette, these produce fluorescent radiation in the ultra-violet and visible parts of the spectrum. These radiations are principally responsible for producing the image on the film.

Further examples of electromagnetic radiation relevant to radiography include:

- the emission of light from image intensifiers when bombarded with X-rays
- the emission of light from cathode ray tubes and television monitors when the phosphors are bombarded by electrons
- the emission of light from fluorescent tubes to allow us to view radiographs
- the emission of X-rays and γ-rays from certain radioisotopes which allow imaging or treatment of organs
- the emission of light from sodium iodide crystals (in gamma cameras and CAT scanners) when bombarded with γ-rays or X-rays
- the emission of light from photostimulable plates when scanned using a laser beam
- the use of a laser beam to 'write' information on to the film in a laser imager.

Summary

In this chapter you should have learnt:

- The properties which are common to all electromagnetic radiations (see Sect. 25.3)
- The different ways in which electromagnetic radiations can react with matter (see Sect. 25.3)
- How electromagnetic radiation can be described as having wave-like properties and how these properties can be used to explain polarisation and interference (see Sect. 25.3.1)
- How electromagnetic radiation can be described as having particle-like properties and the equation which links the photon energy and the wavelength of the radiation (see Sect. 25.3.2)
- The various components of the electromagnetic spectrum and the principal interactions of the radiations with matter (see Sect. 25.4)
- The electromagnetic radiations which are of importance to radiography (see Sect. 25.5).

SELF-TEST

a. List the general properties of all electromagnetic radiations.

b. Define the following terms which may be used to describe electromagnetic radiations:
   (i) cycle
   (ii) wavelength
   (iii) frequency
   (iv) amplitude.

c. Give two equations which link the photon energy and the wavelength of electromagnetic radiation. What is the wavelength of the radiation which has a photon energy of 50 keV? What is the photon energy of radiation which has a wavelength of 0.0124 nm?

d. List the main divisions of the electromagnetic spectrum in order of decreasing wavelength.

e. Describe the different types of electromagnetic radiations involved in the production of a radiograph.

f. List five examples other than those used in (e) above to show where electromagnetic radiations are used in radiography.

FURTHER READING

You will find further information on the methods of X-ray production in Chapter 28 and more information on the mechanisms by which X-rays interact with matter in Chapter 30 of this text. In addition you may find chapters of the following texts useful:

Ball J L, Moore A D 1986 Essential physics for radiographers, 2nd edn. Blackwell Scientific Publications, London, ch 14

Curry T S et al 1990 Christensen's Physics of diagnostic radiology. Lea & Febinger, London, ch 1

Gifford D 1984 A handbook of physics for radiologists and radiographers. John Wiley & Sons, Chichester, ch 10

Hay G A, Hughes D 1983 First year physics for radiographers. Baillière Tindall, London, ch 9

Johns H E, Cunningham J R 1983 The physics of radiology, 4th edn. Charles C Thomas, Illinois, USA, ch 1

Ohanian H C 1994 Principles of physics. W W Norton, London, ch 24

Sumner D, Wheldon T, Watson W 1991 Radiation risks: an evaluation. The Tarragon Press, Glasgow, ch 2

Thompson M A 1994 Principles of imaging science and protection. W B Saunders, London, ch 3

26

Elementary structure of the atom

26.1 AIM

The aim of this chapter is to introduce the reader to the elementary structure of an atom. The principal particles which form the nucleus will be identified as also will the factors which determine whether or not the nucleus is stable. The differing electron orbitals and the influence of the electron orbitals on the chemical properties of the material will be discussed. The consequences of transitions of electrons between orbitals will also be identified.

26.2 INTRODUCTION

Any attempt to understand the universe around us must start with the fundamental question *what is matter made of*? The atom as the fundamental building block of matter has therefore been the subject of a great deal of both theoretical debate and experimental study by physicists. Many of the modern theories concerning atomic and subatomic structures are extremely complex and are the subject of a number of textbooks in their own right. However, most of the phenomena which we encounter in radiography can be explained using a relatively simple *planetary model* of the atom. In this model there are solid electrons orbiting a solid nucleus—some phenomena can also be explained using the *quantum physics model* and where this is appropriate this model will be referred to in Insights.

The planetary model of the atom was first described by Rutherford in 1911. It describes an atom consisting of a small positively charged central nucleus around which negatively charged electrons move in defined orbitals. This model can be used to illustrate the carbon atom as shown in Figure 26.1. As we can see from this diagram, the nucleus of this atom consists of *12 elementary particles, 6 protons* and *6 neutrons*. These particles are bound together in a small volume of extremely high density—about three thousand million, million times greater than the density of water. The protons in the nucleus carry a positive charge and the electrons carry an equal negative charge, so this atom is electrically neutral—the neutrons carry no charge. The electrons are arranged in orbitals or shells called *K, L, M* . . . starting from the orbital closest to the nucleus. The *K*-shell can only contain 2 electrons and, in the case of the carbon atom, the *L*-shell contains the remaining 4. Different atoms contain different numbers of protons and neutrons in the nucleus and different numbers of electron configurations as will be discussed later in this chapter. As the particles which make up the atom are very tiny, the atom consists largely of empty space. For example, if an atom were to be enlarged until it was the size of a house, the size of the nucleus would be about the size of a pin-head, although it contains 99.95% of the total mass of the atom.

The masses and charges of the subatomic particles which will be considered in this and later chapters are summarised in Table 26.1.

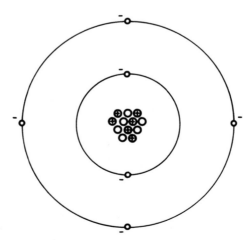

Figure 26.1 The basic structure of a carbon atom. At the centre of the atom is a nucleus which contains 6 protons (positively charged) and 6 neutrons (zero charge)—i.e. the nucleus contains 12 nucleons. 6 electrons (negatively charged) orbit the nucleus in defined orbitals. As the atom contains equal numbers of positive and negative charges the whole atom is electrically neutral.

Table 26.1 Masses and charges of main subatomic particles

Particle	Symbol	Rest mass		Rest energy (MeV)	Charge*	Comments
		(kg)	(amu)†			
Proton	p	1.672×10^{-27}	1.007	938	+1	Nucleons, i.e. present in the atomic nucleus
Neutron	n	1.675×10^{-27}	1.009	939	0	
Alpha particle	α	6.645×10^{-27}	4.003	3725	+2	2 protons and 2 neutrons Ejected in α decay
Electron	e^- or β^-	9.109×10^{-31}	0.00055 or 1/1820	0.511	−1	Form stable discrete orbits around nuclei Ejected from nucleus in β^- decay
Positron	e^+ or β^+	9.109×10^{-31}	0.00055 or 1/1820	0.511	+1	Antiparticle of the electron—produces annihilation radiation when both meet
Pi meson	π^+	2.480×10^{-28}	0.150	139	+1	Keep the nucleus together (π^0 and π^- also exist)
Neutrino	υ	0	0	0	0	Emitted during β-decay and electron capture Very weak attenuation by matter
Photon or quantum	$h\upsilon$	—	—	—	0	Travels at 3×10^8 m·s^{-1} Forms part of the electromagnetic spectrum

* A charge of +1 is $+1.602 \times 10^{-19}$ coulomb.
† 1 *amu* is 1 atomic mass unit which is 1/12 of the mass of a neutral $^{12}_{6}$C atom.

Insight

Rutherford carried out some elegant experimental work connected with the scattering of α-particles by atoms. From this he concluded that the only explanation of the wide scattering angles which he found experimentally was given by assuming that the atom consists of a very heavy positively charged nucleus with orbiting electrons. The alternative model whereby all the subatomic particles were contained in a very small volume was unacceptable because it would produce much smaller scattering angles for the α-particles.

Similar experiments have recently been carried out by physicists to try to establish whether protons and neutrons can be broken into smaller pieces. Unfortunately, if the energy of the projectile is large enough to break up the proton or neutron, then the energy is great enough to create new particles—remember $E = mc^2$—and so it is difficult to tell which are fragments of the proton and which have been created as a result of energy being converted into matter. More subtle experiments use high-energy electrons to bombard the protons and neutrons and measure the angle of deflection of these particles. These angles are again over a wide range suggesting that there are small solid structures within the protons and neutrons. These may be the basic building blocks of the universe; they are known as *quarks* and 18 different types of quark have been identified. Further discussion regarding this search to identify whether there is a smaller structure within the quark is well outside the scope of this text.

26.3 THE ATOMIC NUCLEUS

The number of protons and neutrons in the atomic nucleus determines both the mass and the charge of the nucleus and the configuration of electron orbitals of the atom. There are several important terms, which we will use in this and in ensuing chapters of this text, that require definition at this stage. These terms which will help us to understand atomic structure are defined in Table 26.2.

Table 26.2 Terms used to describe a nucleus

Term	Symbol	Definition
Nucleon		A proton or neutron within a nucleus
Atomic number	Z	The number of protons in the nucleus
Atomic mass number	A	The total number of nucleons in the nucleus
Neutron number	N	The number of neutrons within the nucleus
Nuclide		A nucleus with a specific value of Z and A
Element	E	A nucleus with a given value of Z
Isotope (of an element)		Any nucleus which contains the same number of protons as the given nucleus but has a different mass number
Isobar		Any nucleus which has the same atomic mass number as another nucleus (i.e. has the same value of A)
Radionuclide or radioisotope		Any nuclide or isotope which is radioactive

We can now consider the use of some of the terms in the table. The most common naturally occurring stable *isotope* of carbon has 6 protons and 6 neutrons as shown previously in Figure 26.1. The *atomic number* (Z) of this isotope is therefore 6 and the *atomic mass number* is therefore 12. Thus the whole atom can be written as $^{12}_{6}C$. Thus $^{12}_{6}C$ is an example of a *nuclide*— one which contains 6 protons and 6 neutrons. In general, an element E is written as $^{A}_{Z}E$. An isotope of $^{12}_{6}C$, which is also naturally occurring but less abundant, has 7 neutrons in its nucleus and may be written as $^{13}_{6}C$.

Note that it is not necessarily the case that isotopes of an element are radioactive, as is shown by this example; $^{12}_{6}C$ and $^{13}_{6}C$ are both isotopes of carbon but neither is radioactive.

An isotope of carbon which is radioactive is $^{14}_{6}C$—the well-known *carbon-14*. This again contains the 6 protons which identify it as a carbon nucleus, but this time it contains 8 neutrons. $^{14}_{6}C$ is an example of a *radionuclide* or a *radioactive isotope*. It decays as we shall see in Chapter 27 by beta decay to form $^{14}_{7}N$ (nitrogen) as the *daughter product*.

26.3.1 The stability of the nucleus

At first sight the atomic nucleus would appear to be inherently unstable as the neutrons are uncharged and the protons have a positive charge and so would electrostatically repel each other. This would suggest that the nucleus should fly apart because of the electrostatic forces between the protons.

In practice we find that some nuclei are so stable as to possess no measurable radioactivity ($^{12}_{6}C$ is an example) while others decay with a half-life (see Sect. 4.5) of less than one-millionth of a second. The nucleus must therefore be visualised as a *dynamic* rather than a *static* structure where there are opposing forces acting—forces which tend to hold the nucleus together and forces which tend to disrupt the nucleus. Thus a *stable nucleus* is one where the disruptive forces never win and an *unstable nucleus* is one where they do succeed. This nucleus is said to undergo *radioactive decay*. It is not possible to predict the exact moment when any particular nucleus will decay, as it is a matter of probability rather than certainty. However, if there are a large number of unstable nuclei in a sample, the *law of radioactive decay* (see Sect. 4.3) is obeyed.

The forces which hold the nucleus together are quite unlike the other forces—e.g. gravity—with which we are familiar. They are known as *short-range nuclear forces* and act over distances of about 10^{-15} metres, over which range they are much more powerful than the electrostatic forces between the protons. These forces are shown diagrammatically in Figure 26.2. A strong force of attraction is evident below 10^{-15} m and this changes to a force of repulsion at about 10^{-16} m. The energy expended in keeping the nucleus together is known as the *nuclear binding energy* (*NBE*). If the NBE is divided by the number of nucleons within the nucleus, then a figure of about 8.4 MeV is obtained for most nuclei. This is known as *the binding energy per nucleon*. The binding energy between the nucleons is provided by the transformation of some of the nuclear mass into energy as given by

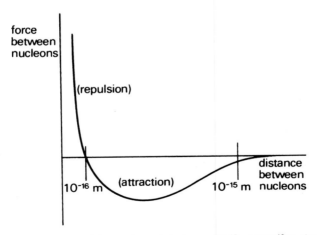

Figure 26.2   If the separation of the nucleons is between 10^{-15} and 10^{-16} m, then a force of attraction exists between the nucleons which helps to hold the nucleus together. If the separation is greater or less than this distance, then the force is a repulsive force.

Einstein's equation $E = mc^2$. Each nucleon has a mass of approximately 931 MeV per atomic mass unit (amu), of which about 8.4 MeV is used for its nuclear binding energy to nearby nucleons. Because of this, the mass of the nucleus is always less than the sum of the masses of the nucleons.

By consideration of the graph in Chapter 27 (Fig. 27.1) it can be seen that, for low atomic numbers, equal numbers of protons and neutrons produce the greatest stability. This leads to the concept of *nuclear shells* which suggests that there is a layering within the nucleus, with maximum stability being produced when a shell is complete. Further discussion of this concept is beyond the scope of this text.

Insight

The π-meson is a particle with a mass between that of an electron and a nucleon and is thought to be responsible for the forces holding the nucleus together. The short-range forces are known as *exchange forces* and result in (for example) an adjacent proton and a neutron changing continually into a neutron and a proton and back again. This interchange may be written as:

$$p_1 + n_1 \rightarrow n_2 + \pi^+ + n_1 \rightarrow n_2 + p_2$$

The π^+-meson has left the original proton p_1, leaving it as a neutron n_2, and then forms a proton p_2 by combining with the original neutron n_1. The proton and the neutron are continuously exchanging their positions. Negative and neutral π-mesons also exist and are exchanged between nucleons.

26.4 ELECTRON ORBITALS

Consider an atom of hydrogen as depicted in Figure 26.3. It is assumed in the planetary model of the atom that the solitary electron is on a circular

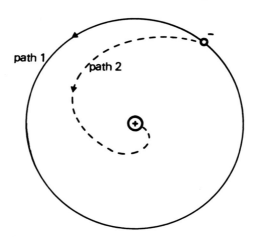

Figure 26.3 A stable, discrete electron orbital (path 1) compared to a 'decaying electron' (path 2) as predicted by the laws of classical physics.

path (path 1) around the nucleus. It may be shown that a body moving in a circle of radius r at a velocity V has an acceleration of V^2/r towards the centre of the circle. According to classical physics, such acceleration would result in the emission of electromagnetic radiation from the electron so that the electron is continuously losing energy and would eventually collide with the nucleus (see path 2). Electrons do not behave in this manner, or atoms as we know them would not exist. The electrons orbit in stable paths (path 1)—*discrete electron orbitals*. Further, these orbitals are grouped in 'shells' where there is a particular number of electrons of approximately the same energy in each orbital. (An explanation of the apparent contradiction of the predictions of classical physics (path 2 and path 1) is given in the Insight below.) The electrons fill up the inner shells first since the energies of the inner shells are less than the outer shells.

Insight

The wave–particle duality of matter (see Sect. 24.6) may be used to explain the existence of discrete electron orbitals. Here it is assumed that an orbiting electron has a de Broglie wavelength which is able to fit around the circumference of an orbital an exact number of times (see Fig. 26.4). This fixes the size of each orbital. The condition necessary for this to occur is that $n\lambda = 2\pi r$ where n is a whole number and r is the mean radius of the orbital. Now λ is the de Broglie wavelength of the electron with momentum p and is given by $\lambda = h/p$.

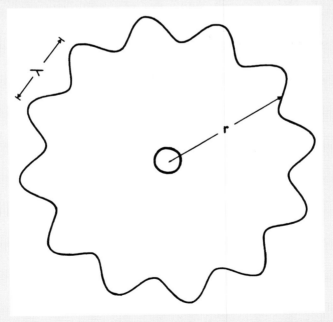

Figure 26.4 The use of the de Broglie wave concept to explain why electrons exist in discrete orbitals.

Thus we can say:

$$\frac{nh}{p} = 2\pi r \quad \text{or} \quad pr = \frac{nh}{2\pi}$$

But pr is the angular momentum of the electron and this must be a multiple of $h/2\pi$. There is now no question of electromagnetic radiation occurring from an orbital electron. This is an example of a situation where modern physics can be used to describe atomic phenomena which are not explicable by classical physics.

Table 26.3   Numbers of electrons in atomic shells

Principal quantum number or shell number (n)	Shell letter	Maximum number of electrons	$2n^2$
1	K	2	2
2	L	8	8
3	M	18	18
4	N	32	32

Table 26.3 shows the maximum number of electrons in each shell from the inner K-shell to the N-shell.

The shell number, n, starts from $n = 1$ for the K-shell and is known as the *principal quantum number*. The chemical properties of an element are controlled by the electron configuration of its atoms. Atoms with filled outer electron shells are chemically inert—neon ($^{20}_{10}\text{Ne}$) has full K- and L-shells as illustrated in Figure 26.5 and so is an inert gas. Fluorine, where the K-shell contains 2 electrons and the L-shell contains 7, is a chemically

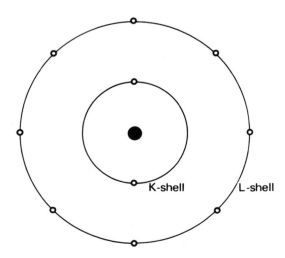

Figure 26.5   An atom of neon showing both K- and L-shells containing their maximum number of permitted electrons. This means that the neon atom is chemically inert.

active *electron acceptor* (the electron fills the vacancy in the *L*-shell) and sodium, where the *K*-shell contains 2 electrons, the *L*-shell contains 8 electrons and the *M*-shell contains 1, is a chemically active *electron donor* (the electron in the *M*-shell is donated, resulting in a filled *L*-shell).

The outer electron shells may contain sub-shells within them. Argon ($Z = 18$) has 2 electrons in its *K*-shell, 8 electrons in its *L*-shell and 8 electrons in the *M*-shell. The *M*-shell has a maximum complement of electrons of 18 and yet argon is chemically inert. An outer sub-shell of 8 electrons is particularly chemically stable, a fact confirmed by the next inert gas, krypton, which has an electron configuration of 2, 8, 18, 8.

26.5 THE PERIODIC TABLE OF ELEMENTS

If the elements are arranged in order of increasing atomic number, it may be shown that their chemical properties—such as valency—and their physical properties—such as specific heat capacity—tend to occur in a periodic manner. Arranging the chemicals in these similar groups produces a *periodic table* as shown in Table 26.4. The chemical similarities of elements in each group may be explained by reference to their electron structure as shown in Table 26.5. It has already been noted that the number of electrons increases with the atomic number and that each electron takes an orbital of the lowest possible energy. This means that inner shells are filled to stable or sub-stable levels before the outer shells accommodate electrons.

There are two rules which determine the way in which electron shells are gradually built up as the atomic number increases:

- An electron shell, n, cannot contain more than $2n^2$ electrons where n is the shell number.
- The outer shell cannot contain more than 8 electrons.

These rules are known as the *Bury–Bohr Rules* after their co-discoverers and ensure that the orbital of minimum energy is filled first.

One additional constraint is required in order that electrons may fill orbitals in the correct manner. This is known as the *Pauli Exclusion Principle* and states that *no two electrons may have precisely the same orbital*.

The two *K*-shell electrons of an atom, for example, are not at precisely the same energy because they orbit the nucleus in opposite directions and hence have slightly different orbitals. These two electrons complete the *K*-shell so that further electrons must start to fill up the *L*-shell (see 'Lithium' in Table 26.5) at a greater distance from the nucleus and so at a higher energy. These *L*-shell electrons all have slightly different energies from each other and the shell is complete when it contains 8 electrons—neon satisfies these conditions where $n = 2$ and so $2n^2 = 8$.

The *K*- and *L*-shells are thus completed in sequence but the *M*-shell (which from the $2n^2$ formula can contain up to 18 electrons), when it

Table 26.4 The periodic table of elements (The atomic mass, 1 amu, equals 1/12th of a neutral $^{12}_{6}C$ atom and the most abundant isotope.)

Group period	0	I	II	III	IV	V	VI	VII	VIII		
1		1.008 H 1									
2	4.003 He 2	6.923 Li 3	9.012 Be 4	10.811 B 5	12.000 C 6	14.003 N 7	15.995 O 8	18.998 F 9			
3	19.992 Ne 10	22.989 Na 11	24.312 Mg 12	26.982 Al 13	27.977 Si 14	30.974 P 15	31.972 S 16	35.453 Cl 17			
4	39.984 Ar 18	39.102 K 19	39.963 Ca 20	44.956 Sc 21	47.948 Ti 22	50.944 V 23	51.944 Cr 24	54.938 Mn 25	55.935 Fe 26	58.933 Co 27	58.71 Ni 28
		63.54 Cu 29	65.37 Zn 30	69.72 Ga 31	72.59 Ge 32	74.922 As 33	78.96 Se 34	79.909 Br 35			
5	83.80 Kr 36	85.47 Rb 37	87.906 Sr 38	88.905 Y 39	91.22 Zr 40	92.906 Nb 41	95.94 Mo 42	(98) Tc 43	101.07 Ru 44	102.91 Rh 45	106.42 Pd 46
		107.87 Ag 47	112.40 Cd 48	114.9 In 49	118.69 Sn 50	121.75 Sb 51	127.60 Te 52	126.90 I 53			
6	131.3 Xe 54	132.905 Cs 55	137.34 Ba 56	**Rare earths** 57–71	178.49 Hf 72	180.9 Ta 73	183.85 W 74	186.2 Re 75	190.2 Os 76	192.2 Ir 77	195.09 Pt 78
		196.97 Au 79	200.59 Hg 80	204.37 Tl 81	207.19 Pb 82	208.98 Bi 83	(209) Po 84	(210) At 85			
7	(222) Rn 86	(223) Fr 87	(226) Ra 88	**Actinides** 89–103	(261) Rf 104	(262) Ha 105					

reaches 8 electrons (argon), then obeys the rule that the outer shell cannot contain more than 8 electrons and so the ninth electron is placed in the *N*-shell (see 'Potassium' in Table 26.5). This process is repeated each time there are 8 electrons in the outer orbital (see 'Rubidium', 'Caesium', 'Francium' etc.).

As mentioned above, the number of electrons in the outer orbital of the atom determines the chemical reactivity of an element. The ability of one atom to join another atom is called *valency* and the electron linkage between them is called a *valency bond*. There are two basic types of valency bond:

Table 26.5 Electron configuration of elements

Element	Symbol	Atomic number	Numbers of electrons in shells						
			K	L	M	N	O	P	Q
Hydrogen	H	1	1						
Helium	He	2	2						
Lithium	Li	3	2	1					
Beryllium	Be	4	2	2					
Boron	B	5	2	3					
Carbon	C	6	2	4					
Nitrogen	N	7	2	5					
Oxygen	O	8	2	6					
Fluorine	F	9	2	7					
Neon	Ne	10	2	8					
Sodium	Na	11	2	8	1				
Magnesium	Mg	12	2	8	2				
Aluminium	Al	13	2	8	3				
Silicon	Si	14	2	8	4				
Phosphorus	P	15	2	8	5				
Sulphur	S	16	2	8	6				
Chlorine	Cl	17	2	8	7				
Argon	Ar	18	2	8	8				
Potassium	K	19	2	8	8	1			
Calcium	Ca	20	2	8	8	2			
Scandium	Sc	21	2	8	9	2			
Titanium	Ti	22	2	8	10	2			
Vanadium	V	23	2	8	11	2			
Chromium	Cr	24	2	8	13	1			
Manganese	Mn	25	2	8	13	2			
Iron	Fe	26	2	8	14	2			
Cobalt	Co	27	2	8	15	2			
Nickel	Ni	28	2	8	16	2			
Copper	Cu	29	2	8	18	1			
Zinc	Zn	30	2	8	18	2			
Gallium	Ga	31	2	8	18	3			
Germanium	Ge	32	2	8	18	4			
Arsenic	As	33	2	8	18	5			
Selenium	Se	34	2	8	18	6			
Bromine	Br	35	2	8	18	7			
Krypton	Kr	36	2	8	18	8			
Rubidium	Rb	37	2	8	18	8	1		
Strontium	Sr	38	2	8	18	8	2		
Yttrium	Y	39	2	8	18	9	2		
Zirconium	Zr	40	2	8	18	10	2		
Niobium	Nb	41	2	8	18	12	1		
Molybdenum	Mo	42	2	8	18	13	1		
Technetium	Tc	43	2	8	18	14	1		
Ruthenium	Ru	44	2	8	18	15	1		
Rhodium	Rh	45	2	8	18	16	1		
Palladium	Pd	46	2	8	18	18			
Silver	Ag	47	2	8	18	18	1		
Cadmium	Cd	48	2	8	18	18	2		
Indium	In	49	2	8	18	18	3		
Tin	Sn	50	2	8	18	18	4		
Antimony	Sb	51	2	8	18	18	5		
Tellurium	Te	52	2	8	18	18	6		
Iodine	I	53	2	8	18	18	7		
Xenon	Xe	54	2	8	18	18	8		

Table 26.5 (*contd*)

Element	Symbol	Atomic number	K	L	M	N	O	P	Q
Caesium	Cs	55	2	8	18	18	8	1	
Barium	Ba	56	2	8	18	18	8	2	
Lanthanum	La	57	2	8	18	18	9	2	
Cerium	Ce	58	2	8	18	20	8	2	
Praseodymium	Pr	59	2	8	18	21	8	2	
Neodymium	Nd	60	2	8	18	22	8	2	
Promethium	Pm	61	2	8	18	23	8	2	
Samarium	Sm	62	2	8	18	24	8	2	
Europium	Eu	63	2	8	18	25	8	2	
Gadolinium	Gd	64	2	8	18	25	9	2	
Terbium	Tb	65	2	8	18	26	9	2	
Dysprosium	Dy	66	2	8	18	28	8	2	
Holmium	Ho	67	2	8	18	29	8	2	
Erbium	Er	68	2	8	18	30	8	2	
Thulium	Tm	69	2	8	18	31	8	2	
Ytterbium	Yb	70	2	8	18	32	8	2	
Lutetium	Lu	71	2	8	18	32	9	2	
Hafnium	Hf	72	2	8	18	32	10	2	
Tantalum	Ta	73	2	8	18	32	11	2	
Tungsten	W	74	2	8	18	32	12	2	
Rhenium	Re	75	2	8	18	32	13	2	
Osmium	Os	76	2	8	18	32	14	2	
Iridium	Ir	77	2	8	18	32	15	2	
Platinum	Pt	78	2	8	18	32	17	1	
Gold	Au	79	2	8	18	32	18	1	
Mercury	Hg	80	2	8	18	32	18	2	
Thallium	Tl	81	2	8	18	32	18	3	
Lead	Pb	82	2	8	18	32	18	4	
Bismuth	Bi	83	2	8	18	32	18	5	
Polonium	Po	84	2	8	18	32	18	6	
Astatine	At	85	2	8	18	32	18	7	
Radon	Rn	86	2	8	18	32	18	8	
Francium	Fr	87	2	8	18	32	18	8	1
Radium	Ra	88	2	8	18	32	18	8	2
Actinium	Ac	89	2	8	18	32	18	9	2
Thorium	Th	90	2	8	18	32	18	10	2
Protactinium	Pa	91	2	8	18	32	20	9	2
Uranium	U	92	2	8	18	32	21	9	2
Neptunium	Np	93	2	8	18	32	23	8	2
Plutonium	Pu	94	2	8	18	32	24	8	2
Americium	Am	95	2	8	18	32	25	8	2
Curium	Cm	96	2	8	18	32	25	9	2
Berkelium	Bk	97	2	8	18	32	27	8	2
Californium	Cf	98	2	8	18	32	28	8	2
Einsteinium	Es	99	2	8	18	32	29	8	2
Fermium	Fm	100	2	8	18	32	30	8	2
Mendelevium	Md	101	2	8	18	32	31	8	2
Nobelium	No	102	2	8	18	32	32	8	2
Lawrencium	Lw	103	2	8	18	32	32	9	2
Rutherfordium	Rf	104	2	8	18	32	32	10	2
Hahnium	Ha	105	2	8	18	32	32	11	2

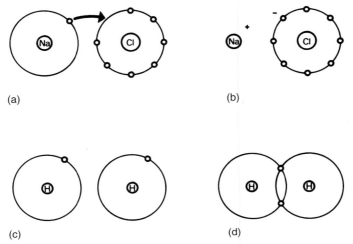

Figure 26.6 An ionic valency bond (or electron valency) is caused by the transfer of an electron from one atom to another—Na to Cl in (a) and (b). A covalent bond (covalency) is formed when two atoms share electrons in the same orbital as shown between two hydrogen atoms in (c) and (d).

- *Ionic bonds*—see Figure 26.6(a) and (b). This type of bond is caused when one or more electrons is transferred from one atom to another thus forming charged atoms (*ions*) which are attracted to one another by electrostatic attraction thus forming the bond. After the electron exchange the shells of each ion appear to be closed.
- *Covalent bonds*—see Figure 26.6(c) and (d). These bonds are formed by the apparent sharing of electrons such that each atom appears to increase its number of electrons thus forming an apparently closed shell.

26.6 ELECTRON ORBITAL CHANGES

The previous sections of this chapter have shown that electrons may only take up fixed or discrete orbitals around an atomic nucleus. We have also discussed the fact that the inner orbitals are filled before the outer orbitals, since this constitutes the lowest energy state of the whole atom. An atom in this state is said to be in its *ground state*, since it cannot have an electron configuration which will produce a lower energy. However, this is not to say that any particular atom at a given moment of time will be at its ground state, since interatomic collisions or interactions with electromagnetic radiations may have raised the energy of one of its electrons so that it is able to take up an orbital of higher energy—the electron will move further away from the nucleus. This process is called *excitation* of the atom. The excited electron is able to return to its original orbital and releases a quantum of electromagnetic radiation in the process. The energy of this quantum is equal to the energy difference between the excited state and the ground state. Alternatively, an orbiting electron may receive sufficient energy to be able to completely escape from the atom—this might happen as result of the interaction of a photon with the electron. This process is called *ionisation* since the remaining atom will now form a positive ion. Both processes are shown diagrammatically in Figure 26.7.

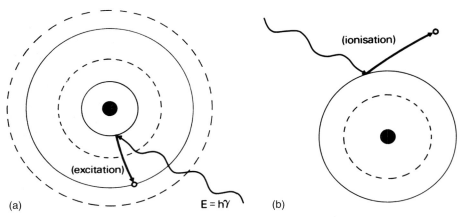

Figure 26.7   An incoming photon interacts with an orbiting electron of an atom. In (a) this photon has sufficient energy to cause excitation and in (b) the photon causes ionisation.

26.7 BINDING ENERGY OF THE ELECTRON SHELLS

Because the various electron shells are positioned at different distances from the atomic nucleus, they experience different forces of attraction from the nucleus. The K-shell is closest to the nucleus and so experiences the greatest force of attraction from the nucleus. It is therefore most difficult to remove an electron from the K-shell—the K-shell has the highest *electron binding energy*. The electron binding energy of a shell is the amount of work which must be done to remove an electron from that shell (it is normally stated in KeV or eV). The L-shell is further away from the nucleus and so experiences less force of attraction. It also experiences some repulsion from the electrons in the K-shell. For this reason the binding energy of the electrons in the L-shell is less than the binding energy of the K-shell for a particular atom. Thus we can say that there is a reduction in the binding energy as we move from the K-shell to the L-shell to the M-shell etc., within a particular atom.

  The reason for the existence of the binding energy is the electrostatic attraction between the nucleus and the electrons in the shells. Thus we would expect to find an increase in the K-shell binding energy with an increase in the atomic number of the element. This is found to be the case in practice.

A knowledge of the binding energy of the various electron shells in different elements is important in radiation physics for the following reasons:

- A knowledge of the binding energies of the different shells allows us to predict the energies of the characteristic radiations which the atom might produce (see Ch. 28 for further details).
- A knowledge of the binding energies of different electron shells within an atom of an element will allow us to determine the likely position of absorption edges during photoelectric absorption (see Ch. 30 for further details).
- If we know the energy of the characteristic radiation from an element and we know the position of absorption edges when radiation is attenuated by this material, then this allows us to explain why elements are relatively transparent to their own characteristic radiation (see Ch. 30 for further details).

Summary

In this chapter you should have learnt:

- The main subatomic particle which can be joined together to produce matter (see Sect. 26.2)
- A basic planetary model of the atom which consists of a nucleus containing protons and neutrons and has electrons in specific orbitals around this nucleus (see Sect. 26.2)
- The basic structure of the atomic nucleus and the reasons for its stability or otherwise (see Sects 26.3 and 26.3.1)
- The configuration of electron orbitals for differing atoms and the factors which determine the maximum number of electrons in an orbital (see Sects 26.4 and 26.5)
- The basic structure of the periodic table of elements and the electron configuration of elements (see Sect. 26.5)
- The meaning of the term *ground state* when applied to an atom and the consequences of raising the energy of the electrons above the ground state (see Sect. 26.6)
- An explanation of the term *binding energy* and a brief outline of areas where a knowledge of the binding energy of electron shells is of importance in radiation physics (see Sect. 26.7).

SELF-TEST

a. With the aid of a diagram, describe the $^{14}_{7}N$ atom.

b. Explain the meaning of the following:
   (i) a nuclide
   (ii) a radionuclide
   (iii) an isotope
   (iv) an isobar

(v) atomic number

(vi) atomic mass number.

c. What is meant by the following terms:
   (i) discrete electron orbital
   (ii) electron shell
   (iii) electron binding energy?

d. List the Bury–Bohr Rules for electron configuration and hence describe the electron configuration of potassium which has an atomic number of 19.

e. Explain what the electron configurations are in the following situations:
   (i) ionic bonds
   (ii) covalent bonds.

f. What is meant by the terms *excitation* and *ionisation* when used to describe changes in electron energy within an atom?

FURTHER READING

Ball J L, Moore A D 1986 Essential physics for radiographers, 2nd edn. Blackwell Scientific Publications, London, ch 4

Curry T S et al 1990 Christensen's Physics of diagnostic radiology. Lea & Febinger, London, part of ch 2

Gifford D 1984 A handbook of physics for radiologists and radiographers. John Wiley & Sons, Chichester, ch 8

Hay G A, Hughes D 1983 First year physics for radiographers. Baillière Tindall, London, ch 2

Hendee W, Ritenour R 1992 Medical imaging physics, 3rd edn. Mosby Year Book, London, ch 2

Johns H E, Cunningham J R 1983 The physics of radiology, 4th edn. Charles C Thomas, Illinois, USA, ch 1

Ohanian H C 1994 Principles of physics. W W Norton, London, ch 29

Sanderson R T 1960 Chemical periodicity. Reinhold Publishing, New York

Sumner D, Wheldon T, Watson W 1991 Radiation risks: an evaluation. The Tarragon Press, Glasgow, ch 2

Thompson M A 1994 Principles of imaging science and protection. W B Saunders, London, ch 3

27

Radioactivity

27.1 AIM

The aim of this chapter is to discuss the various types of radioactive decay which can occur. Within the chapter the relevance of these processes to nuclear medicine will be considered along with a list of clinically useful radionuclides.

27.2 INTRODUCTION

Radioactive decay has already been considered as an example of exponential decay in Chapter 4 where we also looked at concepts like half-life and decay constant (if the memory of these concepts is getting dim please refer to the appropriate section(s) of Ch. 4).

In Chapter 26 we also referred to various terms which may be used to define nuclear structure. This chapter will now look at the changes which may take place in the nucleus during radioactive decay and we will also look at the production of artificial radionuclides.

The term *radioactive* is applied to nuclei which are unstable. In these nuclei the forces disrupting the nucleus are stronger than the forces which hold the nucleus together. The instability of the nucleus is demonstrated by the fact that it changes its internal structure to a more stable form, often (but not always) ejecting a charged particle from the nucleus in the process. Each time a nucleus changes its structure it is called a *radioactive disintegration* or a *nuclear transformation* and may result in a change in the atomic number (and therefore element) or a change in the mass number or a change of both the atomic number and the mass number.

A pictorial representation of the decay process (see Fig. 27.2) is called a *decay scheme*. In addition to this, it is possible for a nucleus to undergo more than one type of transformation (see Fig. 27.12) and this type of decay is called a *branching scheme*.

It is impossible to determine the exact time when a particular nucleus will transform, but the laws of probability may be used to determine the behaviour of a large number of nuclei (see Sect. 4.3 for a discussion of radioactive decay and the Exponential Law).

The unit of radioactivity is the *becquerel* (Bq) where 1 becquerel is 1 nuclear disintegration per second.

Insight

Before the introduction of SI units, radioactivity was measured in curie (Ci). 1 curie was equal to 3.7×10^{10} nuclear disintegrations per second. Thus an activity of 1 Ci is the same as an activity of 3.7×10^{10} Bq or 37 GBq. From this it can be seen that the curie was a much larger unit than the becquerel.

It is often useful to know the specific activity of a sample. This is the activity of radionuclide per unit mass of the sample and so is measured in Bq kg^{-1} or sub-multiples thereof.

27.3 NUCLIDE CHART

It is often useful to draw a graph, plotting the number of neutrons in a nucleus against the number of protons, as all nuclides may be included in this *nuclide chart*. Such a chart is shown in simplified form in Figure 27.1. Note that isotopes (lines of equal atomic number) are given by any vertical

Figure 27.1 A graph of the neutron number (*N*) plotted against the atomic number (*Z*) showing the position of the stable nuclides as a shaded band. *Note* that as the atomic number increases a higher proportion of neutrons to protons is required to achieve stability. Also shown are the directions which a nucleus takes for various forms of radioactive decay (these movements are not to scale).

line on the figure. In such a graph, an angle of 45° to the X-axis represents a situation where the nucleus contains equal numbers of protons and neutrons ($Z = N$).

It is found on such a graph that there is a broad band of nuclides with low atomic numbers at about 45° to the X-axis and these are all stable or only weakly radioactive. Thus for the lighter elements, nuclear stability can be produced with equal numbers of protons and neutrons. From the graph it can be seen that as the atomic number increases, a proportionately larger number of neutrons is necessary to produce nuclear stability. Thus we can say that as the Coulomb repulsion (see Sect. 9.4) between the protons increases, then more neutrons are required to produce the short-range nuclear forces (see Sect. 26.3.1), thus producing the cohesive forces required for a stable nucleus. Nuclei which have atomic numbers greater

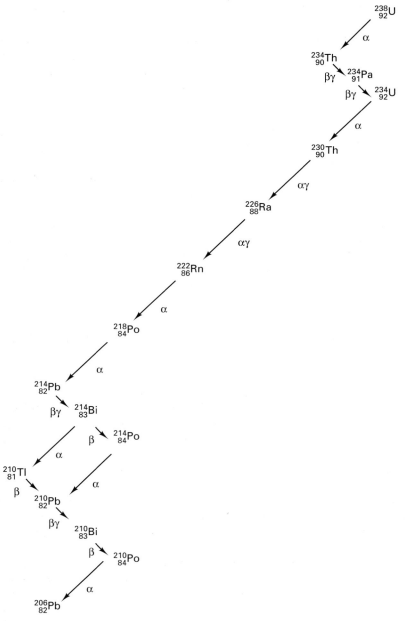

Figure 27.2 The uranium decay series. *Note* that arrows to the right indicate an increase in the atomic number while arrows to the left indicate a decrease. The downward direction of the arrows indicates that the nucleus loses energy with each transformation (downward direction not drawn to scale).

than 83 (bismuth) are so large that it is impossible to produce a stable nuclear configuration.

Nuclides whose combination of neutrons and protons means that they land outside the band of stability shown in Figure 27.1 have nuclei possessing higher energies than those within the band. As a consequence such a nucleus is unstable and tends, on decay, to produce a new nucleus of lower energy which is closer to or within the stable band. The energy difference between the nucleus before and after decay is emitted either as a charged particle or as a quantum (or quanta) of electromagnetic radiation. The decay scheme towards stability may be in the form of a single step (e.g. $^{14}_{6}C$ decays to stable $^{14}_{7}N$ by the emission of a beta particle—see Fig. 27.4) or it may be in the form of a very circuitous route involving many nuclear transformations (e.g. the decay of $^{238}_{92}U$ to $^{206}_{82}Pb$ involves at least 14 steps—see Fig. 27.2). As a general rule, the greater the mass number of the nuclide, the more complicated the decay path to eventual stability.

The effect of different decay modes is illustrated using arrows on Figure 27.1. The direction of the arrow shows the direction of change of position on the chart before and after the decay process. You may find it helpful to refer back to this chart while studying the decay processes in more detail in the following sections of this chapter.

27.4 ALPHA DECAY OR ALPHA PARTICLE EMISSION

For the spontaneous emission of an alpha (α) particle from a nucleus, the nuclide must have an atomic mass number greater than 150. The nucleus must also have *too few neutrons for the number of protons*—a higher neutron : proton ratio would be required to produce nuclear stability. The alpha particle consists of two protons and two neutrons tightly bound together (a helium nucleus). It may be considered as a free particle having high kinetic energy, which is trapped in the nucleus. Thus the daughter nucleus has two protons and two neutrons fewer than the parent nucleus (see Equation 27.1).

The mechanism of production of the α-particle is quite complex. As we have already identified (see Sect. 26.3.1), the nucleus depends on a balance of disruptive electrostatic (Coulomb) forces and attractive forces between the nucleons caused by the short-range nuclear forces. In very large nuclei there is a large amount of electrostatic repulsion between the protons which extends across the whole nucleus. This is balanced by the short-range nuclear force which exists between adjacent nucleons. Thus, if the nucleus becomes elongated, the electrostatic forces dominate and the nucleus becomes even more elongated. This process continues until the nucleus divides into two fragments, the daughter nuclide and the α-particle.

An example of α-decay is the decay of bismuth-212 to thallium-208 with the emission of α-particles. This process is shown in the equation below:

$$^{212}_{83}\text{Bi} \longrightarrow {}^{208}_{81}\text{Tl} + {}^{4}_{2}\alpha \qquad\qquad\text{Equation 27.1}$$

Note that there is a reduction of 4 in the atomic mass number and 2 in the atomic number between parent and daughter product.

This reaction can also be written as shown in Figure 27.3 (the decay of $^{212}_{83}\text{Bi}$ also includes the emission of a β-particle and is discussed later as an example of a branching programme; for simplicity only the α-particle reaction is shown in Figure 27.3 and the percentages shown refer only to the α-particles). Because the daughter product is to the left of the parent nuclide this shows that there is a reduction in the atomic number. The reaction also shows that the difference in energy between the parent nuclide and the daughter nuclide is 6.08 MeV. If we consider only the α-particles emitted we find that approximately 71% of these have an energy of 6.04 MeV and 29% have an energy of 6.08 MeV. In the case of the first group of α-particles, the nucleus is left in an excited state with excess energy of 0.04 MeV which it emits as a γ-ray.

The ejection of an α-particle means that, to preserve momentum, the nucleus must also recoil with an equal and opposite momentum to that of the α-particle. The energy of the recoiling nucleus is typically about 2% of

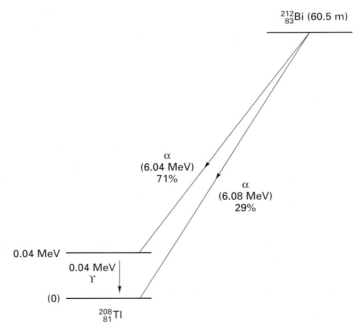

Figure 27.3 An example of alpha particle emission. The nucleus decreases its atomic number and energy as shown.

that of the emitted α-particle. (Recoil also exists for β-decay but is much smaller due to the tiny mass of the β-particle.)

α-particles are intensely ionising but have a very short range in tissue so have little practical application in radiology.

27.5 BETA DECAY OR BETA PARTICLE EMISSION

In the process of beta decay a particle, having a mass equal to that of an electron, is ejected from the nucleus. The ejected particles, however, may have either a positive or negative charge and so, although they are known collectively as beta particles (β-particles), negative beta particles (β⁻) or *negatrons* and positive beta particles (β⁺) or *positrons* both exist. Although the negatron is exactly the same as an electron, in this and subsequent chapters, the term *negatron* will be used to describe the particle which exits from the nucleus of an atom while the term *electron* will be used to describe particles which orbit the nucleus of the atom. Because the processes are different for the production of the negatron and the positron they will be dealt with under separate headings.

27.5.1 Negatron (β⁻) emission

As we can see from Figure 27.1, β⁻-particles are emitted from nuclei which have too many neutrons for nuclear stability. As we saw in Chapter 26, nucleons are being constantly changed from proton to neutron and back within the atomic nucleus. A neutron may be thought of as consisting of a proton and a negatron:

$$n \longrightarrow p^+ + \beta^- \qquad \text{Equation 27.2}$$

It appears that in nuclei which have too many neutrons, there is a finite possibility that a neutron becomes isolated within the nucleus and then decays to form a proton and a negatron. The proton rejoins the nucleus and the negatron is ejected. This transformation results in the atomic mass number remaining unchanged (the combined number of protons and neutrons is still the same) but the atomic number will increase by 1 as one extra proton has been added to the nucleus (this results in the formation of a different element with the consequent rearrangement of electron orbitals to suit the new element).

An example of β⁻-particle decay is shown below where carbon-14 decays to form nitrogen with the emission of a β⁻-particle.

$$^{14}_{6}\text{C} \longrightarrow {}^{14}_{7}\text{N} + \beta^- \qquad \text{Equation 27.3}$$

This can also be illustrated using the methods discussed for alpha

Figure 27.4 An example of pure beta particle (negatron) emission. The nucleus increases its atomic number and loses energy as shown.

particle emission to show the transformation from parent to daughter product. Such a diagram is shown in Figure 27.4.

Note that this time there is an increase in the atomic number so the line is down and to the right. This simple decay process is an example of *pure beta emission* since no other transformations are involved.

Figure 27.5 shows a more complex emission pattern where the parent and daughter nuclei are separated by an energy difference of 2.81 MeV. The β^--particle has an energy of 0.31 MeV and so the nucleus is left in an excited state—2.50 MeV above its ground state. The nucleus emits this energy in the form of two gamma rays, one of energy 1.17 MeV and the other of energy 1.33 MeV. (This will be discussed further when we consider γ-ray emission in a later section of this chapter.)

Figure 27.5 The decay of cobalt-60 as an example of beta decay followed by a gamma decay of the daughter nucleus.

27.5.2 Positron (β⁺) emission

As mentioned earlier, protons are continuously changing into neutrons and back. In these reactions we can consider a proton as consisting of a neutron and a positron.

$$p^+ \longrightarrow n + \beta^+ \qquad\qquad \text{Equation 27.4}$$

If we consider Figure 27.1, we see that positron emission takes place from nuclei which have too many protons to achieve stability. In such cases protons appear to become isolated within the nucleus and then to decay to form a neutron which rejoins the nucleus and a positron which is ejected from the nucleus. In this reaction the atomic mass number will remain the same but the atomic number will decrease by 1 (the total number of protons and neutrons is unchanged but one proton has been converted into a neutron).

An example of such a reaction is the decay carbon-11 to boron as shown below:

$$_{6}^{11}\text{C} \longrightarrow {}_{5}^{11}\text{B} + \beta^+ \qquad\qquad \text{Equation 27.5}$$

If we consider the energy changes which take place within the nucleus as shown in Figure 27.6, we see that the situation regarding energy of the β⁺-particle is not as simple as it is for the β⁻-particle. The energy difference between the parent and daughter nucleus in this case is 1.99 MeV. An energy loss of $2mc^2$ is required to allow the positron to escape from the nucleus—where m is the mass of the positron and c is the velocity of electromagnetic radiation. As the mass of the positron is the same as the

Figure 27.6 An example of positron decay. The nucleus experiences a decrease in the atomic number and loses energy as shown.

mass of the electron, then 1.02 MeV is required to create the positron and eject it from the nucleus and any remaining energy (in this case 0.97 MeV) is given to the positron as kinetic energy.

Insight

A negatron or a positron is influenced by the electrostatic forces which exist between it and the nucleus until it is able to escape from the atom. As a result the kinetic energy of the β⁻-particle is reduced by the force of attraction which exists between it and the nucleus, while the kinetic energy of the β⁺-particle is increased by electrostatic repulsion. Energy and momentum are conserved in this process.

27.5.3 The fate of the positron

An energetic positron emitted by a nucleus will move through the surrounding atoms and will lose kinetic energy because of collisions with them. As its momentum decreases, it is more likely to interact with a free electron in the material. The positron is the *antiparticle* of the electron and when they meet they completely annihilate each other to form two gamma rays of annihilation radiation. This process is shown diagrammatically in Figure 27.7 where the annihilation radiation consists of two photons each of energy 0.511 MeV ejected at 180° to each other. In this way both energy and momentum are conserved. The mutual annihilation of the electron and the positron is an example of the principle of mass–energy equivalence (see Sect. 24.4.1) as given by Einstein's equation $E = mc^2$, and shows that each particle has a mass–energy of 0.511 MeV in agreement with Table 26.1.

The annihilation radiation produced by the reaction may now interact with neighbouring atoms by the processes of Compton scattering and photoelectric absorption (see Ch. 30) and may produce characteristic radiation and Auger electrons (see Sect. 27.6.3) by processes which will be discussed later in this chapter.

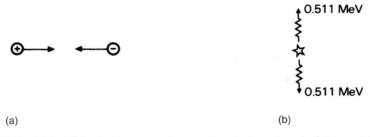

(a) (b)

Figure 27.7 (a) A collision between a positron and an electron where both have a minimal kinetic energy; (b) shows the annihilation radiation where two photons each of 0.511 MeV are produced at 180° to each other.

Insight

The positron and the electron may annihilate each other when the positron still has considerable kinetic energy. In this case the two quanta are not emitted at 180° to each other and each has an energy higher than 0.511 MeV. The excess of energy of the positron is divided equally between each quantum. In each case energy and momentum are conserved. A diagrammatic representation of the process is shown in the figure.

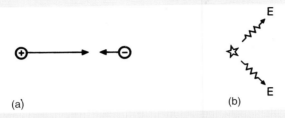

(a)   (b)

(a) A collision between a positron and an electron where the positron has significant kinetic energy; (b) shows the direction of propagation of the annihilation radiation where the photons have energy in excess of 0.511 MeV each.

27.5.4 The neutrino

Consider the carbon-14 reaction which we discussed earlier. Here the carbon-14 decayed to nitrogen where the difference in energy between the parent and the daughter nucleus was 159 keV. As only beta decay takes place we could confidently expect that all the β⁻-particles should have an energy of 159 keV. If we plot a graph of the energy of the beta particles against the numbers emitted we get a graph similar to the β⁻ graph shown in Figure 27.8. The maximum or end-point energy of the β⁻-particles in this case is 159 keV. The graph means that, although only beta decay takes place and although the difference between the parent and the daughter nucleus is 159 keV, some of the β⁻-particles have energies less than 159 keV. Such a situation would appear to suggest that this does not obey the Law of Conservation of Energy (see Sect. 24.4). This difficulty was overcome by Wolfgang Pauli in 1933 when he postulated that another particle—the *neutrino*—is always ejected with a beta particle. He suggested that a neutrino (symbol v) is ejected at the same time as a positron and that an antineutrino (symbol $\bar{v}$) at the same time as a negatron. The *total energy* of the emitted negatron and antineutrino corresponds to the energy difference between the parent and daughter nucleus. How this energy is shared between the two particles will differ for each decay of the nucleus. In this way a continuous distribution of energies is obtained both for the β⁻-particle and the antineutrino as shown in Figure 27.8. Because of the presence of the neutrino and antineutrino we now need to modify some of the equations we considered earlier:

$$\ce{^{14}_{6}C} \longrightarrow \ce{^{14}_{7}N} + \beta^- + \bar{v}$$

$$\ce{^{11}_{6}C} \longrightarrow \ce{^{11}_{5}B} + \beta^+ + v \qquad\qquad \text{Equation 27.6}$$

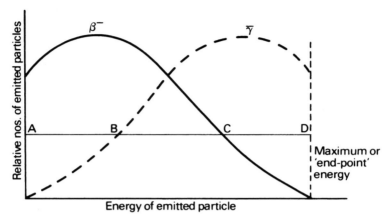

Figure 27.8 The sharing of energy between the beta particle and the neutrino in beta decay—the case shown is for negatron emission.

Insight

Although Pauli postulated the existence of neutrinos and antineutrinos in 1933 the presence of these particles proved difficult to detect until much later. There is now conclusive proof of their existence because of experiments performed using nuclear reactors and particle accelerators. The neutrino and the antineutrino differ in their direction of spin relative to their direction of motion—the neutrino spins anticlockwise and the antineutrino spins clockwise. They are antiparticles and if they are made to collide will produce electromagnetic radiation in the form of annihilation radiation. The reason the particles are so difficult to detect can be seen by considering their three major properties:

- zero rest mass
- zero charge
- extremely small interaction with matter.

Because of these properties it is extremely difficult to detect the presence of neutrinos (or antineutrinos)—they have a HVT (see Sect. 4.8) of many miles in lead!

27.6 GAMMA DECAY OR GAMMA RAY EMISSION

Gamma (γ) rays are part of the electromagnetic spectrum and are similar in many ways to X-rays. γ-rays are emitted from a nucleus which has excess energy whereas X-rays are from electrons as they lose energy (this will be further discussed in Ch. 28). It is possible for γ-rays to have lower energies than X-rays and vice versa. However, the maximum energy possible from γ-rays exceeds that of X-rays.

We discussed in this chapter (see 27.5.1) the fact that cobalt-60 decayed with the emission of a β⁻-particle but the daughter nucleus was left in an excited state. The situation for this daughter nucleus is depicted in Figure 27.9(a). The figure illustrates the energy states of the daughter nucleus by means of horizontal lines above the thick line representing the ground state of the nucleus. In this case, the $^{60}_{28}$Ni nucleus is left at an energy 2.5 MeV above its ground state. It immediately decays to its ground state in two jumps:

- it decays to 1.33 MeV above its ground state by the emission of a 1.17 MeV γ-ray
- it then drops to its ground state by the emission of a second γ-ray of energy 1.33 MeV.

(a)   (b)

Figure 27.9   (a) The excited states of a nickel-60 nucleus which is left in an excited state as the result of the previous decay of a cobalt-60 nucleus. This decays to its ground state by the emission of two gamma photons each representing the difference in energy between the excited states; (b) shows the line spectrum produced by the gamma radiation.

Figure 27.9(b) shows the line spectra of the gamma radiation emitted by the nucleus where each γ-ray has a precise energy corresponding to the discrete energy transformations within the nucleus.

27.6.1 Metastable states and isomeric transitions

In the case of $^{60}_{27}$Co decaying to $^{60}_{28}$Ni the nucleus remains in an excited state before the emission of the γ-rays for a time so short that it is incapable of accurate measurement. However, this is not always the case, and those excited states which last sufficiently long for their durations to be measured are known as *metastable states*. The transition from a metastable state to a more stable state is known as an *isomeric transition*. Such metastable radionuclides prove to be useful in nuclear medicine because of the low dose which they deliver to the patient—the patient gets no dose from

β^--particles emitted before metastability. Technetium-99m (usually written $^{99}_{43}Tc^m$ or less commonly $^{99m}_{43}Tc$) is a radionuclide which is widely used in nuclear medicine. A simplified decay scheme for it is shown in Figure 27.10 and it will be discussed in more detail later in this chapter (see Sect. 27.11.1). The half-life of $^{99}_{43}Tc^m$ is 6 hours and it emits a γ-ray of energy 140 keV when it decays to $^{99}_{43}Tc$. The half-life of $^{99}_{43}Tc$ is so long (2.1×10^5 years) that it can be considered stable for all practical purposes.

The reaction can be written as:

$$^{99}_{43}Tc^m \longrightarrow \ ^{99}_{43}Tc + \gamma \qquad\qquad\text{Equation 27.7}$$

Figure 27.10   An example of the decay of technetium from a metastable to a stable state with the emission of a 140 keV gamma photon.

The next section of this chapter considers the possible effects of gamma emission from the nucleus on the whole atom rather than on the nucleus only.

27.6.2 Internal conversion

When a nuclide is decaying by γ emission there is a competing process within the atom called *internal conversion*. This process results in electrons with discrete energies (unlike the continuous spectrum of energies of negatrons) being emitted from the atom. The process is a result of a direct interaction between the nucleus and an orbiting electron such that the nucleus is able to drop to its ground state by giving all of its excess energy to the electron.

The innermost electrons of the atom have orbitals which pass close to or even through the nucleus. Thus it is a matter of statistical probability whether the excess energy of the nucleus will result in a γ-ray emission from the nucleus or electron emission from the inner shells. The K-shell is situated closest to the nucleus so is most likely to participate in such a reaction followed by the L-, M-shells, etc. The *converted electron* escapes from the atom with an energy equal to the energy donated by the nucleus minus the binding energy of that particular electron. This can be stated:

KE of converted electron = nuclear energy transition − BE

Equation 27.8

The *internal conversion coefficient,* α, is defined as the ratio of the number of nuclear transformations which result in internal conversion to the number which result in γ-ray emission. Thus, α may take a value between 0, resulting in no internal conversions, and infinity, corresponding to complete internal conversion. This can be illustrated by considering the figures for the decay of $^{99}_{43}Tc^m$ to $^{99}_{43}Tc$. Approximately 9% of the nuclear transitions result in internal conversions of electrons from the K-shell, 1.1% from the L-shell and 0.3% from the M-shell. This means that 10.4% of the nuclear transitions result in internal conversions and 89.6% result in γ-ray emission. This gives an internal conversion coefficient (α) for $^{99}_{43}Tc^m$ of 0.116.

27.6.3 X-rays and Auger electrons

If a radioactive decay results in a vacancy occurring within one of the inner electron shells of the atom, then electrons from orbitals further away from the nucleus will perform quantum jumps inwards until there are no inner shell vacancies. Each such quantum jump will result in the emission of electromagnetic radiation from the atom equal to the energy difference between the two shells. For inner shell transitions the energy of this electromagnetic radiation may be in the X-ray part of the spectrum. Such radiation is known as *fluorescent radiation* and its energy is characteristic of the atom concerned.

If we consider the internal conversion process which we have just described and take a situation where a K-shell electron is removed from the atom, the vacancy thus created in the K-shell may be filled from the L-shell (a K_α transition) or from the M-shell (a K_β transition). Such a quantum jump would be accompanied by the emission of a photon of electromagnetic radiation equivalent to the energy difference between the two shells. If it was a K_α transition, there would now be a vacancy in the L-shell and this might be filled from the M-shell, etc. This would again be accompanied by the emission of a photon of electromagnetic radiation equal to the energy difference between the L- and M-shells. This process continues until the atom is able to capture a free electron to fill the vacancy—usually in one of its outermost shells. Until this occurs the atom contains more protons than electrons and so is regarded as a *positive ion.*

This already rather complex situation is further complicated by the fact that some of the photons emitted by such transitions may have sufficient energy to interact with other electrons in the atom and to remove them from their orbitals and eject them from the atom—this process is called the photoelectric effect and may occur if the photon energy is greater than the binding energy of the electron (see Ch. 30 for a more detailed description). The electrons thus ejected are called *Auger electrons* and have discrete energies equal to the photon energy minus the binding energy of the electron. The ejection of an Auger electron from a shell leaves a vacancy in that shell which will be filled by electrons jumping down from orbitals even further away from the nucleus with the release of more fluorescent radiation and perhaps the release of even more Auger electrons.

From the above we can see that the ejection of an electron from one of the orbitals by internal conversion may result in a complicated sequence of orbital quantum jumps accompanied by the release of photons of electromagnetic radiation and the ejection of Auger electrons from the atom. The term *fluorescent yield* is used to describe the fraction of the electron transitions which result in the production of fluorescent radiation.

If we consider $^{99}_{43}\text{Tc}^m$ from the previous discussion, you may remember that 11.6% of the energy from the nucleus results in internal conversion ($\alpha = 0.116$). Of the resulting electron quantum jumps, 80% of the transitions result in fluorescent radiation and 20% result in the production of Auger electrons. Thus the fluorescent yield for technetium is 0.8. Some typical fluorescent radiation energies for $^{99}_{43}\text{Tc}^m$ are:

$$K_\alpha = 18.4 \text{ keV}, \quad L_\alpha = 2.4 \text{ keV}, \quad M_\alpha = 0.2 \text{ keV}.$$

Note: The fact that the electrons emitted by this process carry discrete amounts of energy makes it easy to distinguish them from negatron emission where there is a continuous spectrum of energies.

Insight

For each decay, the total energies for all the fluorescent radiation and of all the electrons emitted from the shells of the atom equal the energy lost by the nucleus in the nuclear transition. This is because the binding energy of each ejected electron is recovered in the fluorescent radiation emitted in the subsequent cascade of orbital jumps. Thus the whole process obeys the Law of Conservation of Energy.

27.7 ELECTRON CAPTURE

If a nucleus of low mass number has too few neutrons for stability but has insufficient excess energy (<1.02 MeV) to eject a positron, then an alternative way by which the nucleus may undergo an isobaric transformation and lose energy is by *electron capture*. In this process the nucleus captures one of the orbiting electrons, the most likely being a capture of a K-shell electron. Sometimes the term 'K capture' and 'L capture' are used to denote the shell from which the electron was captured. A situation where electron capture is the only process involved is shown in Figure 27.11(a) where $^{131}_{55}\text{Cs}$ decays to $^{131}_{54}\text{Xe}$.

In the diagram, the atomic number is reduced by 1 because the capture

(a)   (b)

Figure 27.11 (a) Pure electron capture decay. (b) Electron capture and positron decay occurring in the same nuclide (85% EC and 15% positron decay). Also emitted are the X-rays from the iron-58 atoms and the 0.511 MeV annihilation radiations from the positron–electron annihilations.

of an electron by the nucleus results in one of the protons in the nucleus changing into a neutron. Also note that during the process of electron capture a neutrino is emitted by the nucleus. The processes involved in electron capture may be shown by Equation 27.9.

$$p^{+} + e^{-} \longrightarrow n + \nu \qquad\qquad \text{Equation 27.9}$$

In situations where a low mass nucleus has too few neutrons and an excess energy greater than 1.02 MeV, then the process of electron capture may compete with the process of positron emission. An example of such a competing process is shown in the decay of $^{58}_{27}$Co into stable $^{58}_{26}$Fe in Figure 27.11(b).

Note that both the process of electron capture and the process of positron emission involve the conversion of a proton to a neutron. Thus the atomic mass number remains unaltered but the atomic number is reduced by 1.

As we mentioned earlier in this chapter (Sect. 27.7.2), creating a vacancy in an inner electron shell will result in the emission of characteristic fluorescent radiation from the atom. It is interesting to note that in the case of electron capture this is characteristic of the *daughter product*. This means that the electron orbitals of the daughter product are established *before* the consequent electron transitions occur.

27.8 BRANCHING DECAY PROGRAMMES

If the nucleus is very large, it is possible that it may disintegrate in more than one way. We have already encountered this—although it was not described in detail—in the uranium series in Figure 27.2. In this case $^{214}_{83}$Bi can either decay to $^{214}_{84}$Po by β⁻-particle emission or it can decay to $^{210}_{81}$Tl by α-particle emission.

Another isotope of bismuth, $^{212}_{83}$Bi, decays in a similar branching programme. The decay process for this isotope involves the emission of α-particles of energies 6.04 MeV and 6.08 MeV, γ-rays of energy 0.04 MeV and β⁻-particles of maximum energy 2.25 MeV. The initial decay scheme for the $^{212}_{83}$Bi nuclide is shown in Figure 27.12. *Note* that for simplicity only the first disintegrations are shown. As can be seen from the diagram, both $^{208}_{81}$Tl and $^{212}_{84}$Po have short half-lives and so are also radioactive.

Figure 27.12 A branching decay programme where alpha and beta decay processes compete in the decay of bismuth-212.

27.9 FISSION

As we mentioned in our discussion of α-decay (see Sect. 27.4) the short-range forces holding the nucleus together exist between adjacent nucleons, whereas the Coulomb forces act across the whole of the nucleus. This fact becomes increasingly important as the size of the nucleus increases. A very large nucleus may be pictured as being rather like a liquid drop in which the nucleons are moving about with very high energy and continuously deforming the shape of the nucleus.

During this process, it is possible for the nucleus to become very elongated and then to break into two fragments—usually of fairly similar sizes. Such a phenomenon is known as *spontaneous fission* and can occur for very large nuclei, e.g. thorium-232 is capable of spontaneous fission. As well as the *fission fragments* from such a reaction, one or more neutrons are usually liberated and the whole fission process is accompanied by the release of large amounts of energy.

Neutron-activated fission is a more controllable process than spontaneous fission. This occurs as a result of a heavy nucleus capturing an incoming neutron and then breaking into large fragments in a similar way to spontaneous fission. An example of such a reaction is the disintegration of $^{238}_{92}U$ into two fission fragments of $^{145}_{56}Ba$ and $^{94}_{36}Kr$ if the uranium-238 nucleus is made to absorb a neutron. The fission of the nucleus is normally accompanied by the release of gamma rays and neutrons. Both of the fissile fragments are extremely rich in neutrons and so each will usually release a neutron. The neutrons from both of the above processes can now react with two $^{238}_{92}U$ nuclei resulting in the release of four fissile fragments and four neutrons and so a *chain reaction* can be set up. Such a process is accompanied by the release of large amounts of energy (see Insight below).

Insight

On average, a uranium-238 nucleus will release an energy of 200 MeV on fission. If we consider the complete fission of a 1 kg mass of uranium (this is about the size of a golf ball) we need to consider the energy released by all the uranium atoms in a 1 kg mass. By applying Avogadro's equation (see Sect. 5.6) to this we can calculate that 1 kg of uranium-238 contains 2.5×10^{24} atoms. If each of these atoms releases 200 MeV of energy, the total energy released will be 5.1×10^{26} MeV. This is the same as 8.1×10^{13} joules of energy.

A pictorial representation of the neutron-activated fission process is shown in Figure 27.13. The incoming neutron is captured in Figure 27.13(a) and delivers sufficient energy to the nucleus (Fig. 27.13(b)) to elongate its shape into an ellipsoid. As mentioned earlier, the Coulomb forces across the nucleus are now at an advantage over the short-range nuclear forces and the nucleus further distorts to form a 'peanut' shape (Fig. 27.13(c)) and eventually breaks to form two fragments because of the electrostatic repulsion between the two main nuclear masses. The two fragments fly apart (their kinetic energy accounts for about 80% of the total disintegration energy) and several neutrons and gamma ray photons are usually emitted (Fig. 27.13(d)). The neutrons emitted by this reaction may now interact with other atoms to cause fission and the release of further neutrons and so a chain reaction is set up with the consequent liberation of large amounts of energy. The fissile fragments (Fig. 27.13(e)) are themselves rich in neutrons for their atomic numbers and so will undergo further disintegration to move towards more stable nuclei. This initial process results in the production of β^--particles (with associated γ-rays) which produces a more stable proton/neutron configuration or, if the nucleus is very excited, the ejection of a neutron from the nucleus. These neutrons are known as *delayed neutrons* to distinguish them from the *prompt neutrons* which are emitted at the moment of fission.

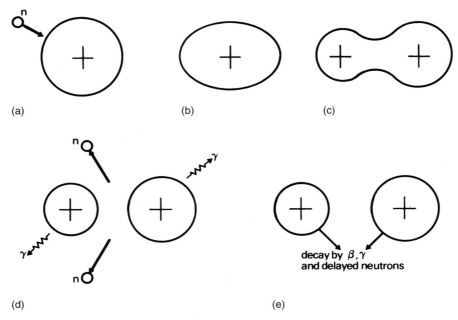

(a)　　　　　　　　　(b)　　　　　　　　　(c)

decay by β,γ
and delayed neutrons

(d)　　　　　　　　　(e)

Figure 27.13 A diagrammatic representation of the of neutron-activated fission (for a fuller explanation of the process, see the text).

Fission products from any type of nucleus are not always the same and may have different relative sizes on each disintegration. Thus a great range of other decay chains is possible from other fissile fragments.

Insight

It is also possible to initiate fission in the nucleus by bombarding it with proton (or with α-particles) or by striking it with high-energy photons. Examples of these are:

- Copper ($^{63}_{29}Cu$), if bombarded with protons, can be made to undergo fission to produce sodium ($^{24}_{11}Na$) and potassium ($^{39}_{19}K$). This process is accompanied by neutron emission.
- Uranium-238 ($^{238}_{32}U$), if it is bombarded by photons of energy equal to or greater than 5.1 MeV, will undergo fission. This latter process is known as *photofission*.

27.9.1 The nuclear reactor

The nuclear reactor (or pile) produces heat energy by controlled fission. The heat generated within the reactor raises the temperature of a coolant which in turn is used to heat water to produce steam. The steam then drives very powerful electric generators.

A simplified diagram of such a reactor is shown in Figure 27.14. The controlled fission is produced by using the neutrons of fissile decay to produce further fission in other atoms. Thus, a sustained reaction can be

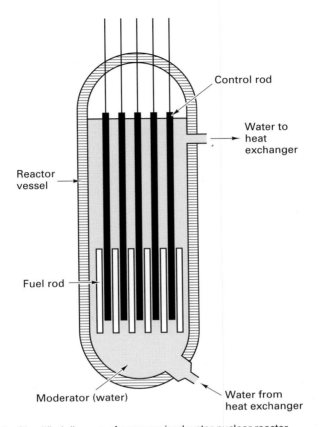

Figure 27.14 Simplified diagram of a pressurised water nuclear reactor.

set up where one neutron released during the fission of a nucleus will interact with another nucleus to produce fission of that nucleus with the release of further neutrons. The *fuel* used in a conventional nuclear reactor is *enriched uranium* which is a mixture of $^{235}_{92}U$ (about 10%) and $^{238}_{92}U$ (about 90%). Controlled fission occurs mainly with uranium-235 because uranium-238 is able to form stable nuclei on the capture of *fast neutrons* (energies greater than 0.5 MeV). Neutrons released by fission are classed according to their energy as shown in Table 27.1.

Table 27.1 Classification of neutrons

Classification	Energy range
Fast	> 0.5 MeV
Intermediate	1 keV–0.5 MeV
Slow	1 eV–1 keV
Thermal	0.025 eV

Uranium-235 is an efficient fissile material for *thermal neutrons*. As can be seen from the table, these have very low energies and so the energies of the neutrons released at the point of fission must be reduced or *moderated*. In most modern reactors, water and/or graphite are used as moderating materials so that neutrons lose some of their energies by reacting with the *moderator* and become thermal and so react with the uranium-235.

The reaction described above can be more than self-sustaining and so it is necessary to control the power generated to prevent *runaway*. If runaway takes place, the reactor can produce sufficient heat to cause explosion of the containment vessel, loss of coolant and vaporisation of the contents of the nuclear pile. This can cause severe radioactive contamination of the environment. By controlling the number of neutrons present, it is possible to control the rate of fission. This is done by inserting boron rods into the nuclear pile—boron readily absorbs neutrons—and so the remaining neutrons are moderated by the graphite to produce thermal neutrons which will react with the uranium-235 nuclei.

To start the reactor, the boron rods are almost completely withdrawn and the neutrons produced by spontaneous fission are sufficient to cause the release of further neutrons to sustain the chain reaction. The reactor is then said to have gone *critical*. The increase in the number of neutrons present near the centre of the reactor core is then quite rapid—an increase of neutron number by 10^{12} in about 30 seconds is typical. The boron rods are gradually reinserted into the pile to absorb neutrons and produce the controlled reaction at the power level required.

Nuclear reactors are important in radiation medicine in that they allow us to insert samples into the neutron flux to allow the manufacture of *artificial radionuclides*.

Insight

In 1986 the operators of the nuclear reactor at Chernobyl near Kiev lost control of the reactor by a somewhat bizarre set of operator errors. As a result, the reactor went hypercritical and power surged to about 100 times its normal value. This caused serious overheating of the core which caused it to explode and start a fire in the graphite moderator. The debris from this explosion contained many by-products of fission and was carried over a large area of northern and western Europe, causing serious radioactive contamination. An area of 30 km radius around the reactor is so seriously contaminated that it has had to be permanently evacuated.

27.10 SUMMARY OF RADIOACTIVE NUCLEAR TRANSFORMATIONS

Table 27.2 is a summary of the types of radioactive decay discussed so far in this chapter. You may find it useful to refer back to this table when considering the production of artificial radionuclides and also in considering the use of radionuclides in medicine.

Table 27.2 Summary of the effects of radioactive decay

Type of decay	Symbol	Effect on nucleus			Effect on atom	Comments
		Z	N	A		
Alpha	α	$Z-2$	$N-2$	$A-4$	Electron orbits change to that of daughter nucleus	Occurs in elements with a mass number greater than 150. Daughter products may undergo further decay by a variety of the processes below
Negatron emission	β^-	$Z+1$	$N-1$	—	Electron orbits change to that of daughter nucleus	Proton changes to neutron in nucleus. Negatron emitted from the nucleus with a spread of energies but the energy of the negatron plus the energy of the antineutrino is constant for a given nuclide. Daughter nucleus may further decay by prompt or delayed γ-ray emission competing with IC
Positron emission	β^+	$Z-1$	$N+1$	—	Electron orbits change to that of daughter nucleus	Neutron changes to proton in nucleus. The positron is emitted with a neutrino and the sum of their energies is constant for a given nuclide. The process only occurs if the energy loss by the parent nucleus can be greater than 1.02 MeV. Positron is annihilated by collision with electron and two photons of annihilation radiation, each of energy 0.511 MeV, are produced. Daughter nucleus may decay by γ-radiation and/or IC
Gamma radiation	γ	—	—	—	No effect on the number of nucleons in the nucleus but the process may compete with IC	Produced by the quantum jump from excited state of the nucleus to a lower energy. Excited states of measurable half-life are defined as *metastable* and the transition is *isomeric*
Internal conversion	IC	—	—	—	Characteristic radiation and Auger electrons emitted	An inner orbital electron of the atom interacts with the nucleus and is ejected from the atom. The electron is given the excess nuclear energy. This creates a vacancy in the shell and results in the emission of characteristic radiation and Auger electrons

Table 27.2 (*contd*)

Type of decay	Symbol	Effect on nucleus			Effect on atom	Comments
		Z	*N*	*A*		
Electron capture	EC	$Z-1$	$N+1$	—	Characteristic radiation and Auger electrons of the daughter nucleus are emitted	An inner orbital electron is captured by the nucleus and changes a proton to a neutron. A neutrino is emitted carrying energy changes of the nucleus. The nucleus may decay spontaneously by γ-ray emission. The vacancy left in the electron orbit results in the emission of characteristic radiation and Auger electrons
Fission	*f*	Size and structure of the fragments may vary			Bonds may be broken or ionisation caused by fragment	Fission may be spontaneous or neutron activated. The nucleus splits producing two or more fragments, γ-rays and neutrons. Controlled fission is used in nuclear reactors (see text) and the neutrons can be used to produce artificial radionuclides

27.11 ARTIFICIALLY PRODUCED RADIONUCLIDES

Radionuclides may be artificially produced by bombarding the nuclei of elements with particles, e.g. neutrons from a nuclear reactor. These particles are captured by the nucleus making it unstable and causing it to decay by one or more of the methods described above.

Many of the artificially produced radionuclides which are relevant to nuclear medicine are produced by bombarding a material with neutrons in a nuclear reactor. The capture of a neutron is immediately accompanied by the ejection of a γ-ray or particle. The daughter nucleus produced by neutron capture is obviously rich in neutrons and so is likely to decay by β⁻-emission. This may be accompanied by γ-emission.

The widespread use of a *technetium generator* in nuclear medicine is an important example of the production of artificial radionuclides and will now be considered in more detail.

27.11.1 The technetium generator

If molybdenum-98 is placed in a neutron stream, the nuclei of the molybdenum atoms can be made to absorb the neutrons to produce molybdenum-99. The capture of a neutron raises the energy of the resulting molybdenum-99 nuclei and each loses this energy by the prompt emission of a γ-ray. The reaction may be shown using the equation below:

$$^{98}_{42}\text{Mo} + n \longrightarrow \, ^{99}_{42}\text{Mo} + \gamma \qquad \text{Equation 27.10}$$

Figure 27.15 Principal features of a technetium-99m generator.

The molybdenum-99/alumina column is in the centre of the generator as shown in Figure 27.15. The molybdenum-99 has a half-life of 67 hours and decays to form technetium-99m by β⁻-particle emission as shown below:

$$_{42}^{99}\text{Mo} \longrightarrow {}_{43}^{99}\text{Tc}^{\text{m}} + \beta^- + \bar{v}$$ Equation 27.11

The $_{43}^{99}\text{Tc}^{\text{m}}$ is eluted (or flushed) from the generator at regular intervals as sodium pertechnetate. This isotope, which is in liquid form, may be used for a number of radionuclide imaging situations. The $_{43}^{99}\text{Tc}^{\text{m}}$ decays to $_{43}^{99}\text{Tc}$ by the emission of a γ-ray of energy 140 keV. The metastable isotope, as we saw earlier in this chapter, has a half-life of 6 hours.

A number of other isotopes used in nuclear medicine can be produced from stable materials when they are bombarded with particles but further discussion about their production is beyond the scope of this book.

27.11.2 Growth of activity

If we consider the molybdenum-98 which has been placed within a neutron stream in a nuclear reactor, then the number of daughter nuclei formed by the capture process increases over a period of time. However, the number of daughter nuclei formed does not increase indefinitely for the following reasons:

- As more of the original nuclei have captured neutrons, there are less left to do the same.
- Daughter nuclei themselves may capture further neutrons and form a different isotope of that element. (In practice, the probability of this happening for most of the isotopes used in nuclear medicine is very low.)
- Daughter nuclei undergo radioactive decay during the irradiation time.

The relative importance of the above processes depends on factors such as the sample material, the half-lives involved, the neutron flux and the neutron energy spectrum. The growth of the activity of the daughter product is in exponential form and is described by the equation:

$$A_t = kF(1 - e^{-\lambda t}) \hspace{4cm} \text{Equation 27.12}$$

where A_t is the radioactivity (measured in becquerel) after a time t
k is a constant for a given sample and a given reactor
F is a measure of the neutron flux (number of neutrons per unit area per second)
λ is the decay constant of the daughter radionuclide formed.

The growth curve of the activity of the daughter nuclide is shown in Figure 27.16 for two levels of neutron flux (note the similarity between these growth curves and the exponential curves obtained when a capacitor is charged through a resistor—Fig. 16.5). In both cases, the activity pro-

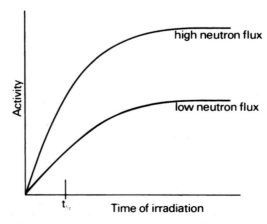

Figure 27.16 A graphical representation of the growth of activity induced by irradiating a suitable sample with neutrons.

duced in the sample reaches a maximum value after about four half-lives. It is usual in most cases, however, to irradiate the sample for only two or three half-lives as this time produces the maximum gain for the time of irradiation.

As can be seen from the graphs, when the activity reaches its maximum value there is a constant value of activity produced even if the sample is further irradiated. This is because equal numbers of daughter nuclei are being produced and decaying each second. This situation is known as *radioactive equilibrium*. Radioactive equilibrium may also occur in decay chains where the daughter nuclide is also decaying into another nuclide (see Insight below).

Insight

Another example of radioactive equilibrium is the decay of $^{99}_{42}\text{Mo}$ into $^{99}_{43}\text{Tc}^{\text{m}}$ that takes place in the technetium generator. The half-life for the $^{99}_{42}\text{Mo}$ is 67 hours and for the $^{99}_{43}\text{Tc}^{\text{m}}$ is 6 hours. If we start the process at a time when there is no $^{99}_{43}\text{Tc}^{\text{m}}$ present, the activity of the $^{99}_{43}\text{Tc}^{\text{m}}$ will rise until it reaches 90% of the activity of the molybdenum. This is shown in section A of the graph in Figure 27.17. The curves for both the isotopes now run in parallel—they are in radioactive equilibrium. Elution of the generator removes all the activity due to the technetium (see 1, 2 and 3 in Fig. 27.17) but it will again return to 90% of the activity of the molybdenum unless two elutions follow each other too rapidly as in 2 and 3. The generator may thus be used as a source of the daughter nuclide for a much longer time than the half-life of the daughter would otherwise permit.

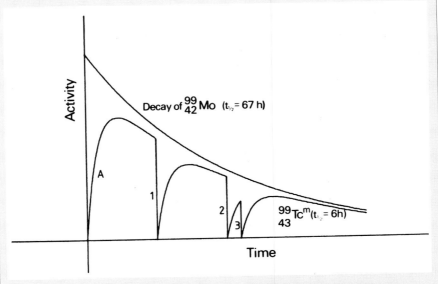

Figure 27.17 An example of radioactive equilibrium. Molybdenum-99 decays with a half-life of 67 h to technetium-99m (half-life = 6 h). At time = 0, the Tc-99m grows in activity (A in the figure)—this is removed by elution from a 'technetium generator' (1, 2, 3), after which the activity grows again. ·

27.12 CLINICALLY USEFUL RADIONUCLIDES

Radionuclides are used to diagnose and to treat certain conditions. When they are used for diagnosis, they may be *labelled* (chemically linked) to a certain *radiopharmaceutical* thus encouraging their uptake by specific body parts. The labelled radionuclide may then be injected into, or ingested by, the patient. Such diagnostic techniques in nuclear medicine have two main uses:

- to provide information on organ physiology, e.g. technetium-labelled DTPA will give information on the rate of excretion of this radionuclide by the kidneys, thus giving information on renal function
- to produce an image of an organ on a gamma camera, e.g. $^{99}_{43}\text{Tc}^m$ as pertechnetate may be injected into the patient to produce images of the skeletal physiology; this is a very useful way of early detection of metastatic spread into bone.

A list of the radioisotopes which are commonly used is given in Table 27.3.

For the diagnostic purposes of imaging or charting organ physiology, only gamma ray emission is useful. This is because particles (α or β) emitted are absorbed very efficiently by the patient's tissues. If the particles are absorbed by the patient and do not reach the imaging or counting device, they contribute radiation dose to the patient but give no diagnostic information.

The ideal radionuclide for imaging should:

- have a short half-life—approximately twice the length of time from injection into the patient to completion of the scan
- emit γ-rays of relatively low energy, so that these are easily detected and do not pose a major hazard to others because of their penetrating power
- emit no particles as part of its decay pattern as these add significantly to the patient dose
- be readily labelled to allow its uptake by specific organs
- be readily excreted by the patient
- be easily generated in the radio-pharmacy.

In many ways $^{99}_{43}\text{Tc}^m$ is the almost ideal radionuclide for scanning purposes.

As can be seen from Table 27.3, other radionuclides can be used for a variety of purposes in medicine. Detailed discussion of their uses is the subject of a specialised text and is beyond the scope of this book. A number of specialist texts on this topic may be found in the list of further reading at the end of this chapter.

Table 27.3 Radionuclides commonly used in medicine

Application	Radio-nuclide	$t_{1/2}$	Decay mode	Gamma energy (MeV)	Max. beta energy (MeV)	Comments
Diagnostic						
Organ physiology	$^{131}_{53}I$	8.04 d	β^-, γ	0.364	0.61	Thyroid uptakes (NaI)
	$^{132}_{53}I$	2.3 h	β^-, γ	0.67 0.78	2.12	Renal function (iodohippurate)
	$^{99}_{43}Tc^m$	6 h	IT	0.140	—	Renal function (DTPA)
Organ imaging	$^{99}_{43}Tc^m$	6 h	IT	0.140	—	Imaging of brain, kidney, liver, lung, skeleton, spleen
	$^{113}_{49}In^m$	90 min	IT	0.390	—	Imaging of brain, kidney, liver
	$^{75}_{34}Se$	121 d	EC	0.14 0.27	—	Imaging of pancreas
	$^{68}_{31}Ga$	68 min	β^+, EC	0.51	1.89	Imaging of tumours and inflammatory lesions
	$^{81}_{36}Kr^m$	13 s	IT	0.19	—	Pulmonary function (ventilation) studies
	$^{133}_{54}Xe$	5.3 d	β^-, γ	0.081	0.34	Cerebral blood flow, pulmonary function (ventilation) studies
Tracers	$^{3}_{1}H$	12.3 y	β^-	—	0.018	Used for a large variety of studies
	$^{14}_{6}C$	5760 y	β^-	—	0.115	
	$^{35}_{16}S$	87.2 d	β^-	—	0.167	Used in the estimation of cellular volumes
	$^{43}_{19}K$	22 h	β^-, γ	0.37 0.61	0.83	
	$^{51}_{24}Cr$	27.8 d	EC	0.32	—	Used for a variety of blood studies
	$^{59}_{26}Fe$	445 d	β^-, γ	1.10 1.29	0.46	
	$^{57}_{27}Co$	270 d	EC	0.112	—	Used for the investigation of pernicious anaemia
	$^{58}_{27}Co$	71 d	β^+, EC	0.51 0.81	0.485	
Therapy						
By injection	$^{32}_{15}P$	14.3 d	β^-	—	1.71	Phosphate used for the treatment of polycythaemia vera
	$^{90}_{39}Y$	62.2 h	β^-	—	2.27	Used as a colloid in the treatment of some lymphatic cancers
By ingestion	$^{131}_{53}I$	8.04 d	β^-, γ	0.364	0.61	Treatment of hyperthyroidism or thyroid cancer
Interstitial	$^{182}_{73}Ta$	115 d	βs, γs	Wide range	Wide range	Localised treatment of cancer by the insertion of needles, tubes or wires of the radionuclide
	$^{192}_{77}Ir$	74 d	βs, γs	Wide range	Wide range	
	$^{137}_{55}Cs$	30 y	β^-, γ	0.662	0.51	

Table 27.3 (*contd*)

Application	Radio-nuclide	$t_{1/2}$	Decay mode	Gamma energy (MeV)	Max. beta energy (MeV)	Comments
Teletherapy	$^{137}_{55}Cs$	30 y	β^-, γ	0.662	0.51	External beams of γ radiation from the radionuclides is used to treat cancers
	$^{60}_{27}Co$	5.3 y	β^-, γ	1.17 1.33	0.31	
Radioimmunoassay						
	$^{125}_{53}I$	60 d	EC	0.027 0.035	—	Used to detect small quantities of hormones

Summary

In this chapter you should have learnt:

- The mechanism for alpha decay and alpha particle emission (see Sect. 27.4)
- Beta decay leading to negatron emission (see Sect. 27.5.1)
- Beta decay leading to positron emission (see Sect. 27.5.2)
- The fate of the positron after emission (see Sect. 27.5.3)
- The fact that a neutrino or an antineutrino forms part of beta emission (see Sect. 27.5.4)
- The mechanism of gamma decay and gamma ray emission (see Sect. 27.6)
- The meaning of metastable nuclei and isomeric transitions (see Sect. 27.6.1)
- The mechanism of the process of internal conversion (see Sect. 27.6.2)
- The mechanisms involved in the emission of X-rays and Auger electrons from the atoms of radionuclides (see Sect. 27.6.3)
- The mechanism of electron capture and the subsequent changes within the atom (see Sect. 27.7)
- The processes involved in nuclear fission (see Sect. 27.8)
- The use of nuclear fission in the nuclear reactor (see Sect. 27.8)
- The mechanisms for the production of artificial radionuclides (see Sect. 27.9)
- The construction and operation of the technetium generator (see Sect. 27.9.1)
- The clinical uses of radionuclides and examples of radionuclides which can be used for each purpose identified (see Sect. 27.10).

SELF-TEST

a. Discuss the conditions necessary for alpha particle emission and describe the mechanism of alpha decay. Give an example of alpha decay.

b. Discuss the conditions necessary for negatron and positron decay and give an example of each—for the purposes of this description, the emission of the neutrino and the antineutrino may be ignored.

c. Discuss gamma ray emission and explain what is meant by *metastable atoms* and *isomeric transitions*.

d. Describe the process of electron capture.

e. Describe what is meant by nuclear fission, distinguishing between spontaneous fission and neutron-activated fission.

f. With the aid of a diagram, discuss the construction and operation of a technetium generator.

g. List the desirable properties of a radionuclide to be used in medical imaging and show how $_{43}^{99}Tc^m$ fulfils these properties.

FURTHER READING

You will find further information on certain aspects of nuclear medicine in Appendix B of this text. In addition you may find sections from the following texts provide useful further reading:

Ball J L, Moore A D 1986 Essential physics for radiographers, 2nd edn. Blackwell Scientific Publications, London, ch 19

Gifford D 1984 A handbook of physics for radiologists and radiographers. John Wiley & Sons, Chichester, ch 9

Hay G A, Hughes D 1983 First year physics for radiographers. Baillière Tindall, London, ch 16

Hendee W, Ritenour R 1992 Medical imaging physics, 3rd edn. Mosby Year Book, London, ch 3

Johns H E, Cunningham J R 1983 The physics of radiology, 4th edn. Charles C Thomas, Illinois, USA, ch 3

Ohanian H C 1994 Principles of physics. W W Norton, London, ch 31

Plaut S 1993 Radiation protection in the X-ray department. Butterworth-Heinemann, Oxford, ch 12

Stockley S M 1986 A manual of radiographic equipment. Churchill Livingstone, Edinburgh, ch 18

Sumner D, Wheldon T, Watson W 1991 Radiation risks: an evaluation. The Tarragon Press, Glasgow, ch 2

Thompson M A 1994 Principles of imaging science and protection. W B Saunders, London, ch 3

Webb S (ed) 1988 The physics of medical imaging. Institute of Physics Publishing, Bristol, ch 6

Young M E J 1967 Radiological physics. Lewis, London, ch 5

PART 5

X-rays and matter

PART CONTENTS

28

The production of X-rays

28.1 AIM

The aim of this chapter is to consider the mechanisms by which X-rays are produced at the target of the X-ray tube. The concept of the X-ray spectrum will be introduced and this chapter will act as a foundation for Chapter 29 where the factors affecting the X-ray spectrum will be considered.

28.2 INTERACTIONS OF ELECTRONS WITH MATTER

In Chapter 22 we discussed the construction of the X-ray tube and the function(s) of its various components. In that chapter we stated that electrons are produced at the filament by thermionic emission, they are accelerated towards the tungsten target and, on impact with the target, they suffer sudden deceleration to produce X-rays and heat. In this chapter we will look in more detail at the processes involved at subatomic level in the target of the X-ray tube.

There are a number of ways in which high-energy electrons from the filament of the X-ray tube may lose their energy when they collide with the atoms of the target. These are:

- the loss of energy by the electrons from the filament because of interactions between them and the outer electrons surrounding the atoms of the target material (see electron 1 in Fig. 28.1)
- the loss of energy by electrons from the filament because of interactions between them and the nuclei of the atoms of the target material (see electrons 2 and 3 in Fig. 28.1)
- the loss of energy by electrons from the filament because of interactions between them and individual inner electrons of the target atoms (see electron 4 in Fig. 28.1).

The interactions between electrons and target atoms may be *elastic* or *inelastic* collisions (see Sect. 5.4) where there is conservation of *kinetic energy* for the former case only. It is also important to realise that an electron from the filament may experience many interactions (typically about 1000) before it is brought to rest within 0.25 to 0.5 mm of the target surface.

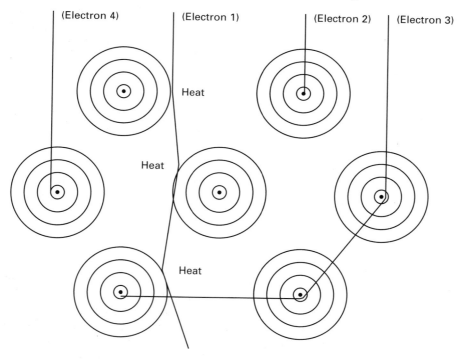

Figure 28.1 Diagrammatic representation of possible interactions between electrons from the filament and target atoms in an X-ray tube. An explanation of the interactions is given in the text.

28.3 INTERACTIONS BETWEEN ELECTRONS FROM THE FILAMENT AND THE OUTER ELECTRONS OF THE TARGET ATOMS IN THE X-RAY TUBE

As you may remember from Chapter 22, the main material of the X-ray tube target is tungsten, which has an atomic number of 74. Thus each target atom is surrounded by 74 electrons in various orbitals. These electrons have the effect of deflecting the approaching electron from the filament because of the electrostatic repulsion between them and the filament electron. Such deflections from the electron's original path are small and so the loss of kinetic energy is small. The kinetic energy lost by the electron is emitted as a photon of electromagnetic radiation. The energy of this photon is such that it falls into the infra-red part of the spectrum and so heat is produced in the target material. If we consider the statistical probability of this process occurring rather than the other two processes identified in Section 28.2, we can see that it has a very high probability of occurring. This is because the other two processes involve an interaction between either the incoming electron and the nucleus or the incoming electron and the inner orbital electrons. The area occupied by the nucleus and the inner electron orbitals is very small compared to the size of the whole tungsten atom and so an incoming electron has a much greater chance of interacting with the whole atom. For the above reasons about 95% to 99% of the energy produced at the target of the X-ray tube is in the form of heat.

28.4 INTERACTIONS BETWEEN ELECTRONS FROM THE FILAMENT AND THE NUCLEI OF THE TARGET ATOMS IN THE X-RAY TUBE

As mentioned at the beginning of this chapter, the interactions of electrons from the filament with the nuclei of the target atoms can be elastic interactions or inelastic interactions. As each of these results in a different outcome they will now be considered separately.

28.4.1 Elastic collisions with the nuclei

The electron has a relatively low mass and a negative charge while the tungsten nucleus has a larger mass (about 334 000 times that of the electron) and a positive charge (74 times that of the electron). Thus the electron is attracted to the heavier tungsten nucleus. As shown in Figure 28.2, the closer the electron travels to the nucleus the more it is deflected from its original path by the attraction of the positive nucleus. Because the mass of the electron is so tiny compared to that of the nucleus, the amount of energy it transfers to it is proportionately small. These events therefore

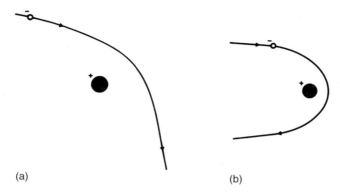

Figure 28.2 The deflection of an electron from the filament when it interacts with the nucleus of a target atom in the X-ray tube; (a) is a small deflection, and (b) is a large deflection.

serve only to produce very tortuous paths for the electrons within the tungsten, without transferring very much energy to the tungsten. The number of such events compared to the number of inelastic collisions—discussed in the next section—increases with the atomic number of the target material and so they are very frequent in tungsten.

28.4.2 Inelastic collisions with the nuclei—production of Bremsstrahlung radiation

Classical physics concluded that when a charged particle changed its velocity this *always* resulted in the emission of electromagnetic radiation. However, we have already seen that this is not the case as the electrons in the Bohr model of the atom are continuously changing their velocity (see Sect. 26.4). We have also seen in the previous section that electrons can undergo elastic collisions with the nucleus which result in no electromagnetic radiation being produced. As shown in Figure 28.2, the electron must accelerate towards the nucleus during its deflection, but despite this acceleration, in only a small percentage of cases is a quantum of electromagnetic radiation emitted. When such a quantum is emitted, the kinetic energy of the electron is suddenly reduced by an amount equal to the energy of the quantum, and so the electron is suddenly slowed down or *braked*. This is an example of an inelastic interaction since the total kinetic energy of the electron and of the nucleus is not conserved because some energy is removed by the emission of the quantum of radiation. The energy of the quantum may be in the X-ray part of the electromagnetic spectrum and the radiation is known as *braking* or *Bremsstrahlung radiation*. The exact energy of this quantum will vary and may be very small if the electron does not lose much energy in its interaction with the nucleus or it may be up to the total kinetic energy of the electron if it is involved in a direct collision with the nucleus (see electron 2 in Figure 28.1).

Note that not every electron passing close to the nucleus will emit such a photon of radiation but only those which are able to undergo a sudden loss of energy by an inelastic interaction with the nucleus.

The Bremsstrahlung process is illustrated in Figure 28.3 where the X-ray photon is emitted at the point P and the electron continues with reduced energy on the pathway shown. The probability of Bremsstrahlung radiation being produced is very small (about 1 to 5% for diagnostic X-ray tubes). The intensity of the radiation produced is related to the atomic number of the target material (Z) and the energy of the electron beam (E) by the equation:

$$I \propto ZE^2 \hspace{5cm} \text{Equation 28.1}$$

In diagnostic X-ray tubes, tungsten is used as the target material as its high atomic number (74) leads to a higher intensity of X-ray production.

The effect on the X-ray spectrum of changing the energy of the electron beam will be discussed in more detail in Chapter 29, but it is worth noting at this stage that the higher electron energies used in linear accelerators mean that there is more efficient X-ray production and that a smaller percentage of the energy is converted into heat.

If the Law Of Conservation Of Momentum (see Sect. 5.4) is applied, then, in order to conserve momentum, the greater the energy of the incident electrons, the more likely the Bremsstrahlung radiation is to be emitted in the same direction as the electrons. Thus, for low electron

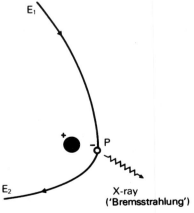

Figure 28.3   The production of Bremsstrahlung X-rays. An electron at point P suddenly loses energy by the emission of an X-ray photon. The electron continues with a reduced energy, E_2.

energy beams the X-rays are directed almost isotropically, in diagnostic X-ray tubes (medium energy range) the central ray of the X-ray beam is at right angles to the electron beam and in linear accelerators (high energy) the useful X-ray beam is transmitted forward through the anode in the same direction as the electrons.

28.5 INELASTIC COLLISIONS WITH THE ELECTRONS OF THE TARGET ATOMS—PRODUCTION OF CHARACTERISTIC RADIATION

As can be seen from Figure 28.1 (see route of electron 4), it is also possible for an electron from the filament to be involved in an inelastic collision with one of the orbital electrons of the target atoms. Such interactions are shown in more detail in Figure 28.4. Depending on the energy transferred to the orbital electron, such collisions may result either in excitation of the atom (see Fig. 28.4(a)) or ionisation of the atom (Fig. 28.4(b)). For excitation to occur, the electron must be given sufficient energy to raise it to its new orbital, whereas for ionisation the electron must be given sufficient energy to overcome its binding energy and thus be liberated from the atom. In the case of ionisation of the target atom, the electron is ejected from its orbital with a given kinetic energy and is often referred to as a *delta ray* (δ-ray). This electron may have sufficient energy to excite or ionise other atoms in its path.

The process of excitation or ionisation causes a vacancy in the electron shell involved—the K-shell in the atom shown in Figure 28.4(b). This

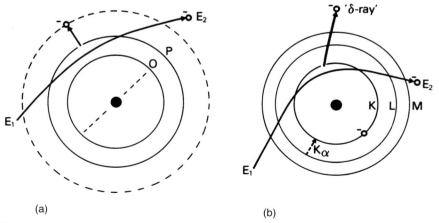

(a)   (b)

Figure 28.4 (a) Excitation, and (b) ionisation caused by the passage of an energetic electron through a tungsten atom. Both processes result in the production of heat and ionisation produces characteristic radiation (K_α radiation is shown in the diagram). E_2 is less than E_1 in both diagrams. *Note* that, for clarity, only the electron orbitals which have a direct bearing on the interaction, are shown.

vacancy is quickly filled by one of the outer electrons undergoing a quantum jump downwards to fill the vacancy and emitting a quantum of electromagnetic radiation in the process. The energy of the quantum emitted is given by:

$$E = E_1 - E_2$$ Equation 28.2

where E_1 is the energy of the electron before the jump and E_2 is the energy of the electron after the jump. As this energy varies for the same transition in different materials it is known as *characteristic radiation* as it is characteristic of the material emitting the radiation.

If we consider Figure 28.5 where a vacancy has been created in the K-shell of the atom, then the most probable jump is from the L-shell with the next probability being a jump from the M-shell followed by the probability of a jump from the N-shell. These are known as K_α, K_β, K_γ transitions and the radiation known as K_α characteristic radiation, etc. If we assume that the vacancy in the K-shell has been filled by a transition from the L-shell, there will now be a vacancy in this shell which can be filled from the M-shell or the N-shell, etc., with the emission of L_α or L_β characteristic radiation. In this way a cascade of electrons will occur with each one emitting a photon of energy given by Equation 28.2. In the diagnostic X-ray tube only the K and L characteristic radiations are of any significance as the others are absorbed by the target material or the glass envelope.

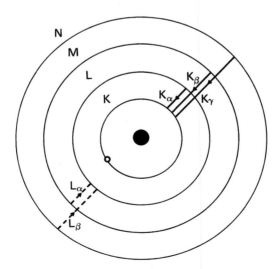

Figure 28.5   The production of characteristic radiation. The K-lines are formed by quantum jumps down to the K-shell. Also note that the energy of the K_α-line must be less than the binding energy of the K-shell. (The significance of this fact is discussed when photoelectric absorption edges are considered in Sect. 30.5.)

As well as the characteristic radiation produced, both excitation and ionisation result in the production of heat within the target—in *excitation* by the absorption of energy by the target as the electron falls back to its original orbital and in *ionisation* by the increased kinetic energy received by the tungsten atoms as they slow down the electrons ejected by the collision.

28.6 THE X-RAY SPECTRUM

So far in this chapter we have considered the production of X-ray quanta by two major mechanisms:

- Energetic electrons from the filament interact with the nuclei of target atoms and are slowed down, thus giving off energy in the form of X-ray quanta—Bremsstrahlung radiation. As we mentioned earlier, the energy of the quantum may be very small if the interaction with the nucleus is small, or it may be up to the energy of the incoming electron if this electron is brought to rest by the nucleus. All energies between the two extremes are possible and so it can be seen that the Bremsstrahlung radiation will form a continuous spectrum (see Sect. 25.5).
- Vacancies created in inner electron orbitals are filled by the electrons from orbitals further away from the nucleus making a quantum jump to fill the vacancy and giving off a photon of radiation in the process. This is the characteristic radiation from the atom. As the energy differences between specific orbitals is constant for an atom this will take the form of a series of line spectra (see Sect. 25.5).

If the overall X-ray intensity is plotted against the energy of the radiation, a summation of the two effects known as the *X-ray spectrum* is produced. Such a spectrum produced at the tungsten target of an X-ray tube is shown in Figure 28.6.

Certain important features of this spectrum are worthy of further discussion:

- The energy of the Bremsstrahlung radiation is expressed in keV and lies somewhere between zero and a maximum value. This maximum photon energy is achieved if an electron which has the maximum kinetic energy gives up all its energy to form a single photon. The value of this photon for a specific beam may be deduced as follows.

Suppose the potential difference across the X-ray tube is $100 \, kV_p$. An electron accelerated across the tube when the peak voltage is applied would have achieved a kinetic energy of 100 keV at its point of contact with the anode. If it now gives up all this energy as a single photon, the energy of the photon will be 100 keV and this will be the maximum photon energy for a tube operating at this kV_p. Similarly, for an X-ray tube

Figure 28.6   An X-ray spectrum as emitted at the anode of an X-ray tube with a tungsten target. (For an explanation of this spectrum, see the text.)

operating at 50 kV$_p$ the maximum photon energy will be 50 keV. Thus it can be seen that *the maximum photon energy is dependent on the potential difference across the tube* (kV$_p$) *but is independent of the material of the target.*

● The Bremsstrahlung radiation is a continuous spectrum. The intensity of the low-energy photons within this spectrum is decreased because of absorption of these photons by the target material—as will be seen in the next chapter, the intensity is further decreased by the filtration of the X-ray beam before it leaves the tube.

● The *average energy* of the X-ray beam is about one-third to one-half of its maximum energy—this is related to the *quality* of the X-ray beam (see Ch. 29).

● The total intensity of the beam—the *quantity of the radiation*—is given by the area under the curve.

● The energies of the K, L, M, etc. lines are always in the same position although the energy of lines from M onwards is so small that it is likely to be totally absorbed in the X-ray tube. These discrete energies form a line spectrum—the exact energy of the line is determined by Equation 28.2.

● The line spectra will not be produced unless the energy of the electron beam from the filament exceeds the binding energy of the appropriate electron shell of the atom. To produce the K-characteristic lines at a tungsten target, electrons must have an energy ≥ 69 keV and to produce L-lines electrons must have an energy ≥ 11 keV. In practice this means that

K-lines are not produced when the potential across the tube is less than $70 \, \mathrm{kV_p}$.

In the spectrograph in Figure 28.6 we have considered the intensity of the radiation plotted against the photon energy. It is sometimes useful to calculate the wavelength of the radiation rather than know its photon energy. As you may remember from Section 25.3.2 the photon energy and its associated wavelength are related by Planck's Equation (see Equation 25.6). From this we can see that the maximum photon energy corresponds to the minimum wavelength. Since the numerical value of the maximum photon energy is the same as the $\mathrm{kV_p}$, we can calculate the minimum wavelength from the equation:

$$\lambda_{min} = \frac{1.24}{\mathrm{kV_p}}$$

Equation 28.3

Insight

Although we have explained the maximum and minimum energies in the continuous spectrum, we have not explained the shape—the distribution of photon energies—of the spectrum. This is quite a complicated process and involves consideration of the chances of photons of various energies being produced, the direction of the radiation emitted and the chances of this radiation being absorbed or scattered within the target.

Consider an ultra-thin target which is constructed in such a way that there are only a few layers of target atoms and so incoming electrons from the filament are only likely to have one interaction and there is negligible attenuation by the target of the radiation produced. In such circumstances the number of photons of each energy produced will be related to the statistical chance of an electron losing that amount of energy in its Bremsstrahlung interaction with the nucleus. As the nucleus of the atom is relatively small compared to the whole atom, the chance of an electron from the filament colliding with it and so producing a maximum-energy photon is equally small. The chance of a filament electron getting close to the nucleus is statistically larger and so there should be more photons produced which have less than the maximum energy compared with the number which have the maximum energy. Thus as we increase the diameter of the circle around the nucleus within which we consider electrons interacting to produce X-ray photons so we increase the statistical possibility of producing photons with that energy—as these electrons are further from the nucleus of the atom, the energy of the photon produced would be smaller.

The production of lower-energy photons is further increased in a target with a finite thickness if we still ignore any radiation attenuation by the target. A target of finite thickness—normally a few millimetres—can really be considered as a series of ultra-thin targets one on top of the other. Because of this, the energy of the electrons reaching the second ultra-thin layer is less due to their energy loss in the first layer—this again favours the production of lower-energy X-ray photons. Thus the deeper we go into the target, the lower the predicted energy of the photons produced.

Because of the two processes described, we would expect the number of photons produced to increase as the photon energy decreases. This is shown by the broken line in Figure 28.7.

In an X-ray tube the target is a few millimetres thick and so we must consider X-rays being produced below the surface of the target. As these photons leave the target they are attenuated by the target atoms. Both scattering and absorption (see Ch. 30) favour attenuation of the lower-energy photons. Thus lower-energy photons are heavily attenuated by the target atoms. The attenuation of the lower-energy photons is

Figure 28.7   A comparison between the continuous spectrum produced if attenuation by the target material is ignored and the actual spectrum produced from a tube target.

increased because they are more likely to be produced deeper in the target material and so have further to travel through the target. This attenuation of the photons produced by the target material produces a continuous spectrum similar to the solid line in Figure 28.7.

The effect of various parameters on the spectrum of radiation emitted from the X-ray tube will form the material of the next chapter.

Summary

In this chapter you should have learnt:

- The three major mechanisms by which electrons from the filament of the X-ray tube may lose energy when they interact with the atoms of the target (see Sect. 28.2)
- The result of interactions between electrons from the filament of the X-ray tube and the outer electrons around atoms of the target material (see Sect. 28.3)
- The result of elastic interactions between electrons from the filament and the nuclei of atoms of the tube target (see Sect. 28.4.1)
- How inelastic collisions between electrons from the filament and the nuclei of atoms of the target of the X-ray tube result in the production of Bremsstrahlung radiation (see Sect. 28.4.2)
- How inelastic collisions between electrons from the filament and the orbital electrons of target atoms may result in the production of characteristic radiation (see Sect. 28.5)
- The graphical representation of the X-ray spectrum and the significant features of this graph (see Sect. 28.6).

SELF-TEST

a. With the aid of a diagram identify the principal interactions which cause the electrons from the filament to lose energy when they interact with the target atoms of the X-ray tube.

b. Describe the mechanism by which Bremsstrahlung radiation is produced at the target of the X-ray tube.

c. Describe the production of characteristic radiation at the target of the X-ray tube and list the conditions necessary for characteristic radiation to be produced.

d. With the aid of a line graph, describe the X-ray spectrum produced at the target of an X-ray tube operating at 100 kV_p. Give an equation to show the relationship between the maximum photon energy and the kV_p across the X-ray tube.

FURTHER READING

You will find that Chapter 29 of this text deals with further detail of the factors which affect the spectrum of X-rays from the X-ray tube. In addition you may find the undernoted chapters from the following texts provide useful further reading:

Ball J L, Moore A D 1986 Essential physics for radiographers, 2nd edn. Blackwell Scientific Publications, London, ch 15

Curry T S et al 1990 Christensen's Physics of diagnostic radiology. Lea & Febinger, London, ch 2

Gifford D 1984 A handbook of physics for radiologists and radiographers. John Wiley & Sons, Chichester, ch 10

Hay G A, Hughes D 1983 First year physics for radiographers. Baillière Tindall, London, ch 10

Hendee W, Ritenour R 1992 Medical imaging physics, 3rd edn. Mosby Year Book, London, ch 5

Johns H E, Cunningham J R 1983 The physics of radiology, 4th edn. Charles C Thomas, Illinois, USA, ch 2

Merideth W J, Massey J B 1977 Fundamental physics of radiology. John Wright, Bristol, ch V

Ohanian H C 1994 Principles of physics. W W Norton, London, chs 28, 31

Thompson M A 1994 Principles of imaging science and protection. W B Saunders, London, ch 3

Webb S (ed) 1988 The physics of medical imaging. Institute of Physics Publishing, Bristol, ch 2

Young M E J 1967 Radiological physics. Lewis, London, ch 3

Factors affecting the X-ray beam quality and quantity

29.1 AIM

The aim of this chapter is to consider the various factors which have an influence on the quantity and/or the quality of the beam of radiation from the X-ray tube.

29.2 INTRODUCTION

In the previous chapter we considered the mechanisms by which X-rays were produced at the anode of the X-ray tube. In this chapter we will consider the various factors which influence the *quantity* and/or the *quality* of the X-ray beam. Before we look at this in any more detail, it is first important to ensure that we understand the meaning of the terms *quantity* and *quality* as applied to a beam of X-radiation.

Definitions

The *quantity* of radiation in an X-ray beam is a measure of the number of photons in the beam. The terms *quantity* and *exposure* are often interchanged in radiography as the higher the quantity or amount of radiation the greater the exposure to a structure. In fact, probably the simplest method of comparing the quantity of two beams of radiation is to compare the exposure received by a structure. As we shall see in Chapter 33, the exposure is measured using the unit of *air kerma*. As the quantity of radiation increases so does the *intensity* of the beam—the intensity is the energy passing through unit area in unit time.

The *quality* of a beam of X-rays is a measure of its penetrating power. As we saw in Section 28.6, the quality of the beam is related to its average photon energy. In Sections 4.7 and 4.8 we saw that a monochromatic beam of radiation is exponentially absorbed by a uniform medium and, so, the penetrating power of two beams may be compared by comparing their half-value thickness—the higher the value of the half-value thickness the more penetrating the beam. Although the beam of X-rays from the tube is not monochromatic, but has a continuous spectrum over a wide range of energies, the half-value layer is a useful way of comparing the penetrating power of X-ray beams.

29.3 THE EFFECT OF mA ON THE X-RAY BEAM

If the current through the X-ray tube (mA) is doubled, for example, the number of electrons flowing across the tube in unit time is doubled. If all the other factors remain unchanged, each electron will have the same chance of creating X-ray photons and so the number of photons of each energy produced per unit time will be doubled. If the mA is halved, the same argument can be used to show that the number of X-ray photons of each energy is also halved. Thus we can say that the quantity of the X-ray

Figure 29.1 The effect of the mA on the X-ray spectrum. *Note* that the *quantity* of the radiation changes—as shown by the alteration of the area under each curve—but the *quality* of the radiation is unaltered—as shown by the maximum photon energy and the peak photon energy being at the same energy for each graph.

beam per unit time (or the beam intensity) is directly proportional to the mA through the tube.

$$I \propto mA \qquad\qquad \text{Equation 29.1}$$

The effect on the X-ray beam of altering the mA is shown in Figure 29.1. Note that the area under the graph for 200 mA is half of the area under the graph for 400 mA. The maximum photon energy and the minimum photon energy are the same in each case and the average photon energy remains unaltered.

Thus we can say that the mA selected for an exposure affects the quantity of the X-ray beam but does not affect the quality of the beam—an increase in the mA will produce an increase in the quantity of radiation from the target.

29.4 THE EFFECT OF kV$_P$ ON THE X-RAY BEAM

The kV_p across the X-ray tube influences the force of attraction experienced by an electron released by the filament as it moves towards the anode. Thus, if the kV_p is increased, then the kinetic energy of the electron at the point when it starts to interact with the target will be increased. As we saw in Section 28.4.2, the efficiency of X-ray production by Bremsstrahlung is proportional to E^2 and so this improved efficiency means that:

$$I \propto kV_p^2 \qquad\qquad \text{Equation 29.2}$$

As we already discussed in Section 28.4.2, increasing the kV_p will also increase the energy of the maximum-energy photons in the beam—if the kV_p is 50 then the maximum photon energy is 50 keV and if the kV_p is 100 then the maximum photon energy is 100 keV. As the average photon energy is approximately 30 to 50% of the maximum photon energy, increasing the maximum photon energy will also increase the average photon energy.

As mentioned earlier, increasing the kV_p will increase the kinetic energy of the electrons from the filament when they reach the target and so this may mean that characteristic radiation is seen on the higher kV_p spectrum but not at the lower value—at 100 kV_p the electrons reaching the target have energies up to 100 keV and so can displace K-shell electrons in tungsten, whereas at 50 kV_p the 50 keV electrons have insufficient energy to displace a K-shell electron from the tungsten atom.

The spectrum produced at 100 kV_p and at 50 kV_p is shown in Figure 29.2 where the changes mentioned above can be identified.

Thus we can say that the kV_p selected for an exposure affects both the quantity and the quality of the X-ray beam produced—an increase in the kV_p will produce an increase in the quantity and the quality of the radiation from the target.

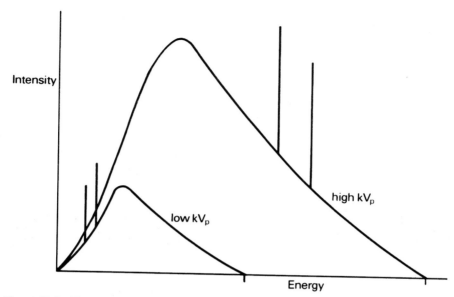

Figure 29.2 The effect of kV$_p$ on the X-ray spectrum. *Note* that the kV$_p$ affects both the *quantity* and the *quality* of the radiation beam. Also note that the lower of the two curves is unable to produce *K*-characteristic radiation although both curves can produce *L*-lines.

29.5 THE EFFECT OF THE TARGET MATERIAL ON THE X-RAY BEAM

As mentioned in Section 28.4.2, the atomic number of the target material has an effect on the X-ray beam from the tube. The higher the atomic number of the target material the more positive the nucleus of the target atom and so the more it attracts the electrons from the filament which pass close to it. Thus the production of X-rays by the Bremsstrahlung process is more efficient and the intensity of the beam is increased. The maximum and minimum photon energies in the beam are not affected by the target material.

The target material also affects the characteristic radiation produced. The energies of the characteristic radiations from a tungsten and a molybdenum target are shown in Table 29.1.

Table 29.1 Comparison of characteristic radiation energies produced from a tungsten target and a molybdenum target

	Energy of K_α characteristic radiation	Energy of L_α characteristic radiation
Tungsten	59.32 keV	8.39 keV
Molybdenum	17.48 keV	2.22 keV

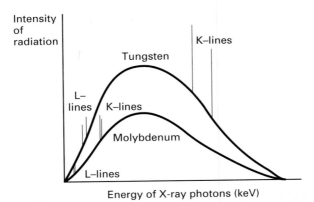

Figure 29.3   The effect of the target material on the X-ray spectrum. *Note* that the lower atomic number of molybdenum means that there is a reduction in the *quantity* of the radiation but the *quality* of the Bremsstrahlung radiation is not affected. The *characteristic radiation* is at a lower photon energy for the target with the lower atomic number.

Thus, although the target material does not affect the quality of the Bremsstrahlung radiation, it does affect the energy of the characteristic radiation and this does have some effect on the overall quality of the X-ray beam—this effect may be enhanced by filtering the radiation with the same material as the target (this will be considered further in Ch. 30 when absorption mechanisms are discussed).

The radiation spectrum from a tungsten and a molybdenum target are shown in Figure 29.3.

29.6 THE EFFECT OF RECTIFICATION ON THE X-RAY BEAM

The type of high-tension rectification of the X-ray generator affects the spectrum of radiation produced at the target of the X-ray tube. This is because of the changing energy of the electron beam striking the target each half-cycle. If we consider full-wave rectification with no capacitor smoothing as produced by the two-pulse generator (see Sect. 20.4), then the potential across the tube varies from zero to the kV_p each half-cycle. Thus the energy of the electrons striking the target varies from zero to a keV with a numerical value equal to that of the kV_p. The maximum photon energy at differing stages in the half-cycle will vary across the same range as the electron energies. We can see how this affects the spectrum produced if we consider Figure 29.4(a) and consider the spectra produced at point B in the voltage waveform and at point C. The time-averaged spectrum for full-wave rectification is shown in Figure 29.4(b). Now consider a constant potential being applied to the X-ray tube during the entire exposure. This would be the same as if voltage B is applied for the whole exposure and so the spectrum for voltage B is labelled in Figure 29.4(b) as the spectrum from a constant-potential unit. Note that for constant potential, the area under the graph is increased and the value of the photon energy of the average photon is also increased.

Thus we can say that the rectification—or the type of X-ray generator—affects both the quantity and the quality of the X-ray beam produced—the nearer the voltage across the tube is to a constant potential the higher the quantity and the quality of the radiation produced at the target.

(a)

(b)

Figure 29.4 (a) The spectrum of radiation produced if a constant potential of value *B* or *C* were applied across the X-ray tube; (b) shows the effect of rectification on the X-ray spectrum where the constant-potential generator produces radiation of higher *quantity* and higher *quality*.

29.7 THE EFFECT OF FILTRATION ON THE X-RAY BEAM

In all the discussion so far we have considered the beam of X-radiation produced at the target of the X-ray tube. Before this radiation can be utilised in radiography or radiotherapy, it must first leave the tube. In leaving the tube the radiation beam must first pass through the glass of the tube insert, the oil in the housing and finally the window of the housing—plus any additional filtration—and it is filtered at each stage of this process. Thus, to consider the beam which will interact with the patient, we need to consider the effect of filtration on the spectrum of radiation produced at the tube target.

Spectrum A in Figure 29.5 shows the distribution of energies emitted from the tube target. This would be the spectrum of the radiation before it leaves the glass envelope of the tube. As we will discuss in Chapter 30, when a beam of radiation passes through any medium, the beam is attenuated by the processes of absorption and scattering. We will see that the lower the photon energy the higher the chance of it being absorbed or scattered. So the passage of the X-ray beam through the glass envelope, the oil and the exit window of the shield results in selective attenuation of the lower-energy photons. Since this filtration is inherent to the tube

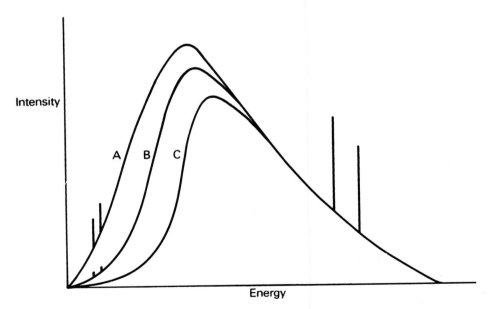

Figure 29.5 The effect of filtration on the X-ray spectrum. Graph A represents the spectrum produced at the target of the X-ray tube; graph B shows how this spectrum is modified because of the inherent filtration of the tube; and graph C shows how the spectrum is modified because of the total filtration. *Note* that filtration causes a reduction in the *quantity* of the radiation but an increase in the *quality*.

construction it is known as the *inherent filtration* of the X-ray tube. The spectrum emitted after the inherent filtration is shown as spectrum B in Figure 29.5.

This beam still contains a significant number of low-energy photons. If these were allowed to interact with the tissues of a patient, they would be absorbed by superficial tissues and so would contribute to the patient dose but would make no contribution to the radiograph—or to the tumour treatment in the case of radiotherapy. The amount of low-energy photons in the spectrum can be significantly reduced by incorporating additional filtration into the beam, near the exit port of the tube, before it interacts with the patient's tissues. Such a spectrum is shown as graph C in Figure 29.5. The inherent filtration of diagnostic X-ray tubes is usually expressed in *mm of aluminium equivalent*, i.e. the inherent filtration is equivalent to the filtration of the beam achieved by the stated number of millimetres of aluminium. The inherent filtration of most diagnostic X-ray tubes is between 0.5 mm and 1.0 mm of aluminium equivalent. The total filtration in the beam is the sum of the inherent filtration and the additional filtration. This total filtration is between 1.5 mm and 2.5 mm depending upon the maximum kV_p at which the tube is designed to operate.

As can be seen from the graphs in Figure 29.5, filtration affects both the quantity and the quality of the X-ray beam—the greater the thickness of the filtration in the X-ray beam the less the quantity but the greater the quality of the X-ray beam emerging from the X-ray tube.

Insight

Aluminium has a low atomic number (13) and so is able to absorb many of the low-energy X-ray photons in a beam of diagnostic energy, by photoelectric absorption (see Ch. 30). High-energy X-ray photons have a low probability of being absorbed or scattered by the aluminium and so are relatively unaffected by the filtration. This makes aluminium the ideal material for filtration of diagnostic energy X-ray beams.

The radiation beam from the therapy X-ray tube has a much higher average energy than the diagnostic beam. This beam is often hardened—low-energy radiations are removed—by the use of a composite filter. An example of this is when the beam is first filtered through copper ($Z = 29$) and then is further filtered through an aluminium filter. The copper is responsible for the initial filtration but transmits some low-energy radiation due to the photoelectric absorption edge of copper. The copper also produces low-energy characteristic radiation as a result of photoelectric absorption in the copper atoms. The function of the aluminium filter is to absorb the radiation transmitted through the copper because of the K-shell photoelectric absorption edge of copper and also to remove the characteristic radiation produced by the photoelectric absorption in the copper. These concepts will be further discussed in the next chapter.

29.8 SUMMARY OF THE FACTORS AFFECTING THE QUANTITY AND QUALITY OF THE X-RAY BEAM

The factors which affect the quantity and/or quality of the beam of X-radiation emerging from a tube are summarised in Table 29.2.

Table 29.2   Factors affecting the quantity and quality of the X-ray beam

Factor	Effect on the quantity of the X-ray beam	Effect on the quality of the X-ray beam
Increase in the tube current (mA)	Produces an increase in the quantity of radiation directly proportional to the increase in mA	The quality of the radiation from the tube is unaffected by the tube current
Increase in the potential difference (kV_p) across the X-ray tube	Produces an increase in the quantity of radiation produced at the target proportional to the kV_p^2	An increase in the kV_p produces an increase in the average energy of the photons in the X-ray beam and so an increase in the beam quality
Target material	An increase in the atomic number of the target material will produce an increase in the quantity of radiation produced directly proportional to the change in the atomic number	A change in the atomic number will produce no change in the quality of the beam produced by the Bremsstrahlung process. A higher atomic number will produce characteristic radiation of higher energy and, if this is in significant amounts, it may increase the quality of the overall spectrum
Rectification	The closer the voltage waveform across the X-ray tube is to a constant potential the greater the quantity of radiation produced	The closer the voltage waveform across the X-ray tube is to a constant potential the higher the quality of radiation produced
Filtration	Filtration reduces the quantity of radiation emerging from the X-ray tube. The reduction is related to the thickness and the atomic number of the filter	Filtration improves the quality of the radiation from an X-ray tube by the selective removal of low-energy photons

Summary

In this chapter you should have learnt:

- The meaning of the terms *quantity* and *quality* as applied to the X-ray beam (see Sect. 29.2)
- The effect of the current through the X-ray tube (mA) on the quantity of the X-ray beam produced (see Sect. 29.3)
- The effect of the potential difference across the X-ray tube (kV_p) on the quantity and the quality of the X-ray beam produced (see Sect. 29.4)
- The effect of the atomic number of the target material on the quantity of the radiation produced and on the characteristic radiation from the target (see Sect. 29.5)
- The effect of the voltage waveform applied to the X-ray tube (rectification) on the quantity and the quality of the X-ray beam produced (see Sect. 29.6)
- The effect of filtration on the quantity and the quality of the radiation beam emerging from the X-ray tube (see Sect. 29.7).

SELF-TEST

a. What is meant by the terms *quality* and *quantity* when used to describe an X-ray beam?

b. With the aid of a graph, discuss the effect of the tube current (mA) on the spectrum of radiation from the X-ray tube.

c. With the aid of a graph, discuss the effect of the potential difference across the X-ray tube (kV$_p$) on the spectrum of radiation from the tube.

d. With the aid of a graph, discuss the effect of the target material on the spectrum of radiation from the tube.

e. With the aid of a graph, discuss the effect of the high-tension rectification on the spectrum of radiation from the tube.

f. With the aid of a graph, discuss the effect of filtration on the spectrum of radiation from the tube.

FURTHER READING

Ball J L, Moore A D 1986 Essential physics for radiographers, 2nd edn. Blackwell Scientific Publications, London, chs 15, 16
Carter P H 1994 Chesneys' Equipment for student radiographers. Blackwell Scientific Publications, London, chs 2, 3
Curry T S et al 1990 Christensen's Physics of diagnostic radiology. Lea & Febinger, London, chs 2, 6
Gifford D 1984 A handbook of physics for radiologists and radiographers. John Wiley & Sons, Chichester, chs 10, 11
Hay G A, Hughes D 1983 First year physics for radiographers. Baillière Tindall, London, ch 10
Hendee W, Ritenour R 1992 Medical imaging physics, 3rd edn. Mosby Year Book, London, chs 5, 6
Hill D R (ed) 1975 Principles of diagnostic X-ray apparatus. Macmillan Press, London, ch 4
Johns H E, Cunningham J R 1983 The physics of radiology, 4th edn. Charles C Thomas, Illinois, USA, ch 2
Merideth W J, Massey J B 1977 Fundamental physics of radiology. John Wright, Bristol, ch V
Ohanian H C 1994 Principles of physics. W W Norton, London, chs 28, 31
Stockley S M 1986 A manual of radiographic equipment. Churchill Livingstone, Edinburgh, ch 8
Thompson M A 1994 Principles of imaging science and protection. W B Saunders, London, ch 9
Webb S (ed) 1988 The physics of medical imaging. Institute of Physics Publishing, Bristol, ch 2

Interactions of X-rays with matter

30.1 AIM

The aim of this chapter is to introduce the reader to the interaction processes which may occur when radiation photons interact with matter. The factors which influence such interaction processes will be discussed. An understanding of the processes is important both for consideration of the production of the radiograph and in the consideration of the biological effects of radiation on tissue.

30.2 OUTLINE OF POSSIBLE INTERACTIONS

When a beam of X-rays interacts with a medium, e.g. an area of patient tissue, there are a number of possible interactions between the photons and

Photon A   Photon C   Photon B

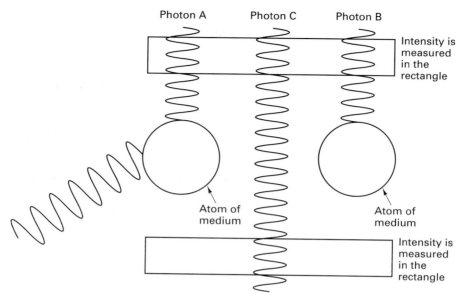

Figure 30.1 Mechanisms of interaction of X-ray photons with matter. Photon A is *scattered*, photon B is *absorbed* and photon C is *transmitted*. *Note* that the number of photons passing through the lower rectangle is less than the number passing through the upper rectangle and so *attenuation* has taken place.

the atoms of the medium. These are outlined in Figure 30.1. If we consider photon (A) we can see that this interacts with an atom of the medium and is deflected from its path—this deflection may or may not be accompanied by a loss of photon energy. This process is known as *scattering*. Photon (B), on the other hand, interacts with an atom of the medium and loses all of its energy to the atom. This process is known as *absorption*. The third photon, photon (C), passes through the material without interacting with any of the atoms. If we measure the intensity of the radiation in a given area before it interacts with the medium and again in a similar area after the interactions, we find that there is a lower intensity of radiation after passing through the medium—*the beam of radiation has been attenuated* (see Sect. 4.7).

Thus we can say:

When a beam of radiation passes through a medium it is attenuated by the processes of absorption and scattering.

The reactions considered above involve an interaction between a photon and an orbiting electron rather than between a photon and the nucleus of the atom—this will be discussed in more detail in the rest of this chapter—and so for an interaction to occur a photon must pass close to the electron orbitals of the atom with which it is capable of interacting. Thus we can consider the atoms in a medium as targets which, if hit, will attenuate a photon from the primary radiation beam.

30.2.1 Probability and cross-sections

The probability of an X-ray photon interacting with a *particular atom* is low, but the very large number of atoms even in a small volume of a solid substance makes the probability of a photon interacting with *some atom* very much greater. In Figure 30.2, a beam of X-rays of area A is incident upon a medium whose atoms appear to the beam to have an area of a. This area is called the *cross-section* of the atom to a particular type of radiation, a typical area being 1.5×10^{-28} m^2. If an X-ray photon hits one of the atoms, it is either absorbed or scattered from the primary beam.

Note that the area a is not the true size of the atom but is the apparent area of the atom likely to interact with the X-ray beam. The value of a depends on a number of things including the atomic number of the material and the energy of the X-ray photon.

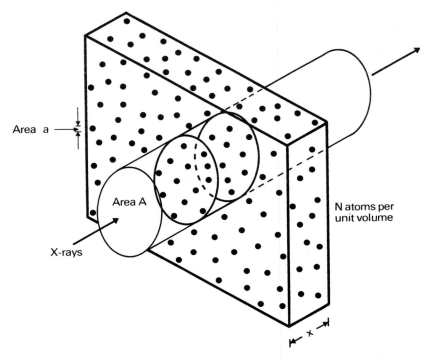

Figure 30.2 Consideration of the area of individual atoms as part of the total irradiated area. If any of the X-ray photons passing through area A hits an atom (area a) then the photon is removed from the beam. As fewer photons will exit from the medium than entered the same area, the beam is said to be attenuated. For further explanation, see the text.

The probability of an interaction occurring can be predicted by dividing the total area of the atoms within the irradiated area by the size of this area. If we consider Figure 30.2 and take it that there are N atoms per unit volume of the material, then the number of atoms in the irradiated cylinder of cross-sectional area A is $N \times A \times x$. Thus the total area of the atoms in the irradiated area is $a(N \times Ax)$ or $aNAx$.

$$\text{The probability of an interaction} = \frac{aNAx}{A}$$

$$= aNx \qquad \text{Equation 30.1}$$

30.2.2 The total linear attenuation coefficient (μ)

As we discussed in Section 4.7, a parallel beam of monoenergetic radiation will undergo exponential attenuation as it passes through a uniform medium. The intensity of the incident beam (I_0) and the intensity after a thickness x are given by the equation:

$$I_x = I_0 e^{-\mu x} \qquad \text{Equation 30.2}$$

where μ is the *total linear attenuation coefficient*. If we now consider Equations 30.1 and 30.2, it can be seen that as the probability of an interaction increases (aNx) the linear attenuation coefficient (μ) will also increase. The total linear coefficient may be defined:

Definition

The *total linear attenuation coefficient*, μ, is the fraction of the X-rays removed from a beam per unit thickness of the attenuating medium.

30.2.3 The total mass attenuation coefficient (μ/ρ)

As we have seen from Equation 30.1, the probability of an interaction between an X-ray photon and a medium containing N atoms is proportional to N. If we consider the medium shown in Figure 30.2 and take a situation where it is heated until it has expanded to a thickness of $2x$, then the number of atoms in the thickness x will be $N/2$ and the linear attenuation coefficient (μ) will also be halved. As the number of atoms per unit volume has halved, the density of the material (ρ) will also have halved. However, the ratio μ/ρ will be the same in both cases. This ratio μ/ρ is known as the *total mass attenuation coefficient* and is defined:

Definition

The *total mass attenuation coefficient*, μ/ρ, is the fraction of the X-rays removed from a beam of unit cross-sectional area by unit mass of the medium.

Insight

Note the use of the term *total* in both of the above coefficients. This is because there is a mass attenuation coefficient due to each of the attenuating processes and so the total linear attenuation coefficient is the sum of the individual linear attenuation coefficients and the total mass attenuation coefficient is the sum of the individual mass attenuation coefficients. Thus:

$$\mu = \tau + \sigma + \pi \qquad \qquad \text{Equation 30.3}$$

where μ is the total linear attenuation coefficient, τ is the linear attenuation coefficient due to the photoelectric effect, σ is the linear attenuation coefficient due to Compton scattering and π is the linear attenuation due to pair production. Similarly:

$$\frac{\mu}{\rho} = \frac{\tau}{\rho} + \frac{\sigma}{\rho} + \frac{\pi}{\rho} \qquad \qquad \text{Equation 30.4}$$

where μ/ρ is the total mass attenuation coefficient, τ/ρ is the mass attenuation coefficient due to the photoelectric effect, σ/ρ is the mass attenuation coefficient due to Compton scattering and π/ρ is the mass attenuation due to pair production.

If we wish to calculate the amount of radiation which would pass through a given *length* of a material, then we would use the linear attenuation coefficient. In most other cases the mass attenuation coefficient would be used as this is unaffected by the state of the medium—it may be solid, liquid or gas as long as the changes in density are taken into account. Thus if we wish to consider the effect of a change, for instance, of photon energy on the transmitted beam, this type of calculation would be undertaken using the mass attenuation coefficient.

The following sections of this chapter will consider the effect on the mass attenuation coefficient of the different types of X-ray interactions and of different attenuating materials. An understanding of these is fundamental to consideration of the formation of the radiograph (see Ch. 32).

30.3 ATTENUATION AND ABSORPTION

The four interaction processes described in the rest of this chapter involve *attenuation* since the intensity of the primary X-ray beam is reduced as a result of each process. In some of the processes, energy is transferred from the photons in the X-ray beam to the atoms of the medium and so *absorption* is said to have taken place. Thus an absorption process must involve the transfer of energy from the photons to the atoms of the material.

In other processes, the photon is deflected from its original path and so is said to be *scattered*. This may involve no transfer of energy to the medium (see coherent or elastic scatter) or it may involve deflection of the photon and a transfer of energy to the medium (see Compton scattering).

As we have already noted, attenuation consists of both absorption and scattering and the contribution of each of the individual processes to the whole is shown in Table 30.1.

Table 30.1 Contribution of each of the attenuation processes to absorption and scatter

Process	Contribution to absorption coefficient	Contribution to scatter
Elastic (coherent) scattering	No contribution to absorption coefficient as no energy is absorbed permanently by the medium	Makes a small contribution to the total scatter in medical radiography
Photoelectric absorption	Usually the energy of the photon is completely absorbed and so this process makes a contribution to the total absorption coefficient	No scattering of the photon occurs as part of the photoelectric process
Compton scattering	Some of the energy of the photon is transferred to the medium during the scattering process and so contributes to the absorption coefficient	This is the major source of scatter in medical radiography
Pair production	Depending on the energy of the photon this process produces partial or complete absorption	This process produces no scattering of the primary beam photons

As can be seen from the table, the *total mass absorption coefficient* will be composed of the mass absorption coefficients from each of the attenuation processes. This may be defined as follows:

Definition

The *total mass absorption coefficient* is the fraction of the energy contained in the X-ray beam which is absorbed per unit mass of the irradiated medium.

30.4 ELASTIC (COHERENT) SCATTERING

When the energy of a photon is considerably less than the binding energies of orbiting electrons of the atoms of the attenuator, the photon may be deflected from its path with no loss of energy after it has interacted with one of the electrons. This process is known as elastic scattering or coherent scattering (sometimes also known as classical scattering or Rayleigh scattering).

In this process the incoming photon interacts with an electron and raises its energy but does not give it sufficient energy to become excited or ionised. The electron then returns to its previous energy level by the emission of a photon which is equal in energy to the incoming photon but is in a different direction—hence scattering has occurred. The photon is scattered predominantly in the forward direction, because elastic scattering cannot occur if the recoil experienced by the atom as a whole during the scattering process is sufficient to produce excitation or ionisation. There is no *absorption* since no energy has been given permanently to the material and the *attenuation*, although present, is small since the majority of the photons are only scattered through a small angle. This is particularly so if the energy of the photon is higher than 100 eV and the atomic number of the attenuator is relatively low. The factors affecting the mass attenuation coefficient due to elastic scattering are shown in Equation 30.5.

$$\frac{\sigma_{coh}}{\rho} \propto \frac{Z^2}{E} \qquad\qquad \text{Equation 30.5}$$

where σ_{coh}/ρ is the mass attenuation coefficient due to elastic scattering, Z is the atomic number of the attenuator and E is the photon energy.

In medical radiography, the effect of elastic scattering can be largely ignored since the average atomic number of tissue is low (approximately 7.4) and the photon energy is too high to allow significant elastic scatter.

Elastic scattering may occur as a result of a photon interacting with the nucleus of an atom of the attenuator but the effect is even less and so may safely be ignored in medical radiography.

Insight

In X-ray diffraction studies of crystals it is the elastic scattering which is responsible for the coherent 'reflections' from the various atomic planes within the crystal lattice. Low-energy, monoenergetic X-rays are used for this purpose but only a small percentage are able to take part in the elastic scattering process.

30.5 PHOTOELECTRIC ABSORPTION

The previous section has shown that elastic scattering has little significance for radiography except at extremely low photon energies. The process of photoelectric absorption, which we will now discuss, is important even at very low energies and continues to be important at the photon energies found in the typical X-ray spectrum for diagnostic radiography.

In photoelectric absorption, the X-ray photon is involved in an *inelastic* collision with an orbiting electron of an atom of the absorber. The photon gives up all its energy to the electron (and thus disappears) and the electron is ejected from the atom. As ejection of the electron from the atom is a necessary part of the process, photoelectric absorption can only take place if the photon energy is equal to, or greater than, the binding energy of the electron.

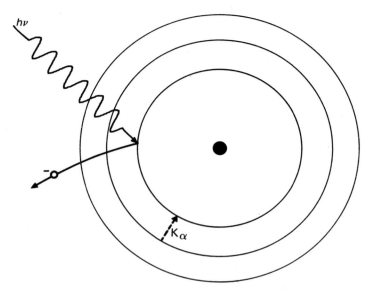

Figure 30.3 The process of photoelectric absorption and the subsequent emission of a quantum of characteristic radiation. The incoming photon (*hv*) is absorbed by the *K*-shell electron which is then displaced from that shell. The vacancy is filled from the *L*-shell with the emission of K_α characteristic radiation.

The process of photoelectric absorption is shown schematically in Figure 30.3, where it is assumed that the X-ray photon of energy *hv* ejects an electron from the *K*-shell of the atom. Some of the energy of the photon is used in overcoming the binding energy of the electron and the rest is given to the electron as kinetic energy. If we assume that the electron has a binding energy of *B*, then the kinetic energy after ejection (it is then referred to as a *photoelectron*) is (*hv* − *B*). The vacancy thus created in the *K*-shell will be filled by electrons in orbitals further from the nucleus performing a series of quantum jumps downwards, producing characteristic radiation (see Sect. 28.5) and the possible emission of Auger electrons (see Sect. 27.6.3) from orbitals further out from the nucleus. As you may remember from Section 28.5, the energy of the characteristic radiation is equal to the difference in energy of the electron before and after the quantum jump. In the case of X-ray photons interacting with atoms of body tissue, this energy difference is very small (normally $2 - 4 \times 10^{-3}$ eV) and so is in the infra-red part of the electromagnetic spectrum.

The probability of a photoelectric interaction occurring at a particular shell depends on the binding energy of the electrons in the shell and the energy of the incoming photon. The probability is zero when the energy of the photon is less than the binding energy of the electron; it is greatest when the photon energy is equal to the binding energy and thereafter decreases rapidly with increasing photon energy. A graph of the mass

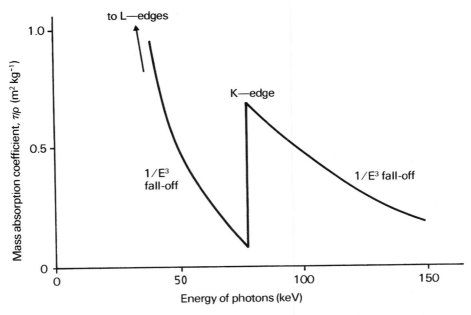

Figure 30.4   The mass absorption coefficient for the photoelectric effect in lead and its variation with photon energy.

absorption coefficient for photoelectric absorption in lead is shown in Figure 30.4 to illustrate these points. The outer orbitals of the atom are affected by the lower photon energies, only to have a reducing absorption as the photon energy increases. When the photon energy reaches the binding energy of the orbital then electrons in that orbital can take part in photoelectric absorption, thus producing a sudden increase in the amount of absorption. Such an increase is shown for the K-shell electrons of the lead atom in Figure 30.4. This sudden increase is known as an *absorption edge* and so Figure 30.4 shows the K absorption edge for the lead atom. Between the absorption edges the mass attenuation coefficient due to the photoelectric effect (τ/ρ) is approximately proportional to $1/E^3$.

Insight

A knowledge of the position of the absorption edges for a material is of importance in radiography in at least two areas.

   • As you may remember from Section 28.5, characteristic radiation is produced when an electron is ejected from an orbital and its place is taken by an electron from an outer orbital. The energy of the characteristic radiation is equal to the energy difference between the two orbitals (in tungsten this is around 59.3 keV). The K-shell binding energy for tungsten is 69.1 keV and so the K-shell absorption edge will appear at this level. As the characteristic radiation has an energy less than this, it will not be heavily absorbed. Thus it can be said that *metallic filters are relatively transparent to their own*

characteristic radiation. This is utilised in the design of the mammography tube; here the radiation is produced at a molybdenum target and is then filtered through a molybdenum filter.
- As we can see from Figure 30.4, photons which have an energy just above the absorption edge are heavily absorbed. When we use a positive contrast agent we wish this to absorb radiation so that we can identify certain structures (e.g. barium sulphate can be used to outline the stomach in a barium meal). The maximum absorption difference (and hence the maximum contrast) between a contrast agent and the surrounding structures will be produced when the photon energy is equal to or just above the absorption edge of the contrast agent.

30.5.1 Photoelectric absorption, attenuation and absorption coefficients

The mass attenuation coefficient for the photoelectric effect (τ/ρ) is related to the atomic number (Z) of the absorber and the photon energy of the radiation (E). A very approximate guide to this relationship is given by the equation:

$$\frac{\tau}{\rho} \propto \frac{Z^3}{E^3} \qquad\qquad \text{Equation 30.6}$$

This equation applies to energies up to about 200 keV. At higher energies the E^3 term approximates to E^2 and eventually to E.

In photoelectric absorption, the X-ray beam is both *attenuated* and *absorbed* since individual photons are removed from the beam (attenuation) and energy is imparted to the absorbing medium (absorption). The absorbed energy is composed of the following parts:

- kinetic energy of the ejected photoelectron
- energy of recoil of the absorbing atom
- the energy of the photons of characteristic radiation and Auger electrons.

The ejected photoelectron is quickly brought to rest by the surrounding atoms and delivers its energy to them in the process. A similar thing happens with the Auger electrons. It is possible, however, for the characteristic radiation to escape from the absorber, especially if the energy of the characteristic radiation is high and it is produced near the surface of the absorber. In such cases, the *mass absorption coefficient* is slightly less than the *mass attenuation coefficient* since not all of the energy of the original photon has been absorbed by the medium. For this difference to be significant, the characteristic radiation must have high photon energy. The effect is thus only important in materials with high atomic numbers. As most of the atoms which make up body tissues have low atomic numbers, it may be considered that the mass absorption coefficient and the mass attenuation coefficient are equal for photoelectric absorption in practical radiography.

When we consider the absorption of X-ray photons to produce a radiographic image we need to look at the linear attenuation coefficient. From Equation 30.6 we can see that, for the photoelectric effect at a given photon energy, this is proportional to the density of the absorber and its atomic number cubed. Bone is approximately twice as dense as soft tissue and its atomic number is also approximately twice that of soft tissue. For these reasons, the linear attenuation coefficient for photoelectric absorption for bone is approximately 16 times that of soft tissue. As the blackening (or optical density) on a radiograph is proportional to the radiation dose it receives, this explains why bones appear lighter than the same thickness of soft tissue.

30.6 COMPTON SCATTERING

In the case of the photoelectric effect, the X-ray photon has an energy close to or just above the binding energy of the electron. If the energy of the X-ray photon is very much higher than the binding energy of the electron, the electron may be regarded as a *free electron*. The reaction between an X-ray photon and a free electron is known as *Compton scattering* and results in the partial absorption of the energy of an X-ray photon which undergoes such scatter. Because the interaction is between a photon and a free electron, the electron density of the material is important in determining the probability of Compton scatter occurring.

The Compton scattering process is shown diagrammatically in Figure 30.5. The incident X-ray photon has an energy $E_1 (= h\nu_1)$ and collides with the electron, which recoils thus taking some of the photon energy. The energy remaining $E_2 (= h\nu_2)$ is the energy of the deflected (or scattered) photon. Since E_2 is less than E_1, then the wavelength of the scattered photon must be greater than the wavelength of the incident photon as shown in Figure 30.5 (see Sect. 25.3.2 for the relationship between photon energy and wavelength). Compton scattering interactions are termed *inelastic* in that the photon energy is not conserved although the total energy of the interaction is conserved.

After a Compton scattering process, the photon may travel in any direction but the electron can only travel in a forward direction relative to the incident photon. Thus in Figure 30.5, θ may be any value, while $\emptyset$ lies between $\pm 90°$ relative to the direction of the incident photon. The division of the energy of the original photon between the electron and the scattered photon depends on the original photon energy (E_1) and the angle through which it has been scattered. It may be shown that in order to preserve both energy and momentum the following equation must be obeyed:

$$\lambda_2 - \lambda_1 = \frac{h(1-\cos\theta)}{mc} \qquad\qquad \text{Equation 30.7}$$

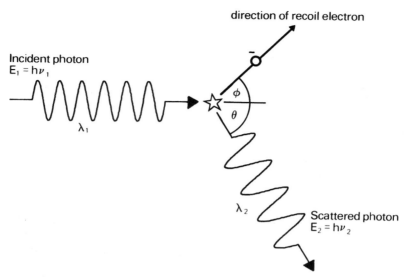

direction of recoil electron

Incident photon
$E_1 = h\nu_1$

λ_1

ϕ

θ

λ_2

Scattered photon
$E_2 = h\nu_2$

Figure 30.5 The process of Compton scattering. The scattered photon has less energy than the incident photon and may be scattered through any angle. The recoil electron is always scattered in a 'forward' direction.

where the quantity $\lambda_2 - \lambda_1$ is called the *Compton wavelength shift*, h is Planck's constant, m is the mass of the electron and c is the velocity of light.

Two important conclusions may be drawn from Equation 30.7:

- $\lambda_2 - \lambda_1$ depends only on h, m, c and θ and so is not dependent on the wavelength of the incident photon or the composition of the attenuating material.

- For a given value of scattering angle, θ, the value of $\lambda_2 - \lambda_1$ is constant. Low-energy photons have longer wavelengths, so that the wavelength change represents a smaller *fractional change* in λ and hence only a slight reduction in the energy of the scattered photons. By applying the same argument, high-energy photons scattered through the same angle will experience a much larger fractional change in their wavelength and energy.

Equation 30.7 shows what happens to the photon wavelengths when scattered through an angle of θ. It does not give any information on the relative probability of a photon actually being scattered through that angle. Mathematical predictions based on quantum mechanics, and practical measurements, have shown that low-energy photons (up to about 100 keV) are scattered in all directions with almost equal probability. High-energy photons (greater than 1 MeV) are scattered predominantly in a forward direction, i.e. they have small scattering angles.

An alternative way of writing Equation 30.7 using the photon energy change instead of the wavelength change is given below:

$$\frac{1}{E_2} - \frac{1}{E_1} = \frac{(1 - \cos\theta)}{511}$$

Equation 30.8

where E_1 and E_2 are in keV.

30.6.1 Compton attenuation, absorption and scatter coefficients

The mass attenuation coefficient for Compton scattering (σ/ρ) is given by the equation:

$$\frac{\sigma}{\rho} \propto \frac{\text{electron density}}{E}$$

Equation 30.9

As shown in the above equation the probability of Compton scattering occurring in unit mass is inversely proportional to the energy of the photon—the amount of Compton scattering occurring in unit mass decreases as the photon energy increases.

It can also be seen from the above equation that the probability is also directly proportional to the electron density. As we saw in Section 5.6, it is possible to use Avogadro's number to calculate the number of atoms per mole of an element ($N_A = 6 \times 10^{23}$ mol^{-1}). We can therefore calculate the number of atoms per unit mass by simply dividing this by the mass number (A) for the element:

$$\text{number of atoms per unit mass} = \frac{N_A}{A}$$

Equation 30.10

The number of electrons in a normal atom is the same as the number of protons and is given by Z—the atomic number (see Sect. 26.3). The electron density is the number of electrons per unit mass and is given by the equation:

$$\text{electron density} = N_A \times \frac{Z}{A}$$

Equation 30.11

If we assume that most elements have approximately equal numbers of protons and neutrons in the atomic nucleus, then the value of Z/A is 0.5. The exception to this rule is hydrogen which contains no neutron in its nucleus and so $Z/A = 1$. Thus hydrogen contains 6×10^{23} electrons per gram (or 6×10^{26} electrons per kilogram) whereas all other substances contain approximately half this value (between 2.5 and 3.5 $\times 10^{23}$ electrons per gram). The lower values are for the heavier elements which have a larger neutron to proton ratio.

Thus we can see from Equation 30.9 that, at a given photon energy, the mass attenuation coefficient due to Compton scattering is very similar for all elements except hydrogen where it is twice as large.

The *mass absorption coefficient* for Compton scattering (σ_a/ρ) represents the average energy transferred to the electron (and hence the medium) as a fraction of the total energy in the beam. As shown in the previous section of this chapter, the higher the energy of the photon, the higher the average energy lost by the photon as a result of Compton scattering. This means that the electron takes more energy in the recoil process as the photon energy increases. As a result of this, the values for the mass absorption coefficient (σ_a/ρ) and the mass attenuation coefficient (σ/ρ) are closer to the same value at higher photon energies than they are at lower photon energies. This situation is shown in the graph in Figure 30.6.

As we have already noted in Equation 30.9, the *mass attenuation coefficient* (σ/ρ) is inversely proportional to the photon energy and so we would expect σ/ρ to decrease as the photon energy increases. This is also shown in Figure 30.6.

Also shown in Figure 30.6 (represented by the broken line) is the *mass scattering coefficient* (σ_s/ρ). This represents the fraction of the total beam energy left to the photons after a Compton scattering event. At the point where the two curves cross (approximately 1.5 MeV) the electrons and the photons share equal amounts of energy. Below this energy the scattered photon carries more energy than the electron and above the energy the reverse is true.

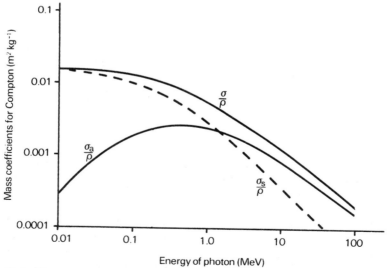

Figure 30.6   The mass attenuation, mass absorption and mass scattering coefficients for Compton scattering. As the energy increases, the absorbed energy (σ_a/ρ) becomes an increasing proportion of the total energy of the interaction (σ/ρ).

When considering the coefficients it is important to remember that the mass attenuation coefficient is a measure of the *total* energy removed from the primary beam, whereas the absorption coefficient and the scattering coefficient are a measure of the *proportion* of energy removed from the beam by the electron and scattered photon respectively.

Since the sum of the energies of the electron and the scattered photon must equal the energy of the incident photon, then we can say:

$$\sigma = \sigma_a + \sigma_s$$

and $\dfrac{\sigma}{\rho} = \dfrac{\sigma_a}{\rho} + \dfrac{\sigma_s}{\rho}$ Equation 30.12

30.7 PAIR PRODUCTION

Pair production results in the formation of a pair of particles—a positron and electron—from a high-energy photon. The process occurs in close proximity to the nucleus and can only occur if the energy of the photon is greater than 1.02 MeV. The process is illustrated in Figure 30.7(a) when the photon is shown approaching the nucleus. When it interacts with the electrical field of the nucleus it may completely disappear giving up all its energy (except for a small amount as recoil energy to the atom) in the formation of an electron and positron (see Figure 30.7(b)). This is an

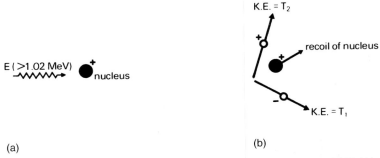

(a)   (b)

Figure 30.7   The mechanism of pair production. (a) A photon of energy ≥ 1.02 MeV approaches the nucleus of an atom of the attenuating material. When the photon passes close to the nucleus it produces a positron and an electron as shown in (b).

example of mass–energy equivalence (see Sect. 24.4.1), since the energy of the photon is converted into the mass of the positron and electron. Any remaining energy of the photon is given to the electron and positron pair as kinetic energy. This can be stated using the following equation:

$$E = (m_0 c^2 + T_1) + (m_0 c^2 + T_2)$$

where E is the energy of the photon, m_0 is the rest mass of positron or electron, c is the velocity of electromagnetic radiation, T_1 is the kinetic energy of the electron and T_2 is the kinetic energy of the positron.

This equation can be further simplified to give:

$$E = 2m_0c^2 + T_1 + T_2$$

If we consider the rest mass of the electron and positron pair then we can calculate that $2m_0c^2$ is equal to 1.02 MeV. This explains why pair production will not take place if the photon energy is less than 1.02 MeV as this amount of energy is required to create the electron and positron pair. The equation may now be written in the form:

$$E \text{ (MeV)} = 1.02 + T_1 + T_2 \qquad\qquad \text{Equation 30.13}$$

This shows that 1.02 MeV of the energy of the photon is used to create the electron and positron pair and the rest is given to the two particles in kinetic energy.

30.7.1 Attenuation, absorption and scatter coefficients for pair production

The linear attenuation for pair production is usually given the symbol π so that the mass attenuation coefficient is π/ρ. This is related both to the photon energy and the atomic number as shown by Equation 30.14 below:

$$\frac{\pi}{\rho} = (E - 1.02)Z \qquad\qquad \text{Equation 30.14}$$

where E is the photon energy in MeV and Z is the atomic number of the attenuation material. *Note* that this is the only process where the amount of attenuation increases with an increase in the photon energy.

The kinetic energies of the electron and positron pair are absorbed by the medium as the particles slow down in it. Thus the energy absorbed by the medium is less than the energy of the original photon and is equal to $(E - 1.02)$ MeV from equation 30.14. However, the positron will eventually collide with an electron and both disappear with the emission of two photons of *annihilation radiation* where each photon has an energy of 0.51 MeV. This is the conversion of matter into energy and is the reverse of pair production. If the two photons of annihilation radiation produced by this reaction are completely absorbed by the material, then the total energy absorbed is given by the relationship $(E - 1.02) + (2 \times 0.51) = E$, i.e. the whole of the energy of the original photon which caused the pair production. There is, however, no certainty that this will happen. In such cases the absorption coefficient (π_a) is less than the attenuation coefficient (π) by a fraction: $(E - 1.02)/E$. This can be rewritten as $1 - (1.02/E)$ and so we have:

$$\pi_a = \frac{\pi(1-1.02)}{E} \qquad \text{Equation 30.15}$$

By analogy with the absorption and scatter coefficient for Compton scatter (see Equation 30.12), in the case of pair production, we may write:

$$\pi = \pi_a + \pi_s$$
$$\frac{\pi}{\rho} = \frac{\pi_a}{\rho} + \frac{\pi_s}{\rho} \qquad \text{Equation 30.16}$$

where π_s is the fraction of the energy carried by the two annihilation photons each of energy 0.51 MeV, so that $\pi_s = 1.02/E$.

However, in all but the most accurate work, it is usual to ignore the scattering coefficient, π_s, since it is usually very small at the photon energies used in therapeutic radiography and so the exact Equation 30.16 is replaced by more approximate relationships which assume that $\pi_s = 0$:

$$\pi = \pi_a$$
$$\frac{\pi}{\rho} = \frac{\pi_a}{\rho} \qquad \text{Equation 30.17}$$

30.8 RELATIVE IMPORTANCE OF THE ATTENUATION PROCESSES IN RADIOGRAPHY

As we have already established in Equation 30.3 and Equation 30.4, at a particular photon energy, some or all of the above processes may be competing to remove photons from the radiation beam. Thus the total linear attenuation coefficient, μ, is the sum of the linear attenuation coefficients due to photoelectric absorption, Compton scattering and pair production. Thus the relationship $I_x = I_0 e^{-\mu x}$ can be rewritten as:

$$I_x = I_0 e^{-(\tau + \sigma + \pi)x} \qquad \text{Equation 30.18}$$

where τ is the linear attenuation coefficient due to photoelectric absorption, σ is the linear attenuation coefficient due to Compton scattering and π is the linear attenuation coefficient due to pair production. From the above equation we can also deduce the relationships given in Equation 30.3 and Equation 30.4:

$$\mu = \tau + \sigma + \pi$$
$$\frac{\mu}{\rho} = \frac{\tau}{\rho} + \frac{\sigma}{\rho} + \frac{\pi}{\rho} \qquad \text{Equation 30.19}$$

By applying the same argument to absorption we can arrive at very similar equations:

$$\mu_a = \tau_a + \sigma_a + \pi_a$$
$$\frac{\mu_a}{\rho} = \frac{\tau_a}{\rho} + \frac{\sigma_a}{\rho} + \frac{\pi_a}{\rho}$$

Equation 30.20

Similarly for scatter, we can write equations:

$$\mu_s = \sigma_s$$
$$\frac{\mu_s}{\rho} = \frac{\sigma_s}{\rho}$$

Equation 30.21

where the contribution to the scattering from pair production is ignored. It should also be remembered that photoelectric absorption contributes to energy absorption but not to scatter.

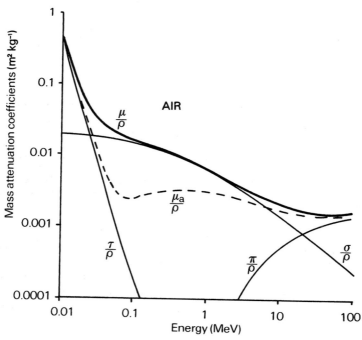

Figure 30.8 Mass attenuation coefficients for air—μ/ρ is the total mass attenuation coefficient, τ/ρ is the mass attenuation coefficient due to photoelectric absorption, σ/ρ is the mass attenuation coefficient due to Compton scattering and π/ρ is the mass attenuation coefficient due to pair production. Also shown (broken line) is the total mass absorption coefficient (μ_a/ρ).

Figure 30.9   Mass attenuation coefficients for lead—μ/ρ is the total mass attenuation coefficient, τ/ρ is the mass attenuation coefficient due to photoelectric absorption, σ/ρ is the mass attenuation coefficient due to Compton scattering and π/ρ is the mass attenuation coefficient due to pair production. Also shown (broken line) is the total mass absorption coefficient (μ_a/ρ).

These points are illustrated in Figures 30.8 and 30.9 where the mass attenuation coefficients for photoelectric absorption (τ/ρ), Compton scattering (σ/ρ) and pair production (π/ρ) are shown for lead and for air. The total mass attenuation coefficients (μ/ρ) are shown as thick lines and the total mass absorption coefficients (μ_a/ρ) are shown as broken lines.

The following important points about the attenuation processes should be noted from the graphs:

- Photoelectric absorption dominates at low energies (up to 50–500 keV depending on the atomic number of the absorber).
- The absorption edges become more pronounced as the atomic number of the absorber increases.

- Compton scattering dominates over a wide range of energies (≈ 500 keV to 5 MeV) in all materials.
- The Compton region is almost identical in all attenuating materials (except hydrogen) because of the similarity of electron density of all materials. Thus the shape of the Compton curve is independent of the attenuator (the curve for σ/ρ is the same shape for both air and lead).
- Pair production is only significant for high energies (≥ 1.02 MeV) and for attenuating materials of high atomic number.
- The significance of the contribution of pair production increases as the photon energy increase above 1.02 MeV. This is the opposite to the effect on the other processes of increasing the photon energy.

30.9 CONCLUSION

As can be seen from the above, the attenuation of an X-ray beam as it passes through a patient's tissues is a complicated affair depending on the energy of the photons, the tissue thickness and the atomic number of the tissue through which the beam passes. In both radiography and radiotherapy we are able to alter the photon energy and this has important consequences for the absorption pattern and the intensity pattern of the beam emerging from the patient. These will be discussed in more detail in Chapter 32 when the formation of the radiographic image is considered.

The significance of the high absorption of materials with high atomic numbers (as shown by the graph for lead in Fig. 30.9) will also be considered in Chapter 34 which considers the topic of radiation protection.

A summary of the interaction processes, which may be useful in subsequent chapters of this text, is given in Table 30.2.

Summary

In this chapter you should have learnt:

- The meaning of the terms *attenuation*, *absorption* and *scattering* as applied to a beam of radiation passing through matter (see Sect. 30.2)
- The factors which control the probability of an interaction taking place between the X-ray photon and an atom of the attenuator (see Sect. 30.2.1)
- The meaning of the terms *total linear attenuation coefficient*, and *total mass attenuation coefficient* and where it is appropriate to use each (see Sects 30.2.2 and 30.2.3)
- The interrelationships between *attenuation* and *absorption* (see Sect. 30.3)
- The mechanism of elastic (coherent) scattering and the factors affecting it (see Sect. 30.4)
- The mechanism of photoelectric absorption and the factors affecting it (see Sect. 30.5)
- The mechanism of Compton scattering and the factors affecting it (see Sect. 30.6)
- The mechanism of pair production and the factors affecting it (see Sect. 30.7)
- The relative importance of each of the attenuation processes in radiography (see Sect. 30.8).

Table 30.2   Summary of interaction processes

Process	Description of interaction	Effect of Z, E	Comments
Elastic scattering	Photon interacts with bound atomic electron. Photon energy is less than the electron binding energy. Photon is re-radiated from the material with no energy loss	$\sigma_{coh}/\rho \propto Z^2/E$	No energy absorption in the medium. Photon scattered in the forward direction. Effect is negligible in biological tissues in radiology because of low Z
Photoelectric absorption	Photon of energy $\geq$ the binding energy of an electron interacts with a bound electron and ejects it from its orbital. Photon disappears as all its energy is absorbed by the electron. KE of the electron $= E -$ binding energy. Atom recoils conserving momentum	$\tau/\rho \propto Z^3/E^3$	Ejected electron loses velocity to surrounding atoms, giving energy to them, i.e. absorption takes place. The electron vacancy created is filled by electrons making quantum jumps and so characteristic radiation is emitted
Compton scattering	Photon behaves like a particle and collides with a free electron. Energy of the incident photon is shared between the electron and the scattered photon	$\sigma/\rho \propto$ electron density/E	Energy of the displaced electron is absorbed by the medium, so Compton process produces attenuation and partial absorption. Electron densities of all materials except hydrogen are similar and so σ/ρ values are largely independent of the type of attenuator
Pair production	Photon of energy greater than 1.02 MeV may spontaneously disappear in the vicinity of the nucleus of an attenuator atom, producing an electron and positron pair. Atom recoils and conserves momentum. Positron eventually annihilated with an electron to form two photons of annihilation radiation each of energy 0.51 MeV	$\pi/\rho \propto (E - 1.02)Z$	Probability of pair production increases with E above 1.02 MeV. Contribution of π_s is very small compared to π and is often ignored

SELF-TEST

a. 'When a beam of radiation passes through matter it is attenuated by absorption and scattering.' What is meant by the terms:
   (i) attenuation
   (ii) absorption
   (iii) scattering?

b. What is meant by the terms *total linear attenuation coefficient* and *total mass attenuation coefficient* and give a different situation where each might be used as a measure of attenuation?

c. Describe the process of photoelectric absorption and give an equation which shows the factors which influence the mass attenuation coefficient due to this effect.

d. Describe the process of Compton scattering and give an equation which shows the factors which influence the mass attenuation coefficient due to this process.

e. Describe the process of pair production and give an equation which shows the factors which influence the mass attenuation coefficient due to this process.

FURTHER READING

Ball J L, Moore A D 1986 Essential physics for radiographers, 2nd edn. Blackwell Scientific Publications, London, ch 16

Curry T S et al 1990 Christensen's Physics of diagnostic radiology. Lea & Febinger, London, chs 4, 5

Gifford D 1984 A handbook of physics for radiologists and radiographers. John Wiley & Sons, Chichester, ch 11

Hay G A, Hughes D 1983 First year physics for radiographers. Baillière Tindall, London, ch 14

Hendee W, Ritenour R 1992 Medical imaging physics, 3rd edn. Mosby Year Book, London, ch 4

Johns H E, Cunningham J R 1983 The physics of radiology, 4th edn. Charles C Thomas, Illinois, USA, ch 5

Merideth W J, Massey J B 1977 Fundamental physics of radiology. John Wright, Bristol, ch VI

Ohanian H C 1994 Principles of physics. W W Norton, London, chs 28, 31

Plaut S 1993 Radiation protection in the X-ray department. Butterworth-Heinemann, Oxford, ch 1

Thompson M A 1994 Principles of imaging science and protection. W B Saunders, London, ch 8

Webb S (ed) 1988 The physics of medical imaging. Institute of Physics Publishing, Bristol, ch 2

Luminescence and photostimulation

31.1 AIM

The aim of this chapter is to introduce the reader to the topics of luminescence, fluorescence, phosphorescence, thermoluminescence and photostimulation. In the case of each of the processes the relevance to diagnostic imaging will be briefly discussed.

31.2 INTRODUCTION

If we irradiate a material with high-energy photons and this causes the material to emit photons of lower energy, then the material is exhibiting the property of *luminescence*. Within the strict laws of physics, the emitted radiation can be in any part of the electromagnetic spectrum (provided that the energy is lower than that of the original radiation beam), but in radiography we are generally more interested in luminescence when the radiation emitted falls in the visible part of the spectrum. Before we can discuss the process in detail there are some basic terms which we need to define.

31.3 LUMINESCENCE, FLUORESCENCE AND PHOSPHORESCENCE

As mentioned above, if we irradiate a material and it emits visible light, then that material is said to exhibit luminescence.

Fluorescence occurs when the light emission ceases almost immediately after the irradiation has stopped (the time interval is about 10^{-8} s). If we consider the use of luminescent materials in radiography (see Sect. 31.5), then it can be seen that we require materials which exhibit fluorescence as this allows us to remove the film from the cassette and process the film immediately after the X-ray exposure has taken place.

Phosphorescence occurs if the material continues to emit light for a significant time after the initial period of radiation. For this reason, phosphorescence is often referred to as *afterglow*. Such a phenomenon is generally not desirable in radiography—if we got significant afterglow then we would have to wait before cassettes could be emptied and refilled with film.

From the above we can say that luminescence occurs when we irradiate a material and the substance produces light. If the production of light ceases within 10^{-8} s of the end of the irradiation, then the process is one of fluorescence; if it continues beyond this point, then we have phosphorescence.

Insight

Fluorescence was first demonstrated in salts of phosphorus and so fluorescent materials in radiography are often referred to as *phosphors*—even although they contain no traces of phosphorus! Some of the phosphors used in intensifying screens (see Sect. 30.5.2) exhibit both fluorescence and phosphorescence. We can encourage fluorescence (and hence discourage phosphorescence) by the addition of *activators* to the phosphor material. This will also be discussed in the rest of this chapter.

31.3.1 Mechanism of fluorescence

The mechanism of fluorescence can be explained by reference to the electron band theory (see Sects 10.3 and 19.2). Fluorescence is caused by an electron in a high-energy state dropping to a lower-energy state and thereby emitting a quantum of radiation. If the wavelength of this quantum is in the range 400–700 nm, then this will form part of the visible spectrum. If we consider a phosphor used in radiography being irradiated with X-ray photons, then the first process necessary is that some of the electrons of the phosphor atoms are involved in photoelectric interactions with the X-ray photons. This raises the energy of the electrons. As already mentioned, the overall efficiency of a phosphor may be improved by the

Conduction Band

E_0

Valence Band

(a)

luminescent centre

E_0 E_1 $-\!\!\!\wedge\!\!\wedge\!\!\wedge\!\!\wedge\!\!\rightarrow E_1 = h\gamma_1$

(b)

Figure 31.1 Mechanism of fluorescence in a crystal; (a) shows the outer electron structure of a pure crystal and (b) shows the effect of an impurity atom on the electron levels. Such impurities enhance fluorescence by the formation of luminescent centres. These impurities are known as activators. The explanation of the fluorescent process will be found in the text.

addition of activators. These impurities encourage the formation of *luminescent centres* within the phosphor—the efficiency of lanthanum oxybromide will be increased by the addition of terbium as an activator. The activators possess discrete electron energy levels which are different from that of the phosphor crystal and these are used to form the luminescent centre. This is shown diagrammatically in Figure 31.1 where (a) shows the electron energy level arrangement in a pure crystal and (b) the arrangement in a crystal with a luminescent centre. These centres will produce fluorescence more efficiently than the pure crystal.

The sequence of events occurring within the crystal is as follows:

- An X-ray photon undergoes a photoelectric interaction with an electron of one of the crystal atoms.
- The photoelectric interaction liberates the electron and gives it some kinetic energy so that it is free to move within the conduction band. This leaves a 'hole' in the valence band.
- The energetic electron, on passing close to other atoms, excites and ionises these atoms and so more electrons are raised into the conduction band (leaving holes in the valence band).
- Some of the electrons so liberated will lose small amounts of energy which will allow them to adjust their energy to the energy level of the luminescent centres.
- At the same time some of the holes in the valence band will have their energy raised to allow them to reach the lower energy level of the luminescent centre.
- Some of the electrons at the upper level of the luminescent centre will perform a quantum jump to neutralise the holes at the lower level of the

centre. This is shown diagrammatically in Figure 31.1(b) where the energy of the emitted photon is $E_1 = h v_1$, where v_1 is the frequency of the emitted photon and h is Planck's constant.

- The difference in energy between the upper and lower levels in the luminescent centre controls the photon energy E_1 and hence the *colour* of the emitted (fluorescent) light.
- As more electrons enter the luminescent centres than are involved in the initial photoelectric interactions, the number of fluorescent photons is greater than the number of absorbed photons.

As can be seen from the above, the process of fluorescence occurs as a number of stages and inefficiency at any one stage can affect the efficiency of the whole process. This allows us to compare the operation of different phosphors by comparing efficiency at each of the stages.

The *quantum detection efficiency* (QDE) is a measure of the percentage of the quanta (e.g. X-rays) incident on the phosphor which are stopped by the phosphor.

The *quantum conversion efficiency* (QCE) is a measure of the percentage of the quantal energy stopped by the phosphor which is converted into light photons.

The *scintillation efficiency* (ScE) is a measure of the percentage of the quantal energy incident on the phosphor which is converted into useful light photons.

As the scintillation efficiency is a measure of the overall process, it is affected by changes in the quantum detection efficiency or the quantum conversion efficiency—if the quantum detection efficiency is 50% and the quantum conversion efficiency is 20%, then the scintillation efficiency will be 10% (ScE = QDE × QCE).

These measures of efficiency are shown in Table 31.1 for two phosphors used in radiography.

Table 31.1 Measures of the efficiency of two phosphors used in radiography (the photon energy of the incident radiation was 60 keV)

Phosphor	Quantum detection efficiency	Quantum conversion efficiency	Scintillation efficiency
Calcium tungstate	13%	5%	0.65%
Gadolinium oxysulphide	51%	20%	10.2%

31.3.2 Mechanism of phosphorescence

Phosphorescence is caused by the presence of *electron traps* within the crystal structure of the phosphor. The mechanism is as follows:

- An X-ray photon undergoes a photoelectric interaction with an electron of one of the crystal atoms.
- The photoelectric interaction liberates the electron and gives it some kinetic energy so that it is free to move within the conduction band. This leaves a 'hole' in the valence band.
- The energetic electron, on passing close to other atoms, excites and ionises these atoms and so more electrons are raised into the conduction band (leaving holes in the valence band).
- Some of the electrons so liberated will lose small amounts of energy which will cause them to fall into the electron traps.
- These electrons get stuck in the traps until they are released as a result of interatomic vibrations if the traps are sufficiently near the conduction band (see trap A in Fig. 31.2).
- Some of these electrons will find luminescent centres and light will be produced by the process described for fluorescence.

Figure 31.2   The production of phosphorescence or 'afterglow'. An electron enters trap A as a result of energy absorbed from the radiation beam striking the material. This electron can subsequently enter the conduction band as a result of thermal agitation and hence produce fluorescent photons as shown. (The electron in trap B will only be released if the material is heated and this will be discussed in thermoluminescence.)

Because there is a measurable length of time when the electron is 'stuck' in the electron trap, the luminescence will occur after the irradiation of the material has ceased. This is phosphorescence or afterglow. The pheno-menon diminishes exponentially from the time of cessation of the irradia-tion. Such a process is generally regarded as a nuisance in radiography since the phosphor may still 'remember' the previous image when a new one is being produced. This is especially the case for television phosphors.

31.4 MECHANISM OF THERMOLUMINESCENCE

If we refer to Figure 31.2 we can see that trap B is too 'deep' below the conduction band for the electrons in it to leave and enter the conduction band. This is a typical arrangement for a thermoluminescent material, e.g. lithium fluoride. This material contains deep traps in the forbidden energy gap between the valence and conduction bands. The mechanism of thermoluminescence is as follows:

- An X-ray photon undergoes a photoelectric interaction with an electron of one of the crystal atoms.
- The photoelectric interaction liberates the electron and gives it some kinetic energy so that it is free to move within the conduction band. This leaves a 'hole' in the valence band.
- The energetic electron, on passing close to other atoms, excites and ionises these atoms and so more electrons are raised into the conduction band (leaving holes in the valence band).
- Some of the electrons so liberated will lose small amounts of energy which will cause them to fall into the electron traps.
- These electrons get stuck in the traps (see trap B in Fig. 31.2). If the substance is subsequently heated, the electrons will gain energy as a result of interatomic vibrations and can move up to the conduction band.
- Some of these electrons will find luminescent centres and light will be produced by the process described for fluorescence.
- Thus the intensity of the light emitted from the thermoluminescent material is proportional to the amount of radiation incident on the material. This is the basis of thermoluminescent dosimetry which will be discussed in Chapters 33 and 34 of this text.

31.5 FLUORESCENT SCREENS IN RADIOGRAPHY

Fluorescent screens are used in a number of situations in radiography but probably the most common use is as intensifying screens in the X-ray cassette. Figure 31.3 shows an open cassette showing the position of the back and the front intensifying screen. It helps to understand the function of such screens if we know the basic construction.

31.5.1 Construction of an X-ray intensifying screen

Figure 31.4 shows a cross-section through a typical intensifying screen.

The *base material* of the screen is usually a flexible white plastic. Its function is to give support to the rest of the screen.

The film side of the base is coated in the *substratum layer*. The function of this layer varies depending on the type of intensifying screen. In a *fast intensifying screen* it has the function of reflecting the light from the phosphor layer forward on to the film and so increasing the speed of the screen. In a *high-resolution intensifying screen* the substratum layer has an

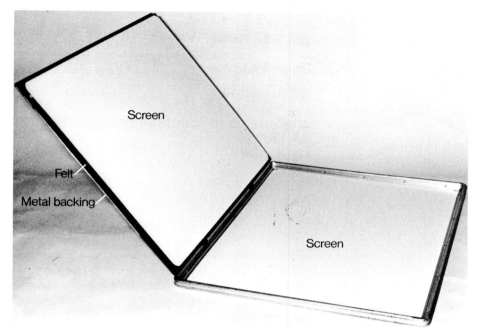

Figure 31.3 The structure of a radiographic cassette. The film is placed between the two screens prior to the X-ray exposure being made.

absorbative function—it absorbs the light from the back of the phosphor layer thus preventing it being reflected forward to the film. This increases the resolving power of the screen but diminishes its speed.

The *phosphor layer* is responsible for converting the X-ray photon energy to light photons. It usually consists of phosphor material crystals (e.g. gadolinium oxybromide activated with terbium) suspended in a clear binder. A colour tint may be added to this binder or it may have carbon microgranules added to it. Both will cause selective absorption of the more oblique light rays from the phosphor crystals and therefore increase the resolution of the screen (but, once again, this improvement is produced at the expense of a loss of speed).

Finally, the *supercoat* is a clear layer of varnish which protects the

Figure 31.4 A cross-section through a typical X-ray intensifying screen (not drawn to scale).

phosphor layer from abrasion and contamination. This layer is usually smooth so that there is close contact between the film and the intensifying screen. Some screen manufacturers add clear microspheres to this layer. This improves the resolution of the screen and also ensures that the film and screen separate easily in daylight film handling devices.

31.5.2 Phosphor materials used in intensifying screens

The traditional material for the phosphor of X-ray intensifying screens was calcium tungstate ($CaWO_4$). This produced light mainly in the blue part of the visible spectrum which allowed a good match with monochromatic film emulsions. However, as can be seen from Table 31.1, the scintillation efficiency for calcium tungstate is fairly low (0.65%) and so it has been replaced over the last 20 years by more efficient phosphors in the form of 'rare earths'.

The first generation of rare earth phosphors were terbium-activated gadolinium oxysulphide (Gd_2O_2S: Tb) or lanthanum oxysulphide (La_2O_2S: Tb). These emitted a line spectrum with the peak emission in the green part of the visible spectrum. This necessitated a switch from monochromatic (blue-sensitive) film emulsions to orthochromatic (green-sensitive) film emulsions. The spectral characteristics of the two phosphors and the corresponding film emulsions are shown in Figure 31.5.

The second generation rare earth phosphors are now more common. These are again activated with terbium and are the oxybromide salts of lanthanum (LaOBr: Tb) or gadolinium (GdOBr: Tb). These have the

Figure 31.5 The fluorescent spectrum of a rare earth screen (line spectra) compared to the spectrum from a calcium tungstate screen (continuous spectrum). Also shown as broken lines are the photographic sensitivities of conventional (monochromatic or blue-sensitive) and extended (orthochromatic or green-sensitive) film.

advantage of fluorescence in predominantly the blue part of the visible spectrum and so they may be used with monochromatic film emulsions.

31.5.3 Comparison of intensifying screens

A detailed comparison of different intensifying screens is beyond the scope of this text and is covered by one of the radiographic photography texts listed at the end of this chapter. However, some of the basic terminology is useful in understanding the formation of the radiographic image which we will cover in Chapter 32.

X-ray photons incident on the intensifying screens cause the screens to fluoresce and the light from this fluorescence will create an image on the film emulsion. At first this may seem a rather inefficient process as the scintillation efficiency of most phosphors is less than 10%. However, it should be remembered that one captured X-ray photon can cause the emission of thousands of light photons. Because the light photons have lower energy, they are much more likely to undergo photoelectric interactions with the crystals of the photographic emulsion. In a typical situation about 99% of the image on the film is created by the action of the light from the screens and about 1% by the direct action of the X-ray photons on the photographic emulsion.

As a general rule, provided we use the same phosphor material, an increase in the screen speed will cause a reduction in the resolution of the system. In a modern diagnostic imaging department it is therefore necessary to have intensifying screens of differing speeds for differing imaging situations. The speed of different screens may be compared by comparing their intensification factors thus:

$$\text{intensification factor (IF)} = \frac{E}{E_S} \qquad \text{Equation 31.1}$$

where E is the exposure without screens and E_S is the exposure required to produce the same image using screens. Thus if 100 mAs is required to produce a certain image density without screens and the same density is produced by 2 mAs when using screens, the intensification factor of these screens is 50. Intensification factors of up to 50 were available for calcium tungstate screens, while intensification factors of up to 500 are available for rare earth screens.

Insight

In many cases in a modern imaging department the speed of an imaging system is stated by quoting the *speed class*. This takes account of the speed of the intensifying screen and the film—the speed class of the system can be altered by altering the speed of either the intensifying screen or the film.

31.6 FURTHER EXAMPLES OF FLUORESCENCE

Four further examples of fluorescence applicable to diagnostic imaging will now be briefly considered (more detailed descriptions may be found in specialist textbooks on X-ray equipment):

- If we use an image intensifier in fluoroscopy, then this contains an input phosphor and an output phosphor. The input phosphor is usually made of caesium iodide and absorbs X-ray photons and re-emits the energy as light photons. The light photons fall on a photocathode which will emit electrons when bombarded by light. The electrons are accelerated and focused on to an output phosphor where their energy is used to create light photons by the fluorescent effect. The net result of this is that the image is intensified by about 5000 times between the input phosphor and the output phosphor.
- In the television monitor the phosphor on the face of the monitor is bombarded by electrons. Such high-energy electrons are capable of causing the phosphor to fluoresce, thus producing the image on the television monitor.
- Scintillation counters made of sodium iodide crystals coupled with photomultiplier tubes can be used to detect small amounts of X-rays and γ-rays. The intensity of the fluorescence from the crystal is measured by the photomultiplier tube and this is proportional to the intensity of the radiation hitting the crystal. Such devices are used in nuclear medicine, CT scanners and osteoporosis scanners.
- Radiographic viewing boxes contain fluorescent tubes. An electrical discharge in the gas in the tube causes the emission of ultra-violet radiation. This is absorbed by a suitable phosphor coated on to the inside of the tubes which then emits light.

31.7 PHOTOSTIMULATION

The process of photostimulation is very similar to the process of thermo-luminescence. A suitable material (normally a barium fluorohalide) is irradiated and the following process takes place:

- An X-ray photon undergoes a photoelectric interaction with an electron of one of the crystal atoms.
- The photoelectric interaction liberates the electron and gives it some kinetic energy so that it is free to move within the conduction band. This leaves a 'hole' in the valence band.
- The energetic electron, on passing close to other atoms, excites and ionises these atoms and so more electrons are raised into the conduction band (leaving holes in the valence band).
- Some of the electrons so liberated will lose small amounts of energy

which will cause them to fall into the electron traps between the valence and conduction bands.

- These electrons get stuck in the traps. The material is then scanned with a laser beam and the electrons in the traps will gain energy to move up to the conduction band.
- Some of these electrons will find luminescent centres and light will be produced by the process described for fluorescence.
- Thus the intensity of the light emitted from each area of the material is proportional to the amount of radiation each area received.

This is the basis of photostimulable plates which are used as part of many digital imaging systems.

Summary

In this chapter you should have learnt:

- The meaning of the terms 'luminescence', 'fluorescence' and 'phosphorescence' (see Sect. 31.3)
- The mechanism of fluorescence (see Sect. 31.3.1)
- The meaning of the terms 'quantum detection efficiency', 'quantum conversion efficiency' and 'scintillation efficiency' (see Sect. 31.3.1)
- The mechanism of phosphorescence (see Sect. 31.3.2)
- The mechanism of thermoluminescence (see Sect. 31.4)
- The construction and practical application of intensifying screens in radiography (see Sect. 31.5)
- Other uses of fluorescence in radiography (see Sect. 31.6)
- The mechanism of photostimulation (see Sect. 31.7).

SELF-TEST

a. Distinguish between the terms *luminescence*, *fluorescence* and *phosphorescence*.

b. Describe the mechanism of fluorescence.

c. Describe the mechanism of thermoluminescence.

d. Briefly describe the construction of a typical X-ray intensifying screen.

e. Outline the basic physics of photostimulation.

FURTHER READING

Ball J, Price T 1989 Chesneys' Radiographic imaging. Blackwell Scientific Publications, London, chs 5C, 16, 17
Carter P H 1994 Chesneys' Equipment for student radiographers. Blackwell Scientific Publications, London, ch 7

Curry T S et al 1990 Christensen's Physics of diagnostic radiology. Lea & Febinger, London, chs 9, 13

Foster E 1985 Equipment for diagnostic radiography. MTP Press, Lancaster, ch 8

Hay G A, Hughes D 1983 First year physics for radiographers. Baillière Tindall, London, ch 9

Hendee W, Ritenour R 1992 Medical imaging physics, 3rd edn. Mosby Year Book, London, ch 13

Hill D R (ed) 1975 Principles of diagnostic X-ray apparatus. Macmillan Press, London, ch 16

Jenkins D 1980 Radiographic photography and imaging processes. MTP Press, Lancaster, chs 5, 16

Johns H E, Cunningham J R 1983 The physics of radiology, 4th edn. Charles C Thomas, Illinois, USA, ch 16

Merideth W J, Massey J B 1977 Fundamental physics of radiology. John Wright, Bristol, ch XVII

Roberts D P, Smith N L 1994 Radiographic imaging: a practical approach. Churchill Livingstone, Edinburgh, chs 2, 5

Webb S (ed) 1988 The physics of medical imaging. Institute of Physics Publishing, Bristol, ch 2

The radiographic image

32.1 AIM

The aim of this chapter is to consider the major factors involved in the production of a radiographic image. The chapter will first consider the attenuation patterns in a patient which produce an X-ray image and will then consider how this interacts with a recording medium to produce a radiograph. The chapter also summarises how the selection of exposure factors affects the quality of the radiographic image produced.

32.2 INTRODUCTION

The geometrical factors which contribute to the quality of the radiographic image have already been discussed in some detail in Chapter 2 of this text.

These factors determine the magnification of the image and the amount of geometric unsharpness produced.

The radiographic image depends on more than geometrical considerations, however, and the purpose of this chapter is to consider the other factors which contribute to the image quality. To understand this it is necessary to understand the contribution of photoelectric absorption (see Sect. 30.5) and Compton scattering (see Sect. 30.6) to the final radiographic image.

It is easier to understand the final image quality if we consider image formation as a two-stage process:

- the production of an X-ray image pattern as the beam of radiation is attenuated by the patient
- the production of a radiographic image as this radiation pattern interacts with a recording medium—in our discussion this will be a film/intensifying screen combination.

This chapter will therefore consist of two halves each looking at one of these stages.

32.3 THE X-RAY IMAGE PATTERN

32.3.1 Attenuation of the X-ray beam by the body

We will assume, for simplicity, that the radiation beam from the X-ray tube striking the body is of uniform intensity across the beam. When this beam interacts with the body substance, different materials will cause different amounts of attenuation and, so, a 'pattern of radiation intensities' is transmitted to the imaging device. If all structures in the beam attenuated the radiation by the same amount, there would be no such pattern and as a consequence no image of any structures would be seen on the radiograph.

A simple example of such differential absorption is shown in Figure 32.1 where two separate rectangular blocks of bone and soft tissue are shown interacting with the X-ray beam. The profiles of the incident (I_0) and the transmitted (I_t) radiation intensities are also shown. If we assume—again for simplicity—that the attenuation of the radiation beam is exponential, then we get:

$$I_B = I_0 e^{-\mu(B)d}$$
$$I_T = I_0 e^{-\mu(T)d} \qquad\qquad \text{Equation 32.1}$$

where I_0 is the intensity of the X-ray beam before it enters the patient, $\mu(B)$ is the total linear attenuation coefficient for bone and $\mu(T)$ is the total linear attenuation coefficient for soft tissue. I_B is the intensity of the radiation transmitted through a thickness d of bone and I_T is the intensity transmitted through a similar thickness of soft tissue.

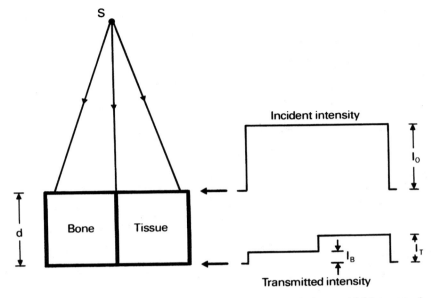

Figure 32.1   A comparison of the attenuation of the X-ray beam by equal thicknesses of bone and soft tissue. *Note* that there is greater attenuation of the X-rays by the bone than by the soft tissue.

As can be seen from Figure 32.1, I_B is less than I_T. This is because $\mu(B)$ is greater than $\mu(T)$. There are two physical reasons for this:

- the density of bone is approximately twice that of soft tissue ($\rho_B = 1.8$; $\rho_T = 1.0$)
- the average atomic number of bone is approximately twice that of soft tissue ($Z_B = 14$; $Z_T = 7.5$).

As we saw in Section 31.2.1, the total linear attenuation coefficient is proportional to the number of atoms present in unit volume and hence the density of the medium. As the density of bone is twice that of soft tissue, then there must be twice as many atoms in unit volume and so, all other things being equal, the linear attenuation coefficient for bone would be twice that for soft tissue.

To appreciate the importance of the difference in atomic number we must consider the attenuation process occurring (see Sects 30.5 and 30.6). The equations for each process are summarised below:

$$\tau \propto \rho \times \frac{Z^3}{E^3}$$

$$\sigma \propto \rho \, \frac{(\text{electron density})}{E} \qquad\qquad \text{Equation 32.2}$$

where τ is the linear attenuation coefficient for the photoelectric effect, σ is the linear attenuation coefficient for Compton scattering, ρ is the density of the attenuator, Z is its atomic number and E is the photon energy. The higher atomic number of bone means that it will greatly attenuate suitable radiation by the photoelectric effect.

As the total attenuation is a combination of both the photoelectric effect and Compton scattering, in the diagnostic energy ranges a given thickness of bone will attenuate radiation at approximately 12 times the level of an equal thickness of soft tissue.

The findings are summarised in Table 32.1.

Table 32.1   Comparisons of X-ray linear attenuation of bone and soft tissue

Attenuator	Photoelectric $\tau \propto \rho \times Z^3/E^3$	Compton scattering $\sigma \propto \rho$ (electron density)$/E$	Total attenuation $\mu = \tau + \sigma$
Bone $Z = 14$ $\rho = 1.8$	Photoelectric absorption is high when the photon energy is low—12 to 16 times greater than soft tissue	Predominates at high photon energies—500 keV to 5 MeV (higher than encountered in diagnostic radiography)	Mainly photoelectric absorption at diagnostic energies
Soft tissue $Z = 7.5$ $\rho = 1.0$	Significant at low energies—25 keV and below	Predominates at photon energies greater than 30 keV	Compton scattering is the dominant process if the average photon energy is greater than about 30 keV (this would be an X-ray beam generated by greater than 60 kVp)

The essential points to be taken from the table are that—in the diagnostic range of photon energies—the higher atomic number of bone results in photoelectric absorption being the main attenuation process, whereas the lower atomic number of soft tissue means that Compton scattering is the main attenuation process. (In the therapy range of photon energies the dominant attenuation processes are Compton scattering and pair production both of which are less dependent on the atomic number of the attenuator.)

A further (and more realistic) example of attenuation is given in Figure 32.2 which simulates the presence of a piece of bone surrounded by soft tissue. A profile of the transmitted radiation intensity is also shown and it can be seen that its minimum corresponds to the maximum thickness of the bone (point A in the figure).

The *fraction* of the incident radiation transmitted through the thickness, d, of bone is $e^{-\mu(B)d}$. Similarly the fraction transmitted through the thickness $D - d$ of soft tissue is $e^{-\mu(T)(D-d)}$. Thus the total fraction can be found by *multiplying* the two fractions so that:

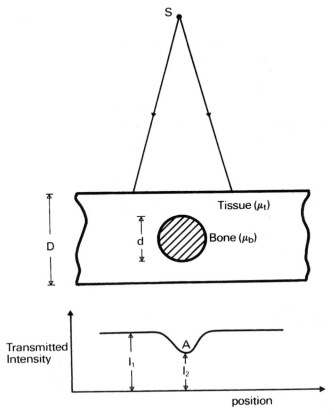

Figure 32.2   A profile of transmitted X-ray intensity obtained from a bone embedded in soft tissue.

$$\frac{I_2}{I_0} = e^{-\mu(B)d} \times e^{-\mu(T)(D-d)}$$

so $I_2 = I_0 e^{-\mu(B)d} \times e^{-\mu(T)(D-d)}$

or $I_2 = I_0 e^{-\mu(T)D - [\mu(B) - \mu(T)]d}$

and $I_1 = I_0 e^{-\mu(T)D}$ Equation 32.3

32.3.2 Scatter and the radiographic image

The sections of this chapter so far have been somewhat over-simplified in that the emerging radiation beam is assumed to be composed only of transmitted primary beam. This would be true if only photoelectric absorption took place but it is not true in the case of Compton scatter where only partial absorption of the photon energy occurs. This scattered radiation may well escape from the patient and reach the image-recording medium. Unfortunately, such scatter will form an image on the radiograph *but the image from scatter forms an overall fog so is not a useful image*. Thus unless the scatter to the radiograph can be limited, serious degradation of the image may occur.

Scatter to the radiograph may be limited in two ways:

- limiting the amount of scatter formed
- stopping the scatter, once formed, from reaching the radiograph.

Each of these will now be considered in turn.

32.3.3 Limiting scatter radiation formation

The amount of scatter radiation formed in the patient depends on the number of atoms involved in scattering interactions. Thus the scatter formation is volume dependent, i.e. *the greater the volume of patient irradiated, the greater the quantity of scatter radiation formed*. One of the major ways in which the radiographer can limit scatter radiation formation is to reduce the volume of tissue irradiated. This can be done by collimation (e.g. using a light beam diaphragm or cones; see Fig. 22.1) or, in some cases, by tissue displacement. Both of the above not only produce an improvement in the image quality but also reduce the radiation dose to the patient by limiting the scatter.

Insight

Most radiographers know from experience that the scatter radiation to the radiograph is increased when the kV_p is increased. This process is a somewhat complicated one. If the kV_p is increased, then the photon energy is increased, and from Equation 32.2 we see that σ/ρ is proportional to $1/E$. Thus with higher-energy photons there are fewer scattering events in a given volume of tissue. However, with higher photon energies, the angle of scatter is smaller and consequently the scatter has higher energy and so is more likely to leave the patient. Thus we have more scatter leaving the patient and the scatter is in a more forward direction and so is more likely to hit the imaging device.

32.3.4 Stopping scatter radiation from reaching the radiograph

The most common way of stopping the scatter radiation, once formed, from reaching the radiograph is to use a secondary radiation grid. Approximately 80–90% of the scatter may be removed by the use of such a grid.

A secondary radiation grid consists of strips of a high atomic number material (e.g. lead) interspersed with strips of a low atomic number material (e.g. carbon fibre). A section through such a grid is shown in Figure 32.3 where the lead strips are shaded. Primary radiation should hit the grid

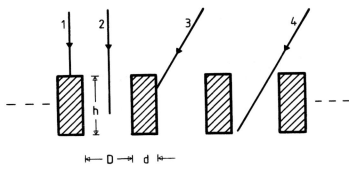

Figure 32.3 The principle of action of a secondary radiation grid—scattered X-rays (3 and 4 in the diagram) are more likely to be absorbed by the lead than the primary rays (1 and 2 in the diagram).

at right angles to its surface (or nearly at right angles) and so should pass readily between the lead strips (see ray 2 in Fig. 32.3). How-ever, some of the primary radiation will also be stopped by the lead strips (see ray 1 in Fig. 32.3). The fraction of the primary beam stopped is given by the ratio $d/(D + d)$ since this is the fraction of the grid area covered by lead—in practice this means that the exposure must be increased when we use a grid.

The scattered radiation is deflected at an oblique angle from the original radiation and so has an increased probability of striking a lead strip and being absorbed (see ray 3 in Fig. 32.3). If the ray is scattered through a very small angle (see ray 4 in Fig. 32.3), it may be able to pass through between the lead strips and strike the imaging device, but such rays do not contribute so much to image degradation as those scattered through larger angles.

Various factors of grid design may be chosen to optimise the performance of the secondary radiation grid for a particular application:

- the *grid ratio* (*r*) is the ratio of the height of the lead strips (*h*) to the width of the space between them (*D*):

$$r = \frac{h}{D} \qquad \text{Equation 32.4}$$

As can be seen by consulting Figure 32.3, either increasing the height of the lead strip or reducing the width of the space between the strips will increase the efficiency of the grid when it comes to absorbing scatter radiation with a relatively small angle of scatter. Thus it can be seen that an increase in the grid ratio will increase the efficiency of the grid. Unfortunately it also increases the amount of primary radiation absorbed by the grid. In most diagnostic imaging departments, grids with ratios of 10 : 1 or 12 : 1 will be encountered.

- the *grid lattice* or *lattice density* is a measure of the number of lines of lead per centimetre. If we consider that the width of the space between the lines is set by the grid ratio then the number of lines per centimetre will affect the thickness of each of the lead lines. Thus grids with a high lattice density (e.g. 30–40 lines per centimetre) have very fine lines and so do not degrade the image.
- If the lattice density of a grid is low, then it is possible to see the grid lines and this detracts from the image quality. One way of overcoming this is to move the grid during the exposure so that the grid lines are blurred out. Such a device is known as a *Potter–Bucky diaphragm*—shortened by most radiographers to 'Bucky'.
- As mentioned earlier, the grid will absorb some of the primary radiation and so it is necessary to increase the exposure when using a grid. The amount by which the exposure must be increased is called the *grid factor* (GF).

$$\text{grid factor } = \frac{\text{exposure with grid}}{\text{exposure without grid}} \qquad \text{Equation 32.5}$$

For most grids encountered in the diagnostic imaging department, the grid factor will be between 2 and 6.

32.3.5 Effect of kV_p on the X-ray image

The effect of the kV_p on the spectrum of radiation from the X-ray tube has already been discussed in Section 29.4 and, as can be seen from Figure 29.2, the average energy of the X-ray spectrum is about one-third to one-half of the maximum photon energy. Thus if 90 kV_p is applied across the X-ray tube, the maximum photon energy will be 90 keV and the average photon energy will be approximately 40 keV. Thus we can apply the various absorption and scattering coefficients to a beam of radiation generated at 90 kV_p that we would apply to a monoenergetic beam of photon energy 40 keV. The effect of increasing the kV_p will be to increase the average photon energy and hence reduce the linear attenuation coefficients of both bone and soft tissue—the radiation beam is more penetrating. From Equation 32.2 it can be seen that increasing the photon energy will reduce the amount of photoelectric absorption (τ) more than it will reduce the amount of Compton scattering (σ) because the photoelectric effect is proportional to $1/E^3$. Thus, as a result of less photoelectric absorption, there is less differentiation in the absorption between bone and soft tissue—there will be less contrast on the resulting radiograph.

As we have already mentioned (see Insight, p. 474) an increase in the kV_p will also result in more scatter radiation to the radiograph, again reducing the contrast.

Increasing the kV_p thus degrades the image contrast in the two ways mentioned above. However, the practical advantages of using a high kV_p are:

- it increases the intensity of the radiation beam thus allowing a reduction in the exposure time
- it results in a higher percentage of the radiation beam being transmitted through the patient, again allowing a reduction in the exposure time
- because a higher percentage of the incident beam is transmitted through the patient, the absorbed radiation dose to the patient is reduced.

Insight

The *best* radiograph is the one which most clearly demonstrates the structures we wish to see! Thus there are some situations where we would use a low kV_p to give a very high contrast in the radiograph (e.g. in mammography). On other occasions we might use a high kV_p to reduce the difference in absorption between structures so that structures of very different radio-opacity can be demonstrated on the same radiograph (e.g. in high-kV chest radiography).

32.4 THE RADIOGRAPHIC IMAGE PATTERN

The X-ray image pattern discussed so far in this chapter may be used to form a visible image—either on a film or on an image intensifier coupled to a television monitor. The intensity of the light emitted from each point on the monitor is proportional to the radiation intensity within the X-ray image but this is not the case for film.

In the case of film exposed in a cassette, the intensifying screens (see Sect. 31.5) will produce light proportional to the radiation intensity and the film is exposed to this light. This light creates a latent image in the film emulsion and this image is made visible when the film is processed. (For details of latent image formation and film processing refer to one of the specialist texts on radiographic photography listed at the end of this chapter.) If we expose a radiographic film to differing amounts of light, we find that increasing the light intensity will increase the blackening on the film—*but the effect is not linear*. The blackening on a film is measured using an instrument called a densitometer which is calibrated to measure *optical density*. We can calculate optical density thus:

$$\text{optical density} = \log_{10}\left(\frac{I_0}{I_t}\right) \qquad\qquad \text{Equation 32.6}$$

where I_0 is the intensity of the light incident on the processed radiograph and I_t is the intensity of the light transmitted through it. If we look at radiographs on a viewing box, it can be seen that the darker the radiograph, the less light is transmitted through it and hence the higher the optical density.

A graph of the optical densities produced by various exposures given to a film is known as the *characteristic curve* for that emulsion.

Insight

Optical density is a logarithmic function and the response of the eye to differing intensities of light is also a logarithmic one. Consider two points where the intensity of light is I_1 and I_2. The contrast is the difference between the two levels of intensity $(I_1 - I_2)$. Because of the logarithmic function of our eyes, our perception of this contrast is given by $(\log_{10} I_1 - \log_{10} I_2)$. However, if we measure two densities D_1 and D_2, then our perception of this contrast is simply the difference between the two densities $(D_1 - D_2)$.

32.5 THE CHARACTERISTIC CURVE FOR AN EMULSION

The characteristic curve for a film emulsion is shown graphically by plotting the densities which result from a known series of *relative photographic exposures*. The use of 'relative' rather than 'absolute' exposures simplifies the scaling of the X-axis and it is usual to plot density against the logarithm of the relative exposure in order to accommodate the wide range of exposures to which the film reacts. Such a graph is shown in Figure 32.4. Certain important features of this graph will now be discussed.

- As can be seen from the graph, even when the logarithm of the relative exposure is zero there is some density on the film. This density is

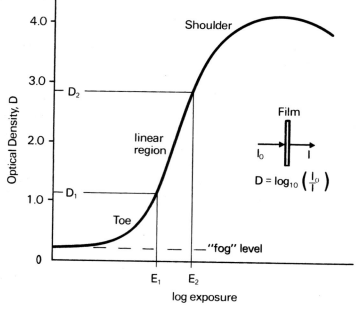

Figure 32.4 A characteristic curve for a radiographic film showing optical density plotted against the log of the relative exposure.

usually referred to as *base plus fog* and results from the blue tint in the film base and a small amount of fog produced by the developing process. The density in this region is usually less than 0.2. (Note that density has no units.)

- There is an initial horizontal portion of the graph where an increase in the exposure produces no increase in the density. This is often referred to as the *threshold* of the curve.
- The *toe* of the characteristic curve represents the region where the emulsion is becoming increasingly more responsive to differences in exposure.
- The *linear region* or *straight line part* of the characteristic curve is the region in which we aim to place most of our radiographic exposures—the reasons for this will be discussed later in this chapter.
- The characteristic curve flattens off at the *shoulder*. This generally occurs at densities between 3 and 4 for X-ray film. As we are only able to see contrast between densities up to just over density 2, then this region is seen by us as black—the film has been overexposed.

32.5.1 Uses of characteristic curves

The characteristic curve for an emulsion has many uses. In this chapter we will concentrate on only three such uses—further details can be found in the section dealing with sensitometry in the specialist texts listed at the end of the chapter.

32.5.2 The use of the characteristic curve for comparing the emulsion contrast

If we refer to Figure 32.4 we can see that an exposure E_1 will produce a density D_1 and an exposure E_2 will produce a density D_2. Image contrast is the difference in density between the two areas. If we now consider a graph for an emulsion where the linear portion forms a steeper angle with the X-axis, then the same exposure difference will produce a bigger density difference on the Y-axis—the second image will produce greater contrast between structures. Thus by measuring the slope of the straight-line portion of the graph we are able to compare the contrast properties of differing emulsions.

32.5.3 Film latitude

The film latitude can be defined as the range of exposures which will produce 'useful densities' on the emulsion. If we consider the useful densities as the ones within which we can see contrast on a standard viewing box, then the useful density range is from 0.25 above base plus fog to 2.0 above base plus fog. These two lines are drawn on Figure 32.5 for two emulsions

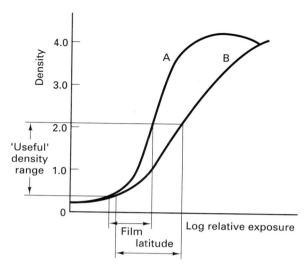

Figure 32.5 Characteristic curves for two film emulsions showing different film latitudes—film B has a wider film latitude than film A.

A and B—note that emulsion A has the steeper straight-line section and thus the higher contrast. As can be seen from the graphs, the range of exposures which will produce useful densities on emulsion B is wider than the range for emulsion A—emulsion B has a wider film latitude. This allows us to see one of the fundamental rules of sensitometry:

Film contrast and film latitude are reciprocal relationships—films with high contrast have narrow film latitude.

32.5.4 Film speed

The speed of a film (or imaging system) determines the amount of exposure required to produce a given density, e.g. if system A requires 24 mAs to produce a given density and system B requires 12 mAs to produce the same density, then we can say that system B is twice as fast as system A.

The speed of different emulsions can be compared using characteristic curves. Consider Figure 32.6. The speed of emulsions is usually compared at a density of 1 above base plus fog. We can see that film B requires a greater exposure (E_2) than film A (E_1). Thus we can say that film A is the faster. We can calculate how much faster by the following formula:

relative speed of A $=$ antilog ($E_2 - E_1$)   Equation 32.7

Note we subtract the two figures ($E_2 - E_1$) because of the logarithmic scale on the X-axis.

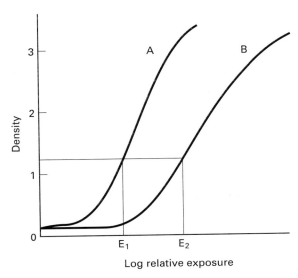

Figure 32.6   Characteristic curve for two film emulsions showing films of different speeds—film B requires more exposure to reach the same density as film A and so is slower.

32.6 PRACTICAL CONSIDERATIONS IN EXPOSURE SELECTION

The interrelationships between the various factors which affect the image quality is a complex one and one which requires considerable skill to master. Since there is a strong subjective element in selecting the 'best' radiograph, no absolute rules can be laid down for exposure factors. In any case, the wide variability in shapes and sizes of patients themselves, together with other practical difficulties (e.g. patients unable to keep still during the exposure) would provide so many exceptions as to make adherence to a strict set of rules impossible. The experience of the radiographer is therefore crucial in the production of radiographs of consistently high standard under all conditions. The following paragraphs of this section should therefore be considered with these general comments in mind.

The value of kV_p selected is crucial in determining the contrast and the average density on the radiograph. This is because the linear attenuation coefficients of various body structures vary with the photon energy of the beam. Thus, selection of too high a kV_p will result in a loss of contrast due to a decrease in the amount of photoelectric absorption. The increased amount of scatter to the radiograph with too high a kV_p will also result in a loss of contrast, although this may be counteracted by the use of a secondary radiation grid and by limiting the radiation beam to the smallest possible field size. On the other hand, if the kV_p selected is too low, this will result in denser body structures (e.g. the bony skeleton) being under-penetrated. Too low a kV_p will also result in an increase in the absorbed dose to the patient.

As we already saw in Section 29.4, the kV_p also affects the amount of radiation from the tube. Thus too low a kV_p results in a radiograph with insufficient density, while too high a kV_p results in a radiograph which is too dark.

The tube current, mA, affects the quantity of radiation from the X-ray tube (see Sect. 29.3). Thus inappropriate selection of mA results in a radiograph lacking in optical density (if mA is too low) or an overexposed radiograph (if mA is too high). While the mA does not affect the contrast of the X-ray beam transmitted through the patient, it must be remembered that the response of the film to exposure is not linear and so both over-exposure and underexposure can lead to a loss in image contrast. It is also important to remember that our ability to perceive contrast is seriously inhibited when the density on the radiograph is much above 2.

Thus the combination of kV_p and mAs determines the optical density on the radiograph. Detailed descriptions of how each can be manipulated to alter the density and contrast on the radiograph is beyond the scope of this text.

Finally the radiographer must choose a suitable film/intensifying screen combination to produce an adequate radiograph. The higher the speed of the combination the smaller the exposure required but this is generally achieved at the expense of a loss of resolution or detail on the radiograph. In choosing the film, the radiographer must also ensure that the film latitude is sufficiently wide to accommodate the range of exposures it is likely to receive. Also the radiographer must ensure that the spectral sensitivity of the film is matched to the spectral emission of the intensifying screen.

Summary

In this chapter you should have learnt:

- How an X-ray beam is attenuated by bone and soft tissue (see Sect. 32.3.1)
- The effect of scatter radiation on the X-ray image and subsequently on the radiograph (see Sect. 32.3.2)
- Methods of limiting the amount of scatter radiation formed (see Sect. 32.3.3)
- Methods of stopping the scatter radiation from reaching the radiograph, including the factors which affect the efficiency of a secondary radiation grid (see Sect. 32.3.4)
- The effect of the kV_p on the X-ray image (see Sect. 32.3.5)
- How the X-ray image pattern is changed to a radiographic image pattern (see Sect. 32.4)
- What is meant by the characteristic curve for an emulsion (see Sect. 32.5)
- The use of characteristic curves for comparing the contrast of different emulsions (see Sect. 32.5.2)
- The use of characteristic curves for comparison of film latitudes (see Sect. 32.5.3)
- The use of characteristic curves for comparison of film speeds (see Sect. 32.5.4)
- Practical considerations when selecting exposure factors (see Sect. 32.6).

SELF-TEST

a. If a uniform beam of radiation is directed at a given thickness of bone and at the same thickness of soft tissue, less radiation will be transmitted through the bone than through the tissue. Explain why this is the case.

b. Discuss the effect of the kV_p selected on the quality of the subsequent radiograph.

c. List three ways in which the amount of scatter radiation reaching the radiograph can be limited.

d. List three items of information which may be calculated from the characteristic curves of two emulsions.

FURTHER READING

Ball J L, Moore A D 1986 Essential physics for radiographers, 2nd edn. Blackwell Scientific Publications, London, ch 17

Ball J, Price T 1989 Chesneys' Radiographic imaging. Blackwell Scientific Publications, London, chs 3, 4, 5B, 11, 12

Carter P H 1994 Chesneys' Equipment for student radiographers. Blackwell Scientific Publications, London, ch 5

Curry T S et al 1990 Christensen's Physics of diagnostic radiology. Lea & Febinger, London, chs 5, 9, 10, 11, 14, 15

Foster E 1985 Equipment for diagnostic radiography. MTP Press, Lancaster, ch 7

Gifford D 1984 A handbook of physics for radiologists and radiographers. John Wiley & Sons, Chichester, chs 11–14

Hay G A, Hughes D 1983 First year physics for radiographers. Baillière Tindall, London, ch 14

Hendee W, Ritenour R 1992 Medical imaging physics, 3rd edn. Mosby Year Book, London, ch 7

Hill D R (ed) 1975 Principles of diagnostic X-ray apparatus. Macmillan Press, London, ch 14

Jenkins D 1980 Radiographic photography and imaging processes. MTP Press, Lancaster, chs 3, 9, 10

Johns H E, Cunningham J R 1983 The physics of radiology, 4th edn. Charles C Thomas, Illinois, USA, ch 16

Merideth W J, Massey J B 1977 Fundamental physics of radiology. John Wright, Bristol, chs XV–XXI

Roberts D P, Smith N L 1994 Radiographic imaging: a practical approach. Churchill Livingstone, Edinburgh, chs 4, 5, 8, 9

Webb S (ed) 1988 The physics of medical imaging. Institute of Physics Publishing, Bristol, ch 2

Dosimetry and radiation protection

33

Radiation dosimetry

33.1 AIM

The aim of this chapter is to introduce the reader to the concepts of exposure, absorbed dose and dose equivalent. The chapter then goes on to consider methods of absolute measurement of radiation dose and different relative methods of dose measurement.

33.2 INTRODUCTION

As we saw in Chapter 1 of this book, we live in an environment where we are continuously subjected to ionising radiations from natural causes such as cosmic rays and naturally occurring radionuclides—in fact about 90% of the average UK radiation dose comes from natural sources. In addition to this there are man-made contributions to the radiation dose as a result of fall-out from weapons testing, leakage from nuclear power plants, manufacture of radionuclides and medical exposure to radiation. All ionising radiations, whether natural or man-made, constitute a hazard. It is assumed that the greater the radiation dose to which the population is exposed, the greater the hazard. The accurate measurement of radiation dose received by the population is therefore important in trying to quantify the hazard.

As can be seen from Figure 1.3, medical radiation constitutes the largest single contribution of the man-made radiation exposure to the population in Britain and so it is important to minimise this radiation dose and hence the total population dose. However, the hazards associated with medical irradiation must be considered against the benefits which the patients get from diagnosis and treatment—this risk–benefit relationship will be discussed in detail in the next chapter.

33.3 UNITS OF EXPOSURE AND DOSE

When an X-ray beam passes through air, it produces excitation and ionisation of the air molecules. The electrons ejected in this first interaction (e.g. during photoelectric absorption) can have sufficient energy to ionise other atoms and so produce more electrons—the delta rays. Such delta rays are responsible for the great majority of ionisations—often referred to as *secondary ionisations*. The net effect on the air is:

- the formation of electrical charges in the air by ionisation
- the absorption of energy by the air as the electrical charges are slowed down by collision with the air molecules (thus producing further ionisation)
- the consequent production of heat energy because of the transfer of energy to the air molecules.

The traditional measure of exposure concerns the first of these effects only and is a measure of the amount of ionisation which occurs in air. The unit of exposure is defined thus:

Definition

The *exposure* at a particular point in a beam of X- or γ-radiation is the ratio Q/m, where Q is the total electrical charge of one sign produced in a small volume of air of mass m.

Thus the units of exposure are coulombs per kilogram ($C \cdot kg^{-1}$) of air. It is important to remember that exposure can only be defined for air and only for X- or γ-radiation.

Exposure rate ($C \cdot kg^{-1} \cdot s^{-1}$) is a measure of the intensity of a beam of given quality since the greater the number of photons at a given energy passing through unit area, the greater the amount of ionisation of air in unit time.

In air, the *proportions* of ionisation, excitation and heat produced by the absorption of radiation are approximately constant and therefore do not depend on the energy of the radiation. The total amount of ionisation produced in air is thus proportional to the energy absorbed from the beam, e.g. the average energy required to produce ionisation in air is about 33 eV, so an X-ray photon of energy 33 keV which is fully absorbed in air produces about 1000 ionisations.

The average atomic number of air is 7.64 which is close to that of muscle at 7.42. For this reason the mass absorption coefficients of air and muscle are very similar. This means that the energy absorbed from an X-ray beam by a given *mass* of air is very similar to the energy absorbed from the beam by the same *mass* of muscle. The energy absorbed both in air and muscle is thus proportional to the exposure measured in air—this is the main reason for the importance of air as a medium in radiation dosimetry as it allows the dose in tissue to be calculated from a knowledge of the air exposure.

33.3.1 Exposure and air kerma

In recent years the term 'exposure' has gradually fallen out of common usage and has been replaced by *absorbed dose in air* or *air kerma* (the initials of *kerma* stand for *k*inetic *e*nergy *r*eleased per unit *ma*ss of *a*bsorber); for instance the maximum permissible radiation leakage rate from the X-ray tube is now quoted in air kerma. The main reason for this is that it is much easier to calculate the absorbed dose in a structure from the air kerma.

33.3.2 Absorbed dose and kerma

The measurement of the quantity of electrical *charge* produced in air by ionisation is not the same as the measurement of the *energy* actually absorbed although the two quantities are proportional to each other.

The energy absorbed by unit mass of the medium is stated as the *absorbed dose* and is defined thus:

Definition

The *absorbed dose* in a medium is the ratio E/m, where E is the energy absorbed by the medium due to a beam of ionising radiation being directed at a small mass m.

The unit of absorbed dose is the *gray* (Gy) and so we can say that *1 gray = 1 joule per kilogram* ($1 \text{ Gy} = 1 \text{ J·kg}^{-1}$).

Note that *exposure* is defined in terms of X- *or γ-radiation* only while *absorbed dose* is defined in terms of *any ionising radiation*. Thus the energies absorbed in a medium due to α-particles, β-particles and neutrons are all measured in gray. However, ultra-violet radiation is capable only of excitation rather than ionisation of the atoms of the medium and so is outside the scope of the definition of absorbed dose.

If all the electrons produced by the primary and secondary ionisations within the medium are stopped within it, then it can be seen that the energy *removed* from the beam of ionising radiation is the same as the energy *absorbed* by the medium (this makes the assumption that all the fluorescent or characteristic radiation is absorbed as is the case in body tissues). However, this does not necessarily apply for a very small volume within the medium—such a volume may be removing energy from the beam but the absorbed energy may be deposited *outside* the volume (but still inside the body) due to the distance travelled by the electrons before coming to rest. This effect is more marked for electrons with high kinetic energy since such electrons travel some appreciable distance before coming to rest—electrons with an energy of 1 MeV travel for about 5 mm in tissue before coming to rest. This effect is illustrated in Figure 33.1 where an incoming X-ray beam of high energy interacts with a volume element V within the medium. Because of the high energy of the X-ray beam, the electrons produced by Compton scatter are scattered in the forward direction, so much of their energy is absorbed outside the volume V. There will also be secondary ionisations resulting in the production of delta rays but, for simplicity, they are not shown in the figure.

In general, if the secondary electrons produced within the volume deposit a total energy E within the medium, and E_{IN} and E_{OUT} are the total energies of the electron entering and escaping from the volume, then the absorbed dose in gray is given by:

$$\text{absorbed dose} = (E + E_{IN} - E_{OUT})/m \qquad \text{Equation 33.1}$$

Figure 33.1 X-rays interacting with atoms in volume V produce electrons which may travel outside V.

where m is the mass of the particular small volume considered. If a larger volume is considered, then this formula can be used to calculate the *average* absorbed dose in that volume.

Electronic equilibrium is said to occur if $E_{IN} = E_{OUT}$ since there is no net loss or gain of electrons over the small volume being considered. If $E_{IN} - E_{OUT}$ is a constant value not equal to zero, there is said to be *quasi-electronic equilibrium*. If the intensity of the radiation is varied, the net loss or gain of electrons will vary in proportion. An example of electronic equilibrium occurs in the free air ionisation chamber which will be discussed later in this chapter.

The absorbed dose expresses the quantity of energy absorbed in the medium due to a beam of ionising radiation passing through it. However, as stated at the beginning of this section, the site of the attenuating events (e.g. photoelectric absorption) may be at some distance from the absorption process because of the distance travelled by the ejected electrons before coming to rest. The quantity which measures the amount of attenuation in a small volume is called the *kerma* (see previous section). Kerma is also measured in gray and may differ significantly from the absorbed dose at any particular position within the medium. The absorbed dose and kerma along the axis of a beam of X-radiation are shown in Figure 33.2. Figure 33.2(a) shows the case where an X-ray beam generated at 100 kV_p is incident upon soft tissue—this type of situation might occur in diagnostic radiography. The electrons released in the primary and secondary ionisations are of relatively low energy and so are absorbed close to the site of the initial attenuating interactions. Hence the kerma and absorbed dose at any particular point along the beam axis are essentially the same and the curves are coincident in the figure. This is not the case if the X-ray beam has high photon energy, since the electrons produced by the initial ionisation have considerable energy and so deposit their energy at some distance from the point of the original attenuation process. As can be seen in Figure 33.2(b), the kerma and the absorbed dose due to 4 MeV X-rays interacting with tissue are not the same. It may be easier to understand these curves if it is remembered that:

- the *kerma* is a measure of the *attenuation*—the number of photoelectric and Compton events
- the *absorbed dose* is a measure of the *energy deposited* in the medium by the primary and secondary electrons being brought to rest.

33.3.3 Effects of different media

Instruments which are used to measure absorbed dose or absorbed dose rate are called *dosemeters* and *dose-rate meters* respectively. Some of these instruments are described in more detail in later sections of this chapter

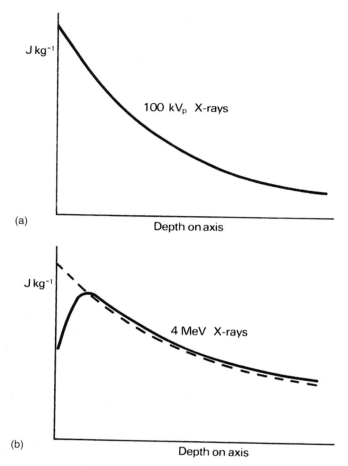

Figure 33.2 Kerma (broken line) and absorbed dose (solid line) for (a) 100 kV$_p$ diagnostic beam and (b) 4 MeV therapy beam. In (a) the two curves are coincident, but they are different in (b) because of the increased energy—and hence increased range—of the secondary electrons.

(see Sect. 33.5 onwards). It is common practice to calibrate these meters to read the absorbed dose or dose-rate in *air* through which the X- or γ-rays are passing. Such a dosemeter may read 0.5 mGy as the total absorbed dose in air at a point within an X-ray beam. *It must not be inferred, however, that this is the absorbed dose which would be received by any other medium if placed in the same position.* For two media to receive the same absorbed dose, they must absorb the same energy from the beam per unit mass (remember 1 Gy = 1 J·kg^{-1}). This is the same as saying that the mass absorption co-efficients (μ_a/ρ) of the two media must be equal. Thus if D_{air} is the absorbed dose in air and D_m is the absorbed dose in a medium when both are irradiated with the same beam of X-rays, then it follows that if the mass absorption coefficients are not equal, this equation may by drawn up:

$$\frac{D_m}{D_{air}} = \frac{(\mu_a / \rho)_m}{(\mu_a / \rho)_{air}}$$

or $D_m = D_{air} \times \dfrac{(\mu_a / \rho)_m}{(\mu_a / \rho)_{air}}$ Equation 33.2

Thus if the mass absorption coefficients of air and the given medium are known at the energy of the X-ray quanta, the absorbed dose in the medium may be calculated using the above equation. In practice, this allows us to measure the absorbed dose in air at a certain point and then calculate the absorbed dose in the patient at the same point without subjecting the patient to a great degree of discomfort.

The mass absorption coefficients of both air and bone vary with photon energy. These variations of the two coefficients are shown in Figure 33.3(a) and the variations in the ratio of the two coefficients are shown in Figure 33.3(b). As can be seen from the graphs, at low photon energies (50 keV is shown with the broken line in Fig. 33.3(a)) the mass absorption coefficient of bone is considerably higher than that of air. This is because, at low energies, the photoelectric effect predominates $(\tau/\rho \propto Z^3/E^3)$ and the atomic number of bone $(Z = 14)$ is approximately double that of air $(Z = 7.64)$. For this reason and because of the large difference in density, we get a high level of contrast between bone and air on a radiograph (this can be seen on the chest radiograph or on radiographs of the paranasal sinuses). At an energy of about 1 MeV, however, the two graphs are very close and the ratio of the two coefficients approaches 1. This is because of the dominance of Compton scattering in this region $(\sigma/\rho \propto$ electron density and the electron density for bone and air is approximately the same). This means that there would be a low level of contrast between the two if they were radiographed using 1 MeV photons. At above about 10 MeV the curves again diverge owing to the greater amount of pair production in bone compared to air $(\pi/\rho \propto Z)$. Thus it is clear that an instrument calibrated to read absorbed dose in air must be used with caution when calculating the absorbed dose in another medium as the relationships between the absorption coefficients vary with the photon energies. This is particularly the case in the *diagnostic range of energies* where absorption is principally by the photoelectric effect which is very sensitive to both atomic number and photon energy.

33.4 QUALITY FACTOR AND DOSE EQUIVALENT

As described in the previous section, the *absorbed dose* measures the energy absorbed per unit mass of the medium when it is subjected to any type of

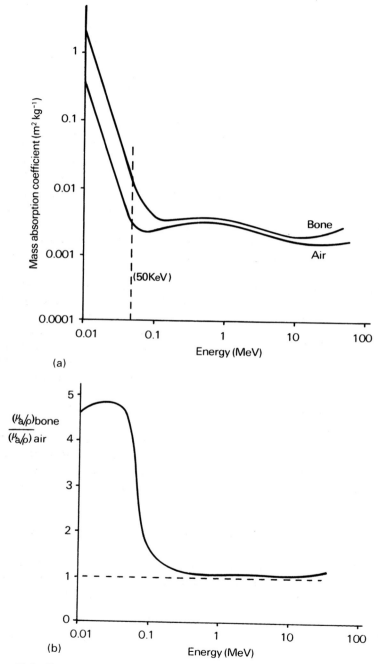

Figure 33.3 The variation with energy of (a) the mass absorption coefficients of air and bone, and (b) the ratio of the two coefficients.

ionising radiation. However, the *biological effects* of the radiation on tissue, for instance, do not depend solely on the absorbed dose, but also on the *type of radiation* and on the *absorbed dose rate*. It is found that α-particles will cause considerably more damage (about 20 times as much) in a biological specimen compared to the same absorbed dose of X-rays. It is also found that radiation delivered as a single large dose will generally cause more biological damage than the same dose fractionated into multiple small doses and delivered over a period of time.

The differences in biological effects of different types of ionising radiations are due to the different densities of ionisations they produce in a sample—radiation which causes large numbers of ionisation per unit length of tract through a material will cause large amounts of biological damage. As you may remember, when an atom is ionised (e.g. by a photoelectric interaction) an electron (negative ion) is released and the atom now becomes a positive ion—an ion pair has been formed. X-rays and β-particles do not produce ion pairs so close together as do the more massive protons or α-particles of the same energy. Thus protons or α-particles are brought to rest quickly within the medium by losing their kinetic energy in the production of many ions over a short distance—an α-particle of energy 1 MeV will only travel 5×10^{-3} mm in tissue, protons will travel 3×10^{-2} mm and β-particles will travel 5 mm before being brought to rest. Because of this, the larger particles break chemical bonds which are very close together and so the chance of repair is reduced. This means that they have a greater biological effect on the specimen. It is also found that neutrons will also produce dense ionisation by the ejection of protons from the nuclei or by nuclear recoil.

The absorbed dose in gray is thus not an accurate measure of the *biological effects* of different types of radiation owing to the very different patterns of ionisation produced. The unit used to measure the overall biological effects of different types of radiation is called the unit of *dose equivalent* and is measured in *sievert* (Sv). The absorbed dose in gray and the dose equivalent in sievert are related to each other as shown in Equation 33.3 below:

$$\text{dose equivalent (Sv)} = Q \times \text{absorbed dose (Gy)} \times N \qquad \text{Equation 33.3}$$

where Q is known as the *quality factor* for the radiation and is related to the number of ion pairs produced per unit length by the radiation. N includes other factors which may affect the biological process, such as the *dose rate*. In many cases the value of N is 1 and so the equation is frequently quoted without the factor N appearing.

Table 33.1 shows the value of the quality factor for different types of radiation.

Note that Q is unity for X-rays and γ-rays so the absorbed dose is the

Table 33.1 Quality factors for different ionising radiations

Type of ionising radiation	Quality factor (Q)
X-rays or γ-rays	1
Electrons or β-particles	1
Thermal neutrons	2.3
Fast neutrons (or neutrons of unknown energy)	10
Protons	10
α-particles	20
Recoil nuclei (e.g. in α-decay)	20
Fission fragments	20

same as the dose equivalent for these radiations. The biological effect of particulate radiations is therefore compared to that of X-rays or γ-rays by means of the value of Q. As can be seen from the table, electrons also have a quality factor of unity. This is because an external beam of electrons will produce secondary electrons with the same ionisation density as X-ray and γ-ray photons. However, α-particles have a Q of 20, indicating that the same absorbed dose will produce 20 times as much biological damage as the same absorbed dose of X-rays.

Since Q is a comparative number, the sievert has the same units as the gray ($J \cdot kg^{-1}$). The quality factor may therefore be considered a *scaling factor* relating the biological effect of the absorbed dose to the same dose of X-rays or γ-rays.

The dose equivalent in sievert has a vital role to play in radiation protection where it is required to consider the sum of the effects of exposure to different types of radiation.

Insight

The dose equivalent is too crude a unit for use in radiobiology as it considers the *average effect(s)* on a group of cells. In radiobiology we wish to look more precisely at individual effects on cells, e.g. impairment of cell reproduction. For this we use the more precise scaling factor *the relative biological effectiveness* (RBE). The RBE compares the absorbed doses of different ionising radiations required to produce the same biological effect. As with the quality factor (Q) these are usually compared to the same dose of X- or γ-radiation.

The remainder of this chapter is concerned with a brief overview of some of the methods used to measure *exposure* and *absorbed doses*.

33.5 ABSOLUTE MEASUREMENT OF ABSORBED DOSE

The absolute measurement of absorbed dose in air due to a beam of X-rays requires very careful techniques and very specialised equipment. It is therefore more suited to a specialised laboratory than to a hospital or university department environment. In the UK, the National Physics

Laboratory, and in the USA, the National Bureau of Standards, calibrate and check specialised dosemeters under carefully controlled conditions. Such dosemeters are termed *absolute standards*. Dosemeters used in hospitals and universities are sent to such centres on a regular basis to be calibrated against the absolute standards—such dosemeters are then known as *secondary standards*. Further dosemeters may be calibrated against these secondary standards—such dosemeters are known as *sub-standards*.

This initial section considers the manner in which an absolute measurement of absorbed dose may be made and the following section (Sect. 33.6) is an overview of the most common of the *relative methods* of assessing absorbed dose.

33.5.1 Calorimetry

A beam of X-rays or γ-rays will be attenuated as it passes through a medium and the attenuation processes (see Ch. 30) will produce many ionisations within the medium. The kinetic energy of the electrons so ejected from their atoms is eventually absorbed by the atoms of the medium. This results in these atoms having an increase in their kinetic energy—heat will be produced in the medium. The medium thus experiences a rise in temperature which is proportional to the heat energy absorbed by the medium and therefore the absorbed dose. In Section 8.3.2 we have shown that:

$$Q = mc(T_2 - T_1)$$

where Q is the heat energy, m is the mass of the body, c is its specific heat capacity and $(T_2 - T_1)$ is the temperature rise experienced by the body.

We also know for the earlier sections of this chapter (see Sect. 33.3.2) that absorbed dose is energy per unit mass of the medium and so:

$$D = \frac{Q}{m}$$

Thus we can produce the equation:

$$D = c\,(T_2 - T_1) \qquad\qquad \text{Equation 33.4}$$

Using the above equation, the absorbed dose may be calculated from the temperature rise produced in an irradiated medium, if we know the specific heat capacity of the medium. This is known as the *calorimetric* method of absorbed dose measurement.

However, the temperature rise produced is very small—1 Gy will produce a temperature rise of about $2 \times 10^{-4}\,°C$ and so the process needs very controlled conditions and is most appropriate when measuring very large absorbed doses of radiation.

The more sensitive method is to collect the charge produced in an ionisation chamber and this is described below.

33.5.2 The free air ionisation chamber

The ions produced by the absorption of an X-ray beam in air may be collected by oppositely charged plates situated in the air. The liberated electrons are attracted towards the positive plate and the positive ions are attracted towards the negative plate. Thus charge, whose magnitude is proportional to the exposure in coulombs per kilogram and the absorbed dose in gray, flows through the chamber.

Certain precautions are necessary, however, to achieve accurate results:

• As shown in Figure 33.4, the central lower disc is surrounded by an annulus which is at earth potential (note that Fig. 33.4 is a section through such a chamber and so the annulus appears as if it were two separate plates). This construction enables an accurate estimation of the volume of air from which the ion pairs are collected as it ensures that the lines of electrical force are at right angles to both the collecting plates. Note that this is not the case at the outer edge of the annulus where the lines of electrical force are bowed outwards thus including an unknown quantity of air beyond the edge of the plates. The volume of air from which the ion pairs are collected may be calculated by knowing the geometry of ABCD. Ion pairs produced outside this volume are still collected by the annulus but do not pass through the meter, M, and its associated electronic amplifier and thus do not contribute to the current indicated by the meter.

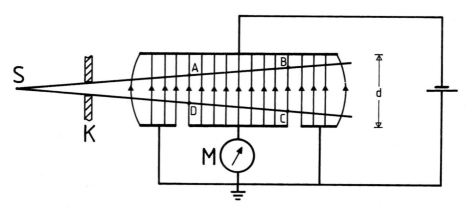

Figure 33.4 A diagrammatic section through the free-air ionisation chamber. S is the source of radiation and K is a collimator. The electrons resulting from the ionisation which takes place in the area ABCD are collected on the collecting plate which is connected to the meter M. This meter measures the total negative charge produced as a result of the radiation.

- Some electrons produced by ionisation in the region ABCD will escape and produce further ionisations over the annulus rather than the central disk. This suggests that the current measured by the meter, M, is too low, but this is not the case because, on average, the same number of electrons from outside the volume of air is gained by the volume. Thus there is *no net loss* of electrons from the volume under consideration—this is a case of electronic equilibrium described earlier (see Sect. 33.3.2).

- The potential difference across the plates must be sufficiently high to collect all the ion pairs produced in the air. If we irradiate a free air ionisation chamber with a steady beam of radiation, the current flowing through the chamber will vary with the potential difference across the plates as shown in Figure 33.5. Below the saturation voltage, some of the positive and negative ions are able to recombine by mutual attraction (germinal recombination) and so are not collected on the plates. At above the saturation level, however, the electrical field strength between the plates is sufficiently large to ensure that the ions are permanently separated and move towards the appropriate plate for collection. In practice, the value of the potential difference chosen depends on the separation of the plates, but is typically of the order of a few hundred volts.

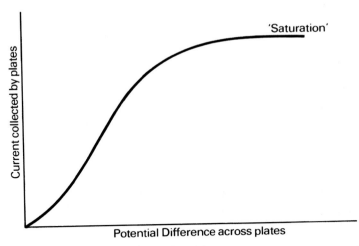

Figure 33.5   The variation of current flowing through the meter M in Figure 33.4 with the applied potential difference across the plates.

- The separation of the plates, *d*, shown in Figure 33.4 must be sufficiently large to enable the production of *all the secondary ionisations in air*—no electron produced during the ionisation process must reach the plates before it produces all the ion pairs of which it is capable. If *d* is too small, then the current measured by the meter, M, will be too low since there are too few ion pairs produced in the air volume and hence the estimate of the exposure or absorbed dose will be too low. The required plate separation depends on the energy of the X- or γ-ray beam, since photons with high energies will produce electrons with correspondingly high energies which will travel further in air—typical values vary from about 20 cm for photon energies up to 250 keV to several metres for photons of energy above 1 MeV. From this it can be seen that the greater the energy of the beam, the more cumbersome the measurement, due to the necessity for greater separation of the plates.

● The total charge in coulomb measured by the free air ionisation chamber is a direct measure of the exposure in $C \cdot kg^{-1}$ and is proportional to the absorbed dose in gray ($J \cdot kg^{-1}$). The mass of the air irradiated depends on the temperature and the pressure of air and must therefore be corrected for the effects of these variations. If ρ_0 is the density of air at a known temperature and pressure, then the mass of the air m_0 in the irradiated volume, v, can be calculated as $m_0 = \rho_0 v$. At a new temperature and pressure (T_1 and p_1) the density changes to $\rho_0 T_0 p_1 / T_1 p_0$ so the mass of the air, m', being irradiated is given by:

$$m' = m_0 \times \frac{T_0}{T_1} \times \frac{p_1}{p_0} \qquad \qquad \text{Equation 33.5}$$

The exposure (in $C \cdot kg^{-1}$) is therefore the ratio of the total charge collected to the mass of air irradiated (m'). The absorbed dose (in Gy) is calculated from the energy absorbed divided by m'—the energy absorbed can be calculated from the charge collected since it takes about 33 eV to produce one ion pair in air.

The ionisation method is not suitable for use with liquids owing to the very rapid germinal recombination of the ions and the relatively high current which flows through many liquids even when they are not being irradiated. A semiconductor (see Sect. 33.6.6) may, however, be used to collect the ion pairs produced by irradiation.

From the above it can be seen that the free air ionisation chamber is suitable for the absolute measurement of exposure and absorbed dose in air. The absorbed dose which would have occurred in another medium placed in the same beam of radiation may be calculated from the mass absorption coefficients as explained earlier in this chapter (see Sect. 33.3.3).

33.5.3 Chemical methods of dose measurement

As we have already established, radiation affects the chemical bonds between atoms of a material through which it passes both by ionisation and excitation of electrons. Because of such processes, it is able to transform a dilute solution of ferrous sulphate, $FeSO_4$, to ferric sulphate, $Fe_2(SO_4)_3$, by rearrangement of the chemical bonds. The number of ferric ions so produced is proportional to the absorbed dose—100 eV of absorbed dose will produce about 15 ferric ions. Thus a chemical measurement of the concentration of the ferric ions may be used as a measure of the absorbed dose.

Such a chemical dosemeter may be calibrated against either of the two preceding methods of absorbed dose measurement. It is included in this section on *absolute methods of dose measurement* because, once the conversion factor between the absorbed dose and the quantity of ferric ions is known, no further calibration is necessary. The process of calibration is therefore similar to the calculation of absorbed dose in the free air ionisation chamber from the knowledge of the energy required to produce an ion pair in air.

The above method of dose measurement is known as the *Fricke dosemeter*, but is only suitable for the estimation of very large doses—in excess of 20 Gy. The limitation is because of the relatively insensitive methods of estimation of the quantity of ferric ions and also because of the effect of chemical impurities. It is, however, particularly suitable for use with high-energy radiation beams and for irregular shapes of irradiated volumes.

33.6 TYPES OF DETECTORS AND DOSEMETERS

So far, in this chapter, we have considered the measurement of absorbed dose by *absolute* methods—these form a standard against which other types of dosemeter can be compared or calibrated. There are many such *relative methods* by which absorbed dose may be estimated, each with some advantages and disadvantages. The most common of these methods are briefly outlined below.

33.6.1 The thimble ionisation chamber

The size and configuration of the free air ionisation chamber discussed so far make it a suitable instrument for the standardisation of radiation dose measurement but totally unsuitable for routine dose measurement in a hospital environment—a plate separation of 5 metres would be required if we needed to measure the dose rate at a patient's skin from a ^{60}Co source!

The thimble ionisation chamber shown in Figure 33.6 circumvents some of these difficulties by, as it were, 'condensing' the air into a solid medium surrounding the central electrode. The cap of the thimble chamber is said to be *air equivalent*, i.e. it is made of a material which has the same atomic number as air (e.g. graphite, bakelite, plastic) and so its absorption properties are the same as the *same mass of air*. The central aluminium electrode has a fixed amount of positive charge put on it from an external source. When the chamber is irradiated, some of the more energetic electrons liberated in the cap will penetrate into the air of the chamber and be attracted to the central electrode. Thus the central electrode will lose some of its positive charge.

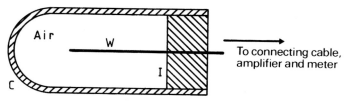

Figure 33.6   Construction of the thimble ionisation chamber. Key: C—cap; W—central wire; I—insulator.

By the choice of suitable materials the thimble chamber can be made to have the same absorbing properties as the same mass of air. Such a device is calibrated for several photon energies against a standard chamber such as the free air chamber described earlier in this chapter, and a correction factor is used to convert the indicated loss of charge from the central electrode to true absorbed dose. The choice of wall thickness of the cap is one of the factors which influence the applied correction, since a thin cap may not produce sufficient electrons entering the chamber while too thick a cap will absorb more radiation than it needs to. *Note* that the vast majority of the electrons used to measure the change in charge or the current through the chamber are produced in the wall of the chamber and not in the air cavity of the chamber, but it is the passage of such electrons into the air cavity which enables the change in charge or the current to be measured. Corrections for variations in the temperature and pressure of the air must be made, as is the case for the free air chamber.

Thimble-type chambers are still extensively used in radiation measurements in hospitals. For example, the calibration of the radiation output from a teletherapy machine is usually accomplished by the use of a thimble chamber connected to an electronic amplification system which measures and displays the charge produced in the chamber during irradiation. However, in order to relate the reading obtained as a result of a given exposure, to the radiation output of the machine (usually expressed in cGy/min), certain correction factors need to be applied. These include the following:

- the reading must be corrected for temperature and pressure
- the reading must be corrected by a factor which relates the reading of this *sub-standard unit* to a *secondary standard unit* calibrated by a national body (e.g. the National Radiological Protection Board)—this correction factor depends on the energy of the radiation
- the correction which requires to be applied to the *secondary standard* to compare it with the *absolute standard*—this is again related to the energy of the radiation
- a factor to convert exposure to absorbed dose at the appropriate radiation energy.

In addition there may be some machine-dependent correction factors such as correction for 'switch on' and 'switch off' errors.

33.6.2 The Geiger–Müller counter

The thimble chamber described in the previous section is an example of an ionisation chamber where the charge collected on the electrodes is proportional to the energy absorbed from the X-ray beam. The Geiger–Müller counter works on the principle of gas multiplication and gives the same magnitude of electrical pulse per absorption event whatever the energy of the absorbed radiation. The structure of a typical Geiger–Müller tube is shown in Figure 33.7(a). A glass envelope contains an inert gas (argon) at low pressure and two electrodes: a positively charged central electrode and a negatively charged mesh cylinder. Ionisation is caused in the gas by the entry of a photon or by the entry of particulate radiation if the window is sufficiently thin to allow particles to enter the envelope. The ions are attracted to the appropriate electrode and, as they pass through the gas, they will gain sufficient energy to eject electrons from the gas atoms if the potential difference between the electrodes is sufficiently great. The electrons so produced continue this process and rapid gas multiplication takes place especially in the vicinity of the central electrode since the field strength is great in this region. The effect of gas multiplication is such that well in excess of 1 million electrons are collected by the central electrode for every single ion produced in the primary absorption process. These 'electron avalanches' form the pulses which allow the system to count the number of initial ionisation events.

The presence of a small quantity of alcohol vapour in the gas helps to 'quench' the gas multiplication process so that it does not become

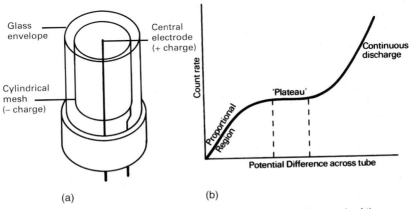

Figure 33.7 (a) Basic construction of the Geiger–Müller tube. (b) The graph of the operating characteristics of such a tube—the tube is operated on its plateau.

continuous. It does this by absorbing the kinetic energy of the positive ions in the gas so that they are prevented from striking the mesh with sufficient energy to release further electrons and so keep the process going indefinitely. Alternatively, the potential difference between the electrodes may be momentarily reduced after an electron avalanche, thus terminating the gas multiplication. In either case, there is a *dead time* after each pulse, where another absorption event, if present, is not recorded. A typical dead time is 5 μs and so the differences between the observed count rates and the real count rates is negligible except at high count rates—at an observed count rate of 1000 per second the true count rate is 1005 whereas at an observed count rate of 100 000 per second the true count rate is 200 000!

The correct potential difference to be applied to a Geiger–Müller tube is determined in practice by plotting a graph of the count rate obtained when a small radioactive source is placed near the tube, against the applied voltage. Such a graph is shown in Figure 33.7(b). Three distinct regions of such a graph exist:

- the *proportional region* where some gas multiplication takes place and the sizes of the electrical pulses are proportional to the energy deposited in the gas by the radiation
- the *plateau region* where the maximum gas amplification takes place and all electrical pulses have the same size irrespective of the energy of the radiation
- the *continuous discharge region* where the electrical field strength is sufficient to ionise the gas atoms and so produce continuous unwanted gas multiplication.

The plateau is usually between 100 V and 1500 V depending on the size of the Geiger–Müller tube.

As can be seen from the above, the Geiger–Müller tube is suitable for detecting the presence of radiation rather than for an accurate estimation of absorbed doses, since the pulses bear no relationship to the energy of the radiation causing them. It is therefore often used as a *contamination monitor* for radioactive spillage or as a method of determining whether or not radiation is present in a specific area.

33.6.3 Scintillation detectors

The operation of a scintillation detector employing a sodium iodide crystal and a photomultiplier tube is described in Appendix B, which considers nuclear medicine in more detail. Any suitable scintillating material may be used, whether solid or liquid, and the principle of operation is that the size of the electrical pulse produced by the photomultiplier is proportional to the energy deposited in the scintillator.

Scintillation plastics have been produced which have an atomic number close to that of air and tissue. These can therefore be termed as being *air equivalent* and so have similar variations of absorption to air, with variations in photon energy. They are therefore useful in estimating absorbed dose in air. Sodium iodide has a much higher atomic number than air and will therefore show a marked variation in absorption with photon energy, especially near its absorption edges (see Sect. 30.5). This requires correction factors to be applied for different photon energies if an accurate estimation of the absorbed dose in air is to be made. This is particularly so for thin crystals, which show a more marked variation in absorption with photon energy, compared with thick crystals.

Scintillation counters are very sensitive devices and are used in many applications in radiography and nuclear medicine, e.g. for the detection of radioactive contamination, for estimation of *in vitro* radioactivity, as radiation detectors on CAT and osteoporosis scanners and as the detection mechanism in gamma cameras.

33.6.4 Thermoluminescent dosimetry (TLD)

The basic physics of thermoluminescence has already been described (see Sect. 31.4). Thermoluminescence may be used to estimate radiation doses by the use of *lithium fluoride* in the form of powder, extruded chips or impregnated Teflon disks or rods. The impurities in the lithium fluoride generate electron traps and the number of electrons which get 'stuck' in these traps is proportional to the absorbed dose in the lithium fluoride. The average atomic number of lithium fluoride is 8.2 so it is close to soft tissue $(Z = 7.5)$ and both have similar absorption variations with photon energy. The small disks do not show up on radiographs and so may be strapped to the part of the body where we wish to measure the absorbed dose. After irradiation, the disks are heated and the amount of light emitted is compared to a standard dosemeter to which a known dose has been given. The dose to the disk can then be calculated by direct proportion. The disks are then annealed and may be reused.

The fact that the disks have a radiolucency similar to tissue, allows us to use them to estimate radiation dose without interfering with the radiograph or radiotherapy treatment. The disks are small, measuring only a few millimetres across, and so may be used to estimate the dose to different structures in the body during a diagnostic or therapeutic procedure.

The role of thermoluminescent dosimetry in personnel monitoring will be considered in the next chapter of this book.

33.6.5 Photographic film

As we have already seen in Section 32.5, photographic film will produce an increase in optical density when it is irradiated. The response, however, is not proportional to the absorbed dose of the emulsion. A calibration graph for the particular film at known radiation doses and specific processing conditions must therefore be produced. This forms a major disadvantage if this is to be used as a method of dose estimation. It is also true that the film emulsion has a higher atomic number than tissue (AgBr has an average atomic number of 41) and so has significantly higher photoelectric absorption at low energies. Therefore the relationship between photographic density and dose must be corrected for the energy of the radiation to allow us to estimate the absorbed dose in tissue.

Photographic film forms the basis of the film badge method of personnel monitoring and its role in this area will be described in more detail in the next chapter. Photographic film is also useful, for instance, in checking the accuracy of the light beam diaphragm on a diagnostic X-ray machine or the accuracy of the jaws on a therapy machine.

33.6.6 Semiconductor detectors

As we saw in Section 19.3, electrons in a semiconductor can readily have their energy raised to that of the conduction band and so can take part in electrical conduction. The absorption of energy from an X-ray photon (either by photoelectric absorption or Compton scattering) can raise an electron to the conduction band energies. This electron causes secondary electrons from the atoms of the material to be raised to the conduction band, by imparting some of its energy to them. If a potential difference is placed across the semiconductor, then these electrons are collected before they have time to recombine. Thus there is a current pulse whose magnitude is proportional to the number of electrons and hence the absorbed dose within the semiconductor. This is similar to the current through an irradiated ionisation chamber and the semiconductor detector can be thought of as a *solid state ionisation chamber*. It has the great advantage over the air ionisation chamber that it produces 10 times as many ion pairs for a given dose of radiation and so is much more sensitive to small doses. This is because only 3 eV is required to produce an ion pair in a semiconductor compared to 33 eV to produce an ion pair in air. The electrical signal obtained from the semiconductor device is thus more accurate—it has a smaller statistical uncertainty—and may, for example, be used to produce very accurate γ-ray spectra.

Semiconductor detectors may be calibrated against a thimble chamber, for example, for a given energy of radiation.

Semiconductor detectors tend to be used for more specialised forms of radiation detection, e.g. a small semiconductor detector may be inserted into the rectum to measure rectal dose.

Summary

In this chapter you should have learnt:

- The definition of exposure and the relationship between exposure and absorbed dose (see Sect. 33.3)
- The definition of and the relationship between absorbed dose and kerma (see Sect. 33.3.2)
- The effects of different media on the absorbed dose (see Sect. 33.3.3)
- The meaning of the terms 'quality factor' and 'dose equivalent' and how their values vary for different types of radiation (see Sect. 33.4)
- Measurement of radiation exposure and absorbed dose by calorimetry (see Sect. 33.5.1)
- Measurement of radiation exposure and absorbed dose by the free air ionisation chamber (see Sect. 33.5.2)
- Measurement of radiation exposure and absorbed dose by chemical dosemeters (see Sect. 33.5.3)
- Measurement of radiation exposure and absorbed dose by the thimble ionisation chamber (see Sect. 33.6.1)
- Detection of the presence of radiation by the Geiger–Müller counter (see Sect. 33.6.2)
- Measurement of radiation exposure and absorbed dose by scintillation detectors (see Sect. 33.6.3)
- Measurement of radiation exposure and absorbed dose by thermoluminescent dosimetry (see Sect. 33.6.4)
- Measurement of radiation exposure and absorbed dose by photographic film (see Sect. 33.6.5)
- Measurement of radiation exposure and absorbed dose by semiconductor detectors (see Sect. 33.6.6).

SELF-TEST

a. Outline the differences between exposure, absorbed dose and dose equivalent in the measurement of radiation and explain why the three units are necessary.

b. List the methods which can be used for the absolute measurement of exposure or absorbed dose of radiation and describe one of those methods in detail.

c. Describe the use of the thimble ionisation chamber in the measurement of exposure or absorbed radiation dose.

d. List six methods which may be used to detect radiation and describe one of those methods.

FURTHER READING

Ball J L, Moore A D 1986 Essential physics for radiographers, 2nd edn. Blackwell Scientific Publications, London, ch 18

Ball J, Price T 1989 Chesneys' Radiographic imaging. Blackwell Scientific Publications, London, ch 5

Curry T S et al 1990 Christensen's Physics of diagnostic radiology. Lea & Febiger, London, ch 21

Foster E 1985 Equipment for diagnostic radiography. MTP Press, Lancaster, ch 15

Gifford D 1984 A handbook of physics for radiologists and radiographers. John Wiley & Sons, Chichester, chs 15–18

Hay G A, Hughes D 1983 First year physics for radiographers. Baillière Tindall, London, ch 17

Hendee W, Ritenour R 1992 Medical imaging physics, 3rd edn. Mosby Year Book, London, ch 8

Johns H E, Cunningham J R 1983 The physics of radiology, 4th edn. Charles C Thomas, Illinois, USA, ch 9

Merideth W J, Massey J B 1977 Fundamental physics of radiology. John Wright, Bristol, chs X, XI, XII

Plaut S 1993 Radiation protection in the X-ray department. Butterworth-Heinemann, Oxford, ch 1

34

Radiation protection

34.1 AIM

The aim of this chapter is to introduce the reader to the basic legal requirements for the safe use of ionising radiation. This will cover the main documents involved and will then look at practical ways in which these are implemented in radiology or radiotherapy departments.

34.2 PURPOSE AND SCOPE OF RADIATION PROTECTION

The purpose of radiation protection is to produce and maintain an environment, both at work and in the outside world, where the levels of ionising radiations pose a minimal acceptable risk for human beings. *Natural ionising radiations* (see Table 34.1) have always existed and our bodies are subject to these radiations at all times. Those natural sources of radiation thus constitute a radiation dose received by the whole population and radiation protection procedures can do little or nothing to reduce this limit. At the beginning of any discussion on radiation protection it is important to realise that our environment can only be described as *relatively safe* from the effects of such radiations. It follows from this that one of the basic tasks of radiation protection is to establish *levels of risk* to the population due to natural and artificial radiation sources and then to take steps to keep these levels of risk as low as possible. The average doses received by the UK population from the various sources of radiation are shown in Table 34.1.

Once the levels of risk from such radiation have been ascertained, appropriate dose equivalent limits (see Sect. 34.7) may be set so that the risk associated with such radiations is no greater (and frequently is much less) than other aspects of life, e.g. the risk of injury as a result of mechanical accident. Establishing such maximum permitted radiation dose levels, and ensuring that staff work within these levels, helps to prevent the suffering and early deaths that were experienced by the pioneering radiation workers who were exposed to very large doses of radiation.

Table 34.1 Average radiation doses to the population in the UK from various sources

Natural/artificial	Source	Percentage of total UK dose	Average annual whole-body dose equivalent (μSv)
Natural radiation	Radon gas from rocks	47	1200
	Gamma rays from rocks	14	350
	Ingested radiation from food and drink	12	300
	Cosmic radiation	10	250
	Radiation from thoron (by-product of radon)	4	100
Artificial radiation	Medical irradiation	12	300
	Nuclear discharges	0.1	2.5
	Occupational exposure (to radiation workers)	0.2	5
	Fallout (from weapons testing)	0.4	10
	Miscellaneous others (e.g. radiation from luminous watches)	0.4	10

A full study of radiation protection would require to cover the following topics:

- radiobiology
- genetics
- statistical analysis of risk
- methods of reducing radiation doses to workers
- the fate and decay patterns of radioactivity released into the environment
- the absorbing power of different materials to different radiations.

Such a vast scope of study cannot be covered in one chapter or even in one book. Only a simplified—but sufficient to allow safe working—treatment of these topics is considered in the remainder of the chapter. For coverage at greater depth the reader is referred to some of the more specialist texts on this topic listed at the end of the chapter.

34.3 IONISING RADIATION REGULATIONS (1985)

The comments above indicate the wide scope of radiation protection and the need for multidisciplinary collaboration in tackling some of the problems. Radiation protection is a developing subject where the acquisition of new knowledge is used to formulate safer procedures and lower radiation doses or risks.

Since joining the EEC (now EC), British radiation protection policy has become subject to centralised policy decisions from Brussels. The *Euratom Directive* (1976) arose from a laudable attempt to standardise and modernise radiation protection practice in all member states. Since this document was prepared, the International Commission for Radiation Protection (ICRP) has produced a number of further publications on this topic. These include ICRP Publication 26 (1977) and ICRP Publication 60 (1990) and contain some substantial changes to the approach to radiation protection seen in earlier publications.

The Euratom Directive has resulted in the UK in the publication of *The Ionising Radiation Regulations* (HSE 1985). These regulations were laid before Parliament in September 1985 and came into operation in the UK on 1 January 1986. They apply to work carried out with ionising radiations in both private and public sectors. The inspectorate of the *Health and Safety Executive* (HSE) is responsible for ensuring that employers comply with the regulations.

The Ionising Radiation Regulations (IRR) is therefore a legal document and so represents a considerable departure from the previous Codes of Practice where radiation workers were expected to comply with certain codes on a *voluntary* basis—under the IRR, an employer may be prosecuted for bad practice *even if no radiation accident has occurred.*

The Ionising Radiation Regulations contain *fundamental requirements* needed to control exposure to ionising radiations, both for radiation workers and for members of the public. Details of acceptable methods of meeting those requirements are give in a supporting document—*Approved Code of Practice* (HMSO 1985). These two documents form the foundations of current radiation protection legislation. The Ionising Radiation Regulations contain 41 Regulations divided into 9 parts, where the general principles of good practice are laid down—in addition there are 10 schedules at the back of the publication which deal with specific points such as the details which the HSE requires from an employer before being able to start work with ionising radiation. The Approved Code of Practice takes the Regulations of the IRR one at a time and indicates acceptable ways by which they may be implemented. In addition to this, there are two documents which have a very specific bearing on medical uses of radiation. These are the *Guidance Notes for the Protection of Persons Against Ionising Radiations Arising from Medical and Dental Use* (NRPB 1988)—this looks at equipment and administrative requirements—and the *Protection of Persons Undergoing Medical Examination or Treatment* (POPUMET) regulations (HSE 1988)—this looks at the knowledge required by those requesting and undertaking radiography. The reader is strongly recommend to study both documents as only a few essential regulations will be considered in this chapter. (See page 537.)

34.4 BIOLOGICAL EFFECTS OF IONISING RADIATION

As we saw in Chapter 30, X- and γ-rays are capable of ionising matter through which they pass—hence the term ionising radiation. The ejection of an electron from an atom or molecule of the material means that *atomic bonds are broken*. This is true even if the electron ejected is from an inner shell, as the resulting cascade of electrons falling into the inner orbitals results in an electron vacancy in the outer, valence shell, and so disrupts the valency bonding between the atoms (see Sect. 26.5).

Such an ejection of an electron from an atom or molecule results in the formation of a negative ion (the electron) and a positive ion (the remaining atom or molecule). If the ions so formed in tissue by the primary or secondary ionisation processes (see Sect. 33.3) are capable of recombining exactly as they were before, then no radiation damage will occur in the tissue. Some such recombinations take place (in about 10^{-11} s) but the breaking of chemical bonds produces free radicals which are chemically highly reactive ions capable of forming new bonds to other ions. Thus new chemicals have been formed within the cells of the tissue. If the original chemical was important to the normal function of the cell then the cell can behave abnormally and so *the radiation has caused biological damage*. A typical sequence of events might run as follows:

1. Photon of ionising radiation absorbed by atom of the cell causing *ionisation*.
2. The ejected electron has sufficient energy to cause ionisation of other atoms in the material—*secondary ionisation* has occurred.
3. Some of the free radicals so produced combine with others to form new chemicals within the cell—a *chemical change* has occurred.
4. This chemical change causes abnormal behaviour of the cell—a *biological change* has occurred.

The effects of the biological changes so caused may be categorised into two headings:

- stochastic effects
- deterministic (non-stochastic) effects.

34.4.1 Stochastic effects

A stochastic effect is one where the probability of the effect occurring is governed by the laws of chance. Thus, for radiation-induced stochastic effects we can say that the greater the radiation dose received, the greater the probability of the effect occurring. This has two important consequences in terms of stochastic effects:

- There is no 'safe dose limit'. All doses of radiation carry some risk. The greater the dose the greater the risk—this allows us to define an acceptable level of risk and hence calculate *maximum permissible doses*.
- Since the probability of the effect occurring is chance related, the *severity of the effect is unrelated to the radiation dose received*. This can be seen more easily if we look at radiation-induced cancers as an example of a stochastic effect. If we increase the dose to a population sample, we will see a corresponding increase in the *number* of radiation-induced cancers but no increase in the *severity* of the cancers produced.

Two important stochastic effects due to exposure to ionising radiation are:

- radiation-induced cancers
- genetic effects.

These will now be discussed in more detail.

34.4.1.1 Radiation-induced cancers

Most radiation-induced cancers develop some years after the radiation was received. This is known as the latent period and may extend up to 30 years.

The risk of inducing a particular type of cancer is measured by comparing the number of cancers produced in the irradiated population sample in excess of those expected in the same size of unirradiated population sample. This is known as the *risk factor* for the particular cancer.

Definition

The *risk factor* is the estimated likelihood of the occurrence of a particular radiation-induced effect per unit dose-equivalent received by each member of the population considered.

If the risk factor for a particular effect is r, then we may express r mathematically as:

$$r = \left(\frac{\text{no. of cases}}{\text{size of population}} \right) / \text{dose-equivalent received by population}$$

Equation 34.1

The units of r are fraction per sievert, i.e. Sv^{-1}.

Insight

The risk factor for radiation-induced leukaemia is estimated at about 2×10^{-3} Sv^{-1}. This means that if members of a population each receive 1 Sv then the fraction of the population developing leukaemia is 2×10^{-3}. Hence, if a population of 1 million individuals were to receive 1 Sv of radiation, then $10^6 \times 2 \times 10^{-3} = 2000$ leukaemias will be likely to occur within that sample. While this may look an alarming number it should be remembered that 1 Sv is a large amount of radiation—about equivalent to the dose received if each member of the sample had 50 000 chest radiographs—so the risk factor although not zero is very small.

The risk factors for most other radiation-induced cancers are of a similar or smaller value than that for leukaemia. Some tissues are, however, more radiosensitive than others. This is particularly true of tissues where the cells are rapidly dividing. The positive side of this is that cancer cells, because of their rapid division, are more susceptible to radiation damage than healthy cells. On the negative side, the fetus is sensitive to radiation damage especially at the early stages of its development. Hence pregnant women, or women who suspect they might be pregnant, should only be X-rayed under very specific conditions (see Sect. 34.6).

As radiation-induced cancers are stochastic effects, the incidence of such cancers in a population sample may be reduced by minimising the radiation dose received.

34.4.1.2 Genetic effects

Genetic effects are caused by radiation-induced damage to the genes or chromosomes in the ova or spermatozoa. Biological damage to the chromosomes occurs due to ionisation and subsequent faulty recombination of the molecules which make up the chromosomes. The biological code contained by the genes on the chromosomes has thus been altered and constitutes an abnormality in the structure of the chromosomes which will be passed on to future generations if reproduction is possible. Thus *the genetically significant radiation dose is the radiation dose to the gonads of persons of reproductive capacity*. Severe genetic effects tend to be eliminated from the population because of the short life span of those affected or their inability to reproduce. However, less severe effects are more likely to become part of the human gene pool as a result of human reproduction. Thus, future generations may be protected from an unacceptably high proportion of defective genes by the reduction of the radiation dose to members of the population who are (or in the case of children, will in future be) of reproductive capacity. In practice this means reducing the contribution of man-made radiations to a minimum, by the use of appropriate radiation protection procedures. The *gonad dose* in radiographic investigations must therefore be reduced as far as possible by the use of good technique and appropriate equipment (see Sect. 34.11.5)

34.4.2 Deterministic (non-stochastic) effects

A deterministic effect of radiation is one:

- whose severity increases with radiation dose (death being the exception to the rule—although the time between the radiation incident and death decreases with an increase in dose)
- for which there is usually a threshold below which the effect will not occur.

Thus we can say that a stochastic effect *may* occur whereas for a deterministic effect, above a certain dose value, the effect *always* occurs. Examples of deterministic effects include erythema (skin reddening) or epilation (hair dropping out).

The radiation doses required to produce such effects are very large and are likely to occur only as the result of radiation accidents. Some such effects with the associated doses are given in Table 34.2.

Insight

The classification of radiation-induced damage into stochastic and deterministic effects is relatively recent. The previous classification was into *somatic effects* and *genetic effects*. Somatic effects referred to damage caused to the individual and genetic effects to damage passed on to future generations. Thus somatic damage includes stochastic and deterministic effects as can be seen from the above discussion.

Table 34.2 Deterministic effects and radiation doses required to produce such effects

Radiation dose (taken as a single dose to the whole body)	Deterministic effect
20 Sv	Death will occur within a matter of hours due to severe damage to the central nervous system
10 Sv	Death likely to occur within a matter of days due to damage to the lining of the gastrointestinal tract. Infection likely to enter the bloodstream and patient will either die of septicaemia or of haemorrhage as a result of the breakdown of the gut lining
5 Sv	Death likely to occur within weeks (unless there is radical medical intervention) due to bone marrow failure
1 Sv	Temporary depression of the blood count but the victim is likely to recover (may develop stochastic effect)

34.5 RISK–BENEFIT, ALARA (ALARP) AND DETRIMENT

In view of the possible adverse effects of radiation on individuals and on future generations, it is logical to suggest that no unnecessary radiation dose should be received by them. Thus no radiological investigation should be undertaken unless there is sound clinical evidence to suggest that the patient is likely to benefit from the investigation. Even when it is decided that the patient is likely to benefit from a radiological procedure, the radiation dose received by staff and patients should be kept as low as possible. Examples of how this can be done have already been covered—patient dose may be reduced by the use of filtration (see Sect. 29.7) and by the use of fast film/screen combinations (see Sect. 31.5) while dose to patients and staff may be reduced by good radiographic technique (see Sect. 34.11.5).

As we have already discussed when we considered stochastic effects, all exposure to ionising radiation carries a risk; the smaller the dose the smaller the risk. Thus all radiographic procedures carry a risk—albeit a small one—that irreversible damage may be done to the patient as a result of the radiation exposure. However, it is necessary to quantify this risk against the potential benefit to the patient as a result of radiography. If we consider a patient with a suspected fracture of the femur, the patient is likely to get a greater benefit out of getting this fracture diagnosed and treated than the extremely small chance that he or she may develop leukaemia in later life as a result of the radiation exposure.

As we have already considered, the risk of radiation-induced injury is decreased when the radiation dose received is reduced. However, it is not practical in a modern society to reduce the radiation dose (and consequently the risk) to zero. A balance must be achieved between the desirability of low radiation doses and the difficulty and cost of achieving these low doses. This leads to the so-called ALARA principle introduced in ICRP 26, which states that doses to patients and staff should be kept *As Low As Reasonably Achievable*. The IRR has a very similar concept, the ALARP principle, which states that radiation doses should be kept *As Low As Reasonably Practicable*.

Radiation exposure reduction due to a particular investigation or technique must therefore be analysed in terms of the benefits likely to be achieved and the difficulty or cost of reducing the detrimental effects of the radiation received to lower levels. An appropriate practical compromise must then be reached between the cost or difficulty against the likely improvement produced. For instance, the use of robotic arms in a hospital radio-pharmacy would undoubtedly reduce the radiation dose received by staff by a small amount but at a very high cost in terms of financial outlay and would also cause considerable inconvenience to the staff involved. On the other hand, the use of lead covering on the benches is a much cheaper solution and is likely to produce a greater reduction in radiation doses. Thus it should be remembered that the high-cost, high-technology solution is not always the most appropriate.

It would often be difficult to choose among various practical solutions to working safely with radiation unless a *quantitative* assessment of the detrimental effects of radiation were possible. The *detriment* due to radiation has a precise mathematical meaning and is defined in ICRP 26 thus:

Definition

The *detriment* is the expectation of harm incurred from an exposure to radiation, taking into account not only the probability of each type of deleterious effect, but also the severity of the effect.

The risk factors discussed above (see Sect. 34.4.2.1) are of value in assessing such detriment.

34.6 RADIOLOGICAL EXAMINATIONS OF WOMEN OF REPRODUCTIVE CAPACITY

The relative sensitivity of the fetus to ionising radiation (see Sect. 34.4) means that it is good radiographic practice to avoid radiological investigations of the lower abdomen of women who may be pregnant unless there are overriding clinical reasons why such investigations must be performed. (In many cases, in the modern diagnostic imaging department, we can get the required information using ultrasound which is a non-ionising type of radiation.)

The ovum also is particularly sensitive to ionising radiation in the 7 weeks prior to ovulation. The risk to the fetus from radiation diminishes as the pregnancy progresses but at no stage is this risk zero. It is therefore important to attempt to ensure that the benefits of a radiological investigation of *a woman who is pregnant or may be pregnant* outweigh the risks involved as outlined in the previous section of this chapter.

The recommendation of the ICRP in 1970 was that *women of reproductive capacity should only be X-rayed within 10 days of the commencement of their last menstrual period* since pregnancy at that time was highly unlikely. This was known as the *Ten-Day Rule*. However, in 1984 the ICRP gave new guidelines as a result of a more accurate estimate of the risks and benefits associated with radiography of the lower abdomen of such women before and after conception. The relevant paragraph reads as follows:

During the first ten days following the onset of a menstrual period, there can be no risk to any conceptus, since no conception will have occurred. The risk to a child who had previously been irradiated in utero during the remainder of a four week period following the onset of menstruation is likely to be so small that there need be no special limitation on exposures required within these four weeks.

In addition to this, the National Radiological Protection Board (NRPB) added some recommendations in 1984, which are summarised below:

- Any woman who has an overdue or missed period should be treated as though she were pregnant.
- If the woman cannot answer 'No' to the question 'Are you, or might you be pregnant?' then she should be regarded as if she were pregnant.
- If the clinical indications are that an exposure should be made where the primary beam irradiates the fetus, then great care must be taken to minimise the number of views and the absorbed dose per view, but without jeopardising the diagnostic value of the investigation.
- Provided good collimation is used, and properly shielded equipment, radiographs of areas remote from the fetus (e.g. chest, skull, hand) may be done safely at any time during the pregnancy. (Reproduced by kind permission of the NRPB.)

The demise of the Ten-Day Rule in favour of the new recommendations does reduce the care which should be taken in limiting the potential radiation dose to the fetus. The change in emphasis of the recommendations is that special precautions need only be taken if the woman is, or may be, pregnant—where 'pregnant' is defined as beginning when a menstrual period is overdue. Other than this, there is no need for special limitations of exposures during a menstrual cycle except for the normal requirements to keep all absorbed radiation doses as low as reasonably practicable. Good radiographic techniques should thus be used at all times to minimise radiation doses for all exposures.

A flow chart showing the progress of a woman of reproductive capacity presenting for a radiographic examination is shown in Figure 34.1.

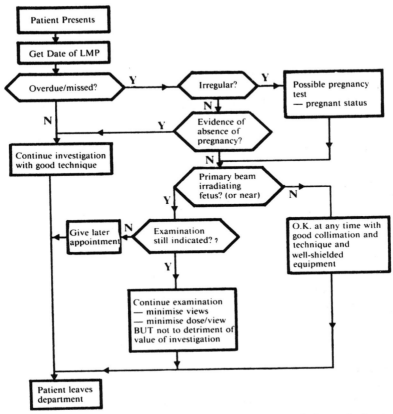

Figure 34.1 A flow chart which can be used to ensure that the radiation protection requirements are met when radiography of women of reproductive capacity is required: LMP = last menstrual period.

34.7 DOSE-EQUIVALENT LIMITS

The Ionising Radiation Regulations (IRR) has followed the recommendations of ICRP 26 in using the term *dose-equivalent limits* (DEL) in preference to the term *maximum permissible dose* (MPD) which was used in the previous Code of Practice. Although many texts still refer to maximum permissible doses, the newer terminology will be used throughout this chapter.

The setting of dose limits for individuals and groups of individuals is an extension of the risk–benefit principle outlined above (see Sect. 34.4.1). In the estimation of such limits, the effects of natural background radiation and radiation to the individual from medical exposure are excluded. This is because the former is largely beyond our control and so no practical purpose is served by its inclusion, and the latter is because individuals irradiated during a medical investigation are assumed to benefit directly from such irradiation. Thus they fall outside the general calculations of risk–benefit.

The limits discussed below should not be considered as constituting boundary lines between safety and danger. Rather, they should reflect levels of risk, either to the individual or to groups within the population, which are comparable to the risks from other activities within society that are already considered to possess an adequate degree of safety—they present an acceptable risk. There is therefore no abrupt increase in hazard if the radiation dose limit is exceeded, only an increasing probability of a stochastic effect occurring after some suitable latent period. If the limit is grossly exceeded, then various prompt deterministic effects will occur.

Insight

The assessment of socially acceptable risk in various occupations and to the general public produces figures in the range 10^{-5} to 10^{-6} per year—it is regarded as an acceptable risk that between 1 in 100 000 and 1 in a million of the population sample may die each year as a result of the hazard involved—the average risk in the UK of death due to an accident at work is approximately 10^{-5}. If we take the figure of 10^{-5} and apply it to Equation 34.1, then the annual dose-equivalent limit (see Sect. 34.7) is 1 mSv if it is assumed that the total risk factor from all stochastic effects is 10^{-2} Sv^{-1}. The use of stochastic effects to derive the dose-equivalent limits is chosen because such effects show no threshold and are therefore more significant than deterministic effects for the lower radiation doses. The dose-equivalent limits are thus chosen to *prevent* deterministic effects and to *limit* the occurrence of stochastic effects to a socially acceptable level.

34.8 EFFECTIVE DOSE

When ICRP 26 was published in 1977 it introduced the concept of *effective dose equivalent* in order to take account of the fact that different organs in the body show different sensitivities to radiation. This concept has been continued in ICRP 60—published in 1990—although the weighting factors (see below) given to the various organs are slightly different from ICRP 26 and the term was changed to *effective dose*. Using the concept of effective dose we can state that a given dose given to an organ of high radiosensitivity carries a higher risk than if the same dose is given to an organ of lower sensitivity. In the former case *a higher effective dose* is received. Each organ is therefore given a *weighting factor* which represents its sensitivity to radiation in relation to that of the whole body when the whole body receives the same dose. Thus the weighting factor can be defined:

Definition

The *weighting factor* (W_t) of a particular tissue or organ is the risk of stochastic effects being induced in the organ when singly irradiated, compared to the total risk of inducing stochastic effects if the same radiation dose is received by the whole body.

Table 34.3   Weighting factors for different tissues irradiated singly

Tissue	Weighting factor (W_t)
Testes and ovaries	0.20
Red bone marrow	0.12
Colon	0.12
Lung	0.12
Stomach	0.12
Breast	0.05
Bladder	0.05
Thyroid	0.05
Liver	0.05
Oesophagus	0.05
Bone surfaces	0.02
Remaining tissues (not listed above)	0.05

The various weighting factors for different tissues are shown in Table 34.3. As can be seen from this table, the testes and ovaries are the most radio-sensitive tissues as they have the highest value of weighting factor. The weighting factors quoted are those from ICRP 60. Notice also that the sum of the weighting factors is unity.

The unit of effective dose is just the same as the unit of dose equivalent (Sv or mSv) since the weighting factors are constants.

The following example shows how the weighting factors given in Table 34.3 are used to calculate the effective dose received from radiography of the chest.

Example

Radiography of the chest produced the following doses: gonads 0.01 mSv, breast 0.05 mSv, red bone marrow 0.005 mSv, thyroid 0.02 mSv, bone 0.005 mSv, stomach 0.05 mSv, liver 0.002 mSv, colon 0.002 mSv and bladder 0.001 mSv. What is the effective dose received by the patient?

We can calculate the effective dose by taking the dose equivalent for each structure and multiplying it by the appropriate weighting factor. Thus we have:

$$
\begin{aligned}
\text{dose equivalent} &= (0.01 \times 0.2) + (0.05 \times 0.05) + (0.005 \times 0.12) + (0.02 \times 0.05) + \\
&\quad (0.005 \times 0.05) + (0.05 \times 0.12) + (0.002 \times 0.05) + (0.002 \times \\
&\quad 0.12) + (0.001 \times 0.05) \\
&= 0.002 + 0.0025 + 0.0006 + 0.001 + 0.00025 + 0.006 + \\
&\quad 0.0001 + 0.00024 + 0.00005 \\
&= 0.01274 \text{ mSv}
\end{aligned}
$$

Thus a chest radiograph produced using the above technique is equivalent to 0.01274 mSv for radiation protection purposes.

34.9 COMMITTED DOSE

When we consider committed dose we are considering the absorbed dose which a person receives as a result of the intake of radioactive material. In such a case the person will continue to receive a dose of radiation as long as any traces of radioactivity remain within the body. The factors which affect the activity remaining in the body are the effective half-life which is related to the physical half-life and the biological half-life as shown in the equation below (this has been discussed in more detail in Sect. 4.6):

$$\frac{1}{t_{\frac{1}{2}(\text{eff})}} = \frac{1}{t_{\frac{1}{2}(\text{phys})}} + \frac{1}{t_{\frac{1}{2}(\text{biol})}}$$

Equation 34.2

where $t_{\frac{1}{2}(\text{eff})}$ is the effective half-life, $t_{\frac{1}{2}(\text{phys})}$ is the physical half-life and $t_{\frac{1}{2}(\text{biol})}$ is the biological half-life. It is not possible to alter the physical half-life of a radionuclide as this depends on the structure of the nucleus, but it may be possible to reduce the biological half-life, e.g. by increasing the rate of excretion of the nuclide from the body. This results in a reduction of the effective half-life as shown by Equation 34.2.

The effective half-life is, however, only one of a number of factors which determine the magnitude of the radiation dose equivalent delivered to the body. Other factors include:

- the concentration of the activity in the organ (measured in $MBq \cdot kg^{-1}$)
- whether the concentration is uniform or localised within 'hot spots' within the organ
- the decay system (see Sect. 27.3) of the radionuclide
- the quality factors (see Sect. 34.4) of the radiations emitted
- the size and shape of the organ
- the weighting factor for the organ.

The decay system is particularly relevant if alpha or beta particles are emitted as they have a very short range in tissue and alpha particles have a high quality factor (20). Gamma rays, however, are exponentially absorbed by the organ and so will contribute a smaller dose to that organ but may contribute a significant dose to other surrounding organs. The higher the energy of the gamma rays the lower the attenuation within the organ.

The *committed dose equivalent* is a quantitative assessment of the effect of a particular intake of radioactivity over the whole of a person's working life. It may be defined as follows:

Definition

The *committed dose equivalent* is the dose equivalent accruing over a period of 50 years following the intake of radioactive material.

The *committed effective dose* is obtained using the weighting factors in Table 34.3, and, once this figure is obtained for a given intake over a given period of time, it is compared with equivalent limits laid down by the IRR for the same period (e.g. annual or quarterly dose limit) for the appropriate category of person (radiation worker, member of the public, etc.). The dose limits stipulated by the IRR are shown in Table 34.4.

Table 34.4(a) shows the dose limits for two categories of radiation workers and also for 'any other person' who is not a radiation worker and therefore has the same dose limits as a member of the general public. Note that in all cases the dose limits for radiation workers under 18 years of age are three-tenths of the adult radiation worker doses, and the dose limits for 'any other person' are one-tenth of the adult radiation worker doses. The whole-body dose limits are expressed in *effective dose* units (including the contributions of the committed dose), whereas the dose limits to individual organs are in *dose-equivalent* units. The use of weighting factors in the determination of effective dose is described above. These are required to calculate the effective whole-body dose.

Table 34.4(b) shows the dose limits specified by the IRR in order to protect the fetus. The dose equivalents shown refer to the maximum value which may be received from *external radiation*, i.e. the committed dose from the intake of radioactive materials is not included. Hence there is a need to

Table 34.4a   Dose limits specified by Ionising Radiation Regulations

Category of person	Effective dose plus committed effective dose for whole body		Dose equivalent plus committed dose	
	Annual	Calendar quarter*	For individual organs—annual	For lens of eye—annual
Radiation workers aged 18 years or more	50 mSv	30 mSv	500 mSv	150 mSv
Trainee radiation workers aged less than 18 years	15 mSv	9 mSv	150 mSv	45 mSv
Any other person	5 mSv	3 mSv	50 mSv	15 mSv

*A calendar quarter covers any of the inclusive periods January–March, April–June, July–September, October–December.

Table 34.4b   Dose-equivalent limits to the abdomen for women of reproductive capacity and pregnant women (radiation workers)

Category	Dose equivalent to the abdomen
Women of reproductive capacity	13 mSv in any consecutive 3-month interval
Pregnant women at work	10 mSv during the declared term of pregnancy

Note: The above limits do not take into account any committed dose to the fetus, so special care must be taken to restrict the intake of radioactive material for a pregnant woman.

restrict the possible intake of radioactivity, especially in working environments where radioactive material is more easily dispersed into the air. *Note that a woman who is not a radiation worker is already subject to the limit of 3 mSv per calendar quarter as shown in Table 34.4(a).*

Insight

It is worth recalling at this point that the unit of dose equivalent, the sievert, is the product of the absorbed dose and the quality factor for the radiation. Now the absorbed dose (measured in Gy) is measured in $J \cdot kg^{-1}$ and so relates to *unit mass*. Thus the total energy absorbed in a man weighing 70 kg who has received a whole-body dose of 3 Gy is $3 \times 70 = 210$ J. For the same person, the lungs might weigh approximately 0.5 kg and so the energy absorbed by the lungs for an absorbed dose of 3 Gy is $3 \times 0.5 = 1.5$ J.

From this it can be seen that the same value of absorbed dose or dose equivalent in different organs does not imply the same total absorption of energy but the same energy per unit mass. The biological effects of the absorbed energy depend on the radiosensitivity of the organ as described above.

34.10 DESIGNATION OF RADIATION WORKERS

If an employee is *likely to receive a dose of ionising radiation which exceeds three-tenths of any relevant dose limit* (IRR Regulation 9) then that person must be designated as a *classified person*, provided that:

- the employee is aged 18 years or more
- the employee has been certified as fit on medical grounds to be designated a classified person
- the employee is informed of being so designated.

For example if an adult employee is likely to receive a whole-body dose in 1 year in excess of 15 mSv (three-tenths of 50 mSv), then he or she must be classified and informed of this fact.

The Approved Code of Practice in paragraphs 64–66 discusses some of the practical ways of implementing the designation of employees as required by IRR Regulation 9. The main points of this discussion are summarised below:

- It is not sufficient to rely on an individual's history of doses received if they are less than the three-tenths limit. The *potential doses* which may be received in a set of circumstances must be assessed.
- The reason for designation may be that the individual works in *controlled areas* (see Sect. 34.11.5) but this is not, on its own, sufficient reason for designation.
- Even if the *Local Rules* (see Sect. 34.11.2), when strictly obeyed, indicate that doses in excess of the three-tenths limit will not occur, persons who work with radiation sources which are capable of producing an overdose in a few minutes will need to be classified. (This has limited

applications in the medical field for diagnostic imaging since it was intended to apply to personnel working with industrial rather than medical sources.)

● When considering the classification of persons in relation to the intake of radionuclides the following factors should be taken into account:

—the potential for any intake to occur

—the likely magnitude of any intake

—the radiotoxicity of any intake.

A person who is a *classified radiation worker* must be subject to *medical surveillance*, with periodic reviews of health at least every 12 months. The health records for such an individual must be kept on a suitable form for at least 50 years from the date of the last entry (IRR Regulation 16). The employer must also arrange for the radiation dose which the classified person receives to be measured using a suitable *personal dosemeter* (see Sect. 34.11.3). Such doses must be measured by an *approved dosimetry service* on the basis of accepted national standards. Again the employer must keep records of all doses recorded for such individuals for at least 50 years after the last entry.

It should be noted that the above discussion does not mean that radiation workers who are not classified should not have dose records and/or medical records kept, but that there is no legal requirement to do so. However, the *radiation protection adviser* (see Sect. 34.11.1) may use personnel and site dose records to justify his designation (or lack of it) both for personnel and for working areas.

Any employee, whether classified or not, whose annual whole-body dose exceeds 15 mSv shall be subject to an investigation to see if the working practices involved are in keeping with the ALARA principle (see Sect. 34.5) or whether improvements may be made which would lead to a reduction in the dose. Records of such investigations must be kept for at least 2 years (IRR Regulation 28).

In a medical environment, employees such as radiographers, medical laboratory scientific officers and medical physics technicians are involved in working with ionising radiations in the fields of diagnostic radiography, therapeutic radiography, nuclear medicine and pathology investigations using radionuclides. Each of these procedures contributes to the radiation doses received by appropriate personnel and these must each be analysed to see if a particular individual needs to become a classified person to conform with the requirements of the IRR. For example, a diagnostic radiographer is subject to ionising radiation from scatter from the patient and the walls of the X-ray room, while a therapy radiographer may receive some radiation through the walls of the treatment room and may receive an unexpected dose if the therapy source sticks in the exposed position after a treatment.

Staff in the nuclear medicine department will receive doses to the hands due to the preparation of radio-pharmaceuticals and the handling of 'flood sources' for gamma cameras. They will also receive a whole-body dose due to being in close proximity to patients who have received diagnostic or therapeutic quantities of radio-pharmaceuticals. Laboratory technicians who perform tests using radioactivity will also receive a dose to their hands and may also receive doses from spills or airborne contamination.

However, it is unlikely that any of those workers will need to be classified, although the radiological monitoring of their received doses and that of their environment is a precaution, and one which may be used to justify their non-classified status.

34.10.1 Dose limitations for employees who have been overexposed to radiation

The Ionising Radiation Regulations 29 and 30 lay down the procedures to adopt if it is known, or suspected, that an employee has been subject to overexposure to radiation. This overexposure may be the result of a single incident or because the total radiation dose received by the person during the period in question exceeds the relevant dose limit for that period— again it must be remembered that this is considered *occupational exposure* and any radiation exposure received by the person due to medical investigation or treatment does not count.

After an overexposure has been reported to the employer he must notify the HSE and the appropriate medical doctor. He must then carry out a detailed investigation into the circumstances of the overexposure. The HSE, the appointed doctor and the employee must receive a copy of the report and it must be kept by the employer for at least 50 years.

The overexposed person may be allowed to continue to work with ionising radiations provided the above notifications and investigations have been carried out, and under any condition(s) which the appointed doctor may specify. The dose limit for the individual for the remainder of the calendar year is given by the appropriate annual dose for the person multiplied by $m/12$, where m is the number of months remaining in the year.

34.11 PRACTICAL RADIATION PROTECTION

As described in the preceding sections of this chapter, radiation protection is based on three general principles:

- Every practice resulting in an exposure to ionising radiation should be *justified* by the advantages it produces.
- All exposures should be kept *as low as reasonably achievable* (ALARA).

- The sum of the doses and committed doses *should not exceed specified limits* (see Table 34.4).

The first two principles show that it is not merely sufficient to observe the current dose limits, since the possible health detriment from a given exposure must be compared to the overall benefit of that exposure and this may result in certain procedures involving ionising radiations being replaced by others which do not, e.g. ultrasound or magnetic resonance scans.

The IRR indicate the legal and procedural framework in which these principles may be achieved in practice. The main requirements are listed below:

- the provision of *suitable environments* for all employees, such that those areas where they are likely to receive a significant radiation dose are suitably restricted and controlled (see Sect. 34.11.5)
- the *designation of employees* into classified and non-classified groups on the basis of the doses which they are *likely to receive*
- the establishing of a suitable personnel monitoring service to ensure that radiation doses received are measured and recorded on a regular basis (whether or not non-classified radiation workers are monitored depends on local circumstances)
- the keeping of health records and radiation dose records for all classified radiation workers for the statutory period required by the IRR (50 years)
- notification to the HSE of all radiation incidents and overexposures, and the writing of reports subsequent to the investigation of these incidents
- the establishment of *environmental monitoring* to establish that the working conditions of the employees and the doses received by the general public are in accordance with the IRR
- the appointment of a *suitably qualified* person as *radiation protection adviser* (RPA) to act in an advisory capacity to the employer to ensure that the IRR is being suitably implemented
- the appointment of suitably qualified persons as *radiation protection supervisors* (RPSs) in each department where work with ionising radiation takes place
- the writing of suitable *Local Rules* for the establishment of safe working practices for employees
- the drawing up of reasonable contingency plans, e.g. what the procedure is in the event of fire in a radiation area.

The designation of workers, personnel record keeping and the notification of incidents and overexposure have been discussed in previous sections of this chapter. The appointment of RPAs and RPSs, the formulation of Local Rules, personnel monitoring methods and the designation of working areas will now be considered in the following sections.

34.11.1 Radiation protection advisers and radiation protection supervisors

Regulation 10 of the IRR states that if an employee is subject to an instantaneous (dose averaged over 1 minute) dose rate which exceeds $7.5\,\mu Sv\cdot h^{-1}$ or where the employer has already created a controlled area (see Sect. 34.11.4), then the employer must appoint one or more radiation protection advisers (RPAs). Any RPA must be *a suitably qualified and experienced person* and is appointed for the purpose of advising the employer as to the observance of the IRR and on all other aspects of the safe use of ionising radiation. The HSE must have been notified of the person's details, including qualifications and experience, at least 28 days before the appointment—or at shorter notice if this is unavoidable. In order that the RPA may perform the advisory role, the employer must provide him or her with an adequate job description, adequate information regarding the activities of the employees and adequate facilities with which to perform his/her duties.

The RPA will be expected to give advice on all of the following:

- dosimetry and monitoring
- the designation and control of restricted areas
- drawing up systems of work and Local Rules
- investigation of radiation incidents
- ensuring adequate training and update of radiation workers
- commenting on the design of new, or modification of old, premises from a radiation protection aspect
- preparation of contingency plans.

The RPA is also involved in the selection of radiation protection supervisors (RPSs), who are persons directly involved in working with ionising radiation on a day-to-day basis. It is normal to have an RPS in each department to ensure safe working practice within that department. Radiation protection supervisors must have sufficient knowledge and experience to allow them to carry out their duties in their department.

34.11.2 Local Rules

Under the IRR, the employer has a legal responsibility to ensure that written Local Rules are produced for departments where employees are involved in work with ionising radiation. These rules must be brought to the attention of all employees working in these departments. In practice, the RPAs have the necessary knowledge and experience to formulate these rules and it is the task of the RPSs to ensure that the rules are known and put into practice by colleagues in their own departments.

The Local Rules for a department should be displayed in a prominent position, or positions, within the department concerned, and should contain the following information:

- the name of the RPS for the department
- a description of each restricted area (see Sect. 34.11.4)
- details of restrictions of access to such areas
- written systems of work detailing the working procedures for the department
- details of any contingency plans.

34.11.3 Personnel monitoring

Personnel monitoring is necessary to measure the radiation doses received by radiation workers in the course of their work to verify that these doses are within the recommended limits. This is known as *personnel monitoring* and acts not only as a check of the actual doses received but also as a scrutiny of the various radiation protection policies formulated by the RPA. It also allows the RPA and the RPSs to identify individuals who habitually have higher doses and counsel such individuals before their neglectfulness reaches serious proportions.

There are two main methods of personnel monitoring currently used in the UK. These are:

- the film badge method
- thermoluminescent dosimetry.

34.11.3.1 The film badge method

This method is based on the principle that the optical density produced by processing on photographic film increases with the amount of radiation received by the film. This principle has already been discussed in Section 33.6.5. The use of plastic, tin and aluminium filters in the badge holder enables the distinction to be made whether the dose was the result of beta particle or low- or high-energy X- or γ-rays. The films may be processed by an approved dosimetry service. Details of the construction of the film badge holder and film are given in Figure 34.2.

The main advantage of the film badge method of monitoring is that the film may be kept as a permanent record of the dose received. It does, however, have the disadvantages that the dose reading takes place some time after the exposure to radiation and that the film is expensive, not reusable and can deteriorate if not stored in proper conditions prior to processing.

34.11.3.2 Thermoluminescent dosimetry (TLD)

Some of the disadvantages of the film badge method of monitoring are overcome by the use of thermoluminescent dosimetry. The basic principles

Figure 34.2 The film-badge holder and film as used in personnel monitoring. The optically sealed film has a fast emulsion on the side facing the front of the badge and a slow emulsion on the other side. If a high exposure to radiation has occurred, the fast emulsion may be removed thus allowing a dose estimation to be made using the slow emulsion. Various filters are used to separate the effects of different types and energies of radiations. Key to structure of the holder: 1—open window; 2—thin plastic filter (0.5 mm); 3—thick plastic filter (2.8 mm); 4—dural (alloy of aluminium) filter (1.0 mm); 5—tin filter (0.7 mm) + lead filter (0.3 mm); 6—cadmium filter (0.7 mm) + lead filter (0.3 mm); 7 is a strip of lead (0.3 mm) which shields filters 5 and 6 to prevent radiation entering the holder through the side of the badge and thus affecting the film under these filters. Beta particles are absorbed by filters 3 onwards. Only high-energy X-rays and γ-rays are able to penetrate the tin + lead filter (5) significantly so that an estimate may be made of the relative amounts of low- and high-energy X- and γ-rays by comparing the photographic densities beneath filters 4 and 5. The cadmium + lead filter (6) is used to estimate exposure to thermal neutrons (for workers in the nuclear industry) because neutron capture by the cadmium nuclei results in gamma photon emission which creates an exposure to the film. (This illustration is reproduced by kind permission of the National Radiological Protection Board, Chilton, Oxon.)

of this process have already been discussed in Section 33.6.4. An example of a TLD badge used for monitoring purposes is shown in Figure 34.3. This badge contains an identified holder which contains two disks of thermo-luminescent material. One disk is positioned behind the open window of the badge and estimates the skin dose while the other disk is behind the plastic dome and is used to estimate the whole-body dose.

Thermoluminescent materials may also be used to measure doses to specific organs, e.g. they can be wrapped round a finger to measure the dose to that finger.

34.11.3.3 Pocket dosemeters

Specialist electronic devices are available which will measure the radiation

Figure 34.3 The thermoluminescent dosemeter badge as supplied by the National Radiological Protection Board (NRPB), Chilton, Oxon. The photograph shows the components of the NRPB thermoluminescent dosemeter for whole-body monitoring: the holder (top left); the insert cover (top right) below which (bottom right) is the insert itself with its two lithium fluoride/PTFE (polytetrafluoroethylene) disks. Each insert is coded by holes punched in it, so enabling computerised record keeping by the NRPB after automatic measuring of the doses received under computer control. The holder has an open window situated over the thin (40 mg·cm^{-2}) disk which is used to estimate the dose received by the skin (e.g. from electrons and low-energy X- and γ-radiation). The thick (90 mg·cm^{-2}) disk is situated under a 700 mg·cm^{-2} thick dome of plastic and is used to estimate the whole-body dose (e.g. that due to high-energy X- and γ-radiation). (Note that the true thickness of the material in cm is obtained by dividing the value of thickness expressed in mg·cm^{-2} by the density of the material in mg·cm^{-3}.) (This photograph is published by kind permission of the National Radiological Protection Board, Chilton, Oxon.)

dose *at the time of exposure* and warn the wearer of any unusually high dose. These may be worn in the pockets of laboratory coats and so are known as *pocket dosemeters*. The dose is usually displayed on a digital readout on the dosemeter.

The final choice as to which is the most appropriate method of personnel monitoring is usually made by the RPA who will assess the risk of receiving an unexpectedly high dose.

34.11.4 Designation of work areas

In order to protect employees and members of the public from unnecessary amounts of radiation when on an employer's property, the IRR (Regulation 8 and Schedule 6) makes a distinction between two types of areas:

Table 34.5 Description of designated areas

Name of designated area	Requirements for designation	Permitted access
Controlled area	a. Area where the instantaneous* dose rate exceeds 7.5 mSv·h⁻¹ b. Area where an adult employee is likely to receive more than three-tenths of any relevant dose limit (e.g. 15 mSv whole-body dose per annum)	a. Classified person b. Any other person under a written scheme of work c. A patient undergoing therapy or diagnostic procedures
Supervised area	An area where any person would be likely to receive in excess of one-third of the value required for designation of a controlled area (e.g. 5 mSv whole-body dose per annum)	Those whose presence is necessary

*Dose rate averaged over 1 minute.

- supervised areas
- controlled areas.

The differences between the two areas are summarised in Table 34.5.

The employer, once having designated an area as a controlled area, must demarcate or otherwise delineate the area by some suitable means, and must restrict access to it. The area may be described with respect to existing walls if this is convenient but this may not always be possible, e.g. in the case of a mobile X-ray unit used in a ward. Access is best restricted using physical barriers, but if the work is of short duration, access may be restricted by continuous supervision, e.g. mobile radiography in a ward. The limitations of access to a controlled area are listed in Table 34.5. Many X-ray departments have dispensed with the 'supervised area' and simply regard the whole of the X-ray room and its protected cubicle as a controlled area.

In the case of mobile X-ray units operating at above 70 kV$_p$ the controlled area is taken as a circle of radius 1.5 metres with the centre of the circle being the focus of the X-ray tube. A similar situation exists for dental units with the circle having a 1-metre radius.

34.11.5 Good radiographic practice

As has already been discussed, it is always important to minimise the radiation doses received by patients and staff. Methods of achieving this are given in Table 34.6 (for patients) and Table 34.7 (for staff). It may be noted that some of the items listed are within the control of the radiographer and some are not. By careful attention to such detail the radiographer should be able to produce radiographs of high diagnostic quality with the lowest practicable radiation dose to the patient.

Table 34.6 Methods of minimising radiation doses to patients

Factors not within the radiographer's control
Filtration of the X-ray beam (see Sect. 29.7)
Rectification (see Sect. 29.6)
Tube shielding (see Ch. 22)

Factors within the radiographer's control
Limitation of field size by the use of collimation
Use of the fastest film/intensifying screen combination consistent with good image quality
Reduction of the number of repeat examinations by the use of good radiographic technique
(positioning, exposure, patient preparation, etc.)
Consistent optimum film processing
Use of the highest practicable kVp
Use of autotimers to control exposure time
Selection of an appropriate secondary radiation grid
Compression of obese patients
Use of digital techniques

In fluoroscopy
Use of properly set image intensifier
Use of automatic collimation
Use of pulsed fluoroscopy
Use of image storage facilities
Use of digital fluoroscopy

Table 34.7 Methods of minimising radiation doses to staff

In radiography
Only those whose presence is required should be in the room during exposures
All staff should stand behind the protective barrier during the exposure
The X-ray tube should have adequate shielding (see Ch. 22)
The use of immobilising devices for restless patients—such patients should not be supported
by radiographers during radiographic examinations

In fluoroscopy
Staff must wear adequate protective clothing as indicated in the Local Rules and Systems of
Work
The use of automatic collimation
Staff should stand as far away as possible from the primary beam
Lead rubber shielding should be incorporated in the image intensifier to reduce dose from
scattered radiation

Fluoroscopy results in higher radiation doses than conventional radiography and therefore good technique is even more essential to keep radiation doses to a minimum. The use of a modern fluoroscopic unit with pulsed fluoroscopy, image storage, automatic collimation and digitisation of the image all result in a reduction of the radiation doses to patients and staff.

34.11.6 Room design

For radiation protection purposes the function of the X-ray room is to provide an enclosure for the X-ray unit and so limit the access to the radiation area. The room should also provide adequate shielding to the rest of the environment from the radiation produced. In addition, provision is made for a barrier inside the room behind which staff may be protected from the radiation while they operate the units—in therapy treatment rooms, the equipment is operated from outside the treatment room. If there is more than one X-ray tube operating off the generator in a diagnostic room, there must be a visual indication (usually a warning light) to indicate which tube is in circuit and so is capable of producing radiation if energised.

The level of radiation protection given by barriers and walls is usually stated in terms of their *lead equivalent.*

Definition

The *lead equivalent* of an absorbing material is the thickness of lead which would absorb the same amount of radiation as the given material when exposed to radiation of the same type and quality.

The lead equivalent thus gives a basis for comparing one barrier to another at a given beam energy.

In the diagnostic range of beam energies (up to 150 keV) the photo-electric absorption within lead is significant owing to its high atomic number (see Sect. 30.5). For this reason, many barriers (e.g. doors) in the diagnostic X-ray room incorporate a few millimetres of lead laminated with wood, to give adequate radiation protection. Lead-glass windows are often fitted to such barriers to enable a visual contact to be maintained. The protection afforded by such a window must be at least the same amount as the protective barrier itself and there must be no gaps where the radiation is able to penetrate. The siting of such a barrier to protect the staff must be such that the radiation must be scattered at least twice (thus greatly reducing its intensity) before reaching the opening in the barrier.

Wall thicknesses between X-ray rooms and adjacent areas must be such that any transmitted radiation will not produce a dose in excess of 0.1 mSv per week (this leads to a maximum dose of 5 mSv per year which is the maximum dose for the general public). This figure must be calculated for all walls, floors, ceilings, and windows of the X-ray rooms and is calculated by applying a *use factor*. The use factor is an estimation of the time when the radiation beam will be pointing towards that area. As a result of this calculation, the maximum dose received by a person sited on the far side of the barrier may be estimated and it must not exceed 0.1 mSv per week—in previous legislation there was also an *occupancy factor* which looked at the fraction of time a person was likely to spend in this area, but this factor has now been discontinued.

The materials used in the construction of the walls and floor of the X-ray room may contain lead sheeting or there may be sufficient thickness of other materials, such as concrete, to provide adequate absorption of the primary and scatter radiation produced in the room. The lead equivalent of a concrete wall 15 cm thick is approximately 1.5 mm within the diagnostic energy range—this reflects the superior absorption of lead compared to concrete in this energy range. The lead equivalent of such walls may be increased by the use of *barium sulphate plaster* as a thin coating on the walls—this is because of the high atomic number of barium (56).

As the beam energy increases, the advantage of lead over concrete diminishes as there is a gradual shift from the predominance of photo-electric absorption to the predominance of Compton scattering. Thus the lead equivalent of a barrier will increase with an increase in the photon energy—a greater thickness of lead will be required to give the same level of protection as the barrier. In the region of 1 MeV the Compton scattering process predominates and lead has no real advantage over concrete since all materials have similar mass attenuation coefficients due to the Compton process. Thus many of the barriers used in radiotherapy departments are made of large thicknesses of concrete.

In conclusion, the design of a room, its wall thickness and the barriers must be such that the radiation dose received by patients, staff and members of the public are kept to a minimum in accordance with the ALARA principle. Further details of the design of diagnostic and therapy rooms will be found in specialised publications on this topic.

Summary

In this chapter you should have learnt:

- The purpose and scope of radiation protection (see Sect. 34.2)
- An outline of ionising radiation regulations (see Sect. 34.3)
- The biological effects of ionising radiation (see Sect. 34.4)
- The stochastic effects of ionising radiation including radiation-induced cancers and genetic effects (see Sect. 34.4.1)
- The deterministic (non-stochastic) effects of ionising radiation (see Sect. 34.4.2)
- Risk-benefit, ALARA (ALARP) and detriment as applied to ionising radiation (see Sect. 34.5)
- Special precautions in the radiological examination of women of reproductive capacity (see Sect. 34.6)
- Dose-equivalent limits in radiation protection (see Sect. 34.7)
- The definition of effective dose and how this is used in radiation protection (see Sect. 34.8)
- The definition of committed dose and how this is used in radiation protection (see Sect. 34.9)
- The requirements for the designation of radiation workers (see Sect. 34.10)
- Dose limitations for employees who have been overexposed to radiation (see Sect. 34.10.1)
- Practical radiation protection measures (see Sect. 34.11)
- The appointment and work of RPAs and RPSs (see Sect. 34.11.1)
- Local Rules and their uses in radiation protection (see Sect. 34.11.2)
- Methods of personnel monitoring (see Sect. 34.11.3)
- Designation of work areas in radiation protection (see Sect. 34.11.4)
- Good radiographic practice and its role in radiation protection (see Sect. 34.11.5)
- The requirements for room design in radiography and radiotherapy (see Sect. 34.11.6).

SELF-TEST

a. Outline the sequence of events which can lead to ionising radiations having a biological effect on tissue.

b. Compare and contrast *stochastic* and *deterministic* effects of radiation.

c. If all the organs of the body receive an effective dose of 2 mSv, what is the effective whole-body dose?

d. List the factors to be considered when estimating the committed dose from an ingested radioactive material.

e. What are the annual whole-body radiation dose limits for the following categories of personnel:
   (i) a radiation worker over 18 years of age
   (ii) a trainee radiation worker under 18 years of age
   (iii) a member of the public who is not a radiation worker
   (iv) a female radiation worker of reproductive capacity
   (v) a pregnant radiation worker?

f. Define a *classified radiation worker* and list the restrictions on the appointment of such a person.

g. List the three general principles of radiation protection.

h. Compare and contrast the role of the radiation protection adviser and the radiation protection supervisor.

i. List three methods of personnel monitoring and give the advantages and disadvantages of one of these methods.

j. List the requirements for the designation of a controlled area and list the persons who have access to such an area.

k. List the factors which a radiographer may use to limit the radiation dose to the patient during a diagnostic radiography procedure.

FURTHER READING

Ball J L, Moore A D 1986 Essential physics for radiographers, 2nd edn. Blackwell Scientific Publications, London, chs 17, 20
Ball J, Price T 1989 Chesneys' Radiographic imaging. Blackwell Scientific Publications, London, ch 5A
Carter P H 1994 Chesneys' Equipment for student radiographers. Blackwell Scientific Publications, London, ch 5

Curry T S et al 1990 Christensen's Physics of diagnostic radiology. Lea & Febinger, London, ch 21

Foster E 1985 Equipment for diagnostic radiography. MTP Press, Lancaster, ch 14

Gifford D 1984 A handbook of physics for radiologists and radiographers. John Wiley & Sons, Chichester, chs 15–18, 47–49

Hay G A, Hughes D 1983 First year physics for radiographers. Baillière Tindall, London, chs 16, 17

Health and Safety Executive (HSE) 1985 The ionising radiation regulations. HMSO, London

Health and Safety Executive (HSE) 1988 The ionising radiation (protection of persons undergoing medical examination or treatment) regulations. HMSO, London

Hendee W, Ritenour R 1992 Medical imaging physics, 3rd edn. Mosby Year Book, London, chs 7, 8, 27–30

HMSO 1985 Approved code of practice. The protection of persons against ionising radiation arising from any work activity. HMSO, London

Jenkins D 1980 Radiographic photography and imaging processes. MTP Press, Lancaster, ch 3

Johns H E, Cunningham J R 1983 The physics of radiology, 4th edn. Charles C Thomas, Illinois, USA, chs 7, 9, 15, 17

Merideth W J, Massey J B 1977 Fundamental physics of radiology. John Wright, Bristol, chs XLII–XLV

National Radiological Protection Board (NRPB) 1988 Guidance notes for the protection of persons against ionising radiations arising from medical and dental use. HMSO, London

Ohanian H C 1994 Principles of physics. W W Norton, London, ch 31

Plaut S 1993 Radiation protection in the X-ray department. Butterworth-Heinemann, Oxford

Sumner D, Wheldon T, Watson W 1991 Radiation risks: an evaluation. The Tarragon Press, Glasgow

Thompson M A 1994 Principles of imaging science and protection. W B Saunders, London, chs 18–21

Webb S (ed) 1988 The physics of medical imaging. Institute of Physics Publishing, Bristol, ch 15

NB At the time of printing it is proposed that the POPUMET (1988) Regulations be replaced by The Ionising Radiation (Medical Exposure) Regulations (1999). From the consultative documents it is suggested that these regulations will be implemented from 1 January, 2000. The reader is recommended to consult this document when published. The information released for consultation can be found at http://www.doh.gov.uk/popumet.htm. The document and its impact on radiation protection will be considered in detail in the next edition of this text.

Appendices, Tables and Answers to self-tests

Appendix A

MATHEMATICS FOR RADIOGRAPHY

This Appendix on the revision of mathematics is directed primarily at those whose mathematics is a little weak. However, many of the worked examples shown are chosen from topics in radiography.

For those studying for examinations, the following remarks may be of help. Examiners frequently complain of cramped, untidy mathematics which is difficult to follow. What they are hoping to see in the answer is a clear statement of the problem and an easy-to-follow development of the mathematics used to obtain the solution. This may be more important (and hence gain more marks) than simply obtaining the correct numerical answer. In fact, the correct answer simply recorded on its own with little or no supporting mathematical reasoning will not achieve many marks—remember that the examiner cannot know how you achieved the final answer unless you tell him/her. In practice, you should use phrases and sentences to tell the examiner how you have progressed from one step of the problem to the next as you move towards the eventual solution. This should also help you to think more clearly about what you are doing and also to check the integrity of your final answer—this is probably even more important with the widespread use of pocket calculators. A study of the worked examples in this Appendix should clarify these points.

A.1 ALGEBRAIC SYMBOLS

The letters of the English and Greek alphabet (see Table D at the end of this book) are often used to represent the magnitude of an unknown quantity. For example, an electrical potential difference may be represented by V volts, an angle by θ (i.e. 'theta') degrees or radians and an energy by E joules. Such a practice enables the symbols to be used in place of the actual numerical values of the quantities, and is of great practical use in the solving of equations (see App. A.4).

A.1.1 Suffixes

Suffixes are used to denote a specific value of a particular quantity. If we use the symbol I to denote the intensity of radiation from a particular source, then I will depend upon the distance from the source at which the intensity is measured (Ch. 3). We may call a particular distance x, say, and denote the intensity of this distance by I_x—meaning *'the intensity at x'*. For another distance y, the corresponding value of intensity is I_y.

Similarly, if a quantity N changes with time, t, the value of N at any given time may be denoted by N_t.

Suffixes are used, then, to avoid ambiguity and are used as such in many chapters of this book.

A.2 FRACTIONS AND PERCENTAGES

Although fractions are not commonly used in radiographic calculations since they have been largely replaced with decimals, nevertheless a knowledge of how to manipulate fractions mathematically is useful in calculations involving Ohm's Law (see Ch. 10) and capacitors (see Ch. 16). For this reason a section on fractions and percentages is still included in this Appendix.

A.2.1 Percentages

If a quantity increases in value by 50 per cent (%), then it is meant by this that it has become greater by one-half of its previous value. Thus, if the electric current passing through an X-ray tube was 200 mA, then an increase of 50% would bring this to 300 mA. Alternatively, it may be said that the new value is 150% of the original value.

In general terms, if a is the original value of a quantity and b is its new value, then:

- the *percentage change* $= 100 \times \dfrac{b-a}{a}$

- $\dfrac{100b}{a}$ is the 'percentage of b compared to a'

- $y\%$ of a is just $\dfrac{y}{100} \times a$.

Examples

a. Original value = 60; new value = 80

The percentage change is then $100 \times \dfrac{20}{60} = 33\frac{1}{3}\%$ and the new value is $100 \times \dfrac{80}{60} = 133\frac{1}{3}\%$ of the original.

b. A quantity has reduced by 25%. What is the new value if it was 600 originally?

25% of 600 is just $\dfrac{25}{100} \times 600 = 150$, so that the new value is $600 - 150 = 450$.

A percentage is a special case of a fraction, where one number is divided by another. The following sections describe how fractions may be added together and multiplied.

A.2.2 Addition of fractions

Suppose we have the fraction a/b, where a and b represent general numbers. Now the addition or subtraction of a/b to another fraction c/d rests on the fact that we can take any fraction and multiply top and bottom by the same factor (k, say) *without* altering its value,

i.e. $\dfrac{a}{b} = \dfrac{ka}{kb}$ (because the ks cancel).

It is the appropriate selection of k for each fraction which makes for the easy addition of fractions. For example, suppose we have:

$$\frac{2}{3} + \frac{5}{6}$$

If we multiply $\frac{2}{3}$ by 2 (top and bottom), we shall have a fraction expressed in sixths, just like the second fraction.

i.e. $\dfrac{2}{3} + \dfrac{5}{6} = \dfrac{2 \times 2}{2 \times 3} + \dfrac{5}{6} = \dfrac{4}{6} + \dfrac{5}{6} = \dfrac{9}{6} = 1\dfrac{1}{2}$

Notice that we multiplied only the first fraction—we need not do the same thing to the second. This method is often very quick, particularly when only two or three simple fractions are involved, and is in fact entirely equivalent to the more general method of using the lowest common denominator (LCD), as illustrated in the following example:

$$\frac{2}{3} + \frac{3}{4} - \frac{5}{6} = \frac{4 \times 2 + 3 \times 3 - 2 \times 5}{12} = \frac{8 + 9 - 10}{12}$$

$$= \frac{7}{12}$$

Here, the LCD of the denominators 3, 4 and 6 is 12 and is therefore used as the overall denominator on the right-hand side. The individual denominators are then divided into 12, the result being multiplied by the respective numerator and summed (observing the correct signs) as shown in the example.

Exercise A.1 (answers at the end of this appendix)

a. $\dfrac{11}{12} - \dfrac{5}{6}$

b. $\dfrac{7}{9} + \dfrac{2}{3}$

c. What is 20% of 50?

d. $\dfrac{2}{3} - \dfrac{1}{4} + \dfrac{3}{5}$

e. $\dfrac{7}{11} + \dfrac{2}{9} - \dfrac{2}{3}$

f. What is the percentage change if a quantity increases from 80 to 90?

A.3 MULTIPLYING AND DIVIDING

A.3.1 Positive and negative numbers

It is obvious that $1 \times 8 = 8$, but what are -1×8, -1×-8 and 8×-1?

To avoid having to work out such problems from first principles every time, a simple rule has been developed which we may call Rule 1.

Rule 1
When multiplying or dividing two numbers together:

> **Two (+)s make a (+).**
> **Two (–)s make a (+).**
> **A (+) and a (–) make a (–).**

i.e. only when the signs are dissimilar is the result negative.

Examples

a. $-3 \times 4 = -12$

b. $14 \div -7 = -2$

c. $\dfrac{-40}{-4} = 10$

d. $-2 \times -4 \times -3 = 8 \times -3 = -24$

Exercise A.2

a. $28 \div 7$

b. $\dfrac{-36}{6}$

c. $\dfrac{144}{-4}$

d. -13×-3

e. $-7 \times \dfrac{-8}{-2}$

A.3.2 Fractions

The *multiplication* of two or more fractions is just a matter of simplification by cancellation (where possible) and then multiplying all the numerators together to form the new numerator, and all the denominators together to form the new denominator.

Examples

a. $\dfrac{2}{3} \times \dfrac{7}{5} = \dfrac{14}{15}$ (no cancellation possible)

b. $\dfrac{2}{3} \times \dfrac{9}{4} = \dfrac{{}^{1}\cancel{2}}{\cancel{3}_{1}} \times \dfrac{\cancel{9}^{3}}{\cancel{4}_{2}} = \dfrac{3}{2}$

The *division* of two fractions is straightforward provided that the following rule is obeyed.

Rule 2
When dividing by one or more fractions, turn those in the denominator upside down and multiply.

Let us say, by way of illustration, that we wish to divide 4 by $\frac{1}{2}$,

i.e. $\dfrac{4}{\dfrac{1}{2}}$

Applying Rule 2, we turn $\frac{1}{2}$ upside down and multiply:

$$\dfrac{4}{\dfrac{1}{2}} = 4 \times \dfrac{2}{1} = 8$$

Is this the answer we would expect intuitively? Well, the problem may be expressed as 'how many halves are there in 4?', and then it is obvious that the answer is 8. Some more examples to clarify the method:

a. $7 \div \dfrac{14}{9} = 7 \times \dfrac{9}{14} = \dfrac{9}{2}$

b. $\dfrac{\dfrac{3}{8}}{\dfrac{7}{11}} = \dfrac{3}{8} \times \dfrac{11}{7} = \dfrac{33}{56}$

c. $\dfrac{\dfrac{4}{9}}{\dfrac{-8}{27}} = \dfrac{4}{9} \times \dfrac{-27}{8} = -\dfrac{3}{2}$

d. $\dfrac{\dfrac{2}{3}}{\dfrac{4}{7} \times \dfrac{3}{5}} = \dfrac{2}{3} \times \dfrac{7}{4} \times \dfrac{5}{3} = \dfrac{35}{18}$

Exercise A.3

a. $\dfrac{\dfrac{-4}{11}}{\dfrac{7}{22}}$

b. $\dfrac{\dfrac{2}{9}}{\dfrac{7}{3} \times \dfrac{-2}{11}}$

c. $\dfrac{\dfrac{1}{3} \times \dfrac{2}{9}}{\dfrac{9}{1} \times \dfrac{1}{2}}$

A.3.3 Brackets

A bracket links two or more quantities together such that the bracket and its contents may be treated mathematically as a single quantity. If we wish to *remove* the brackets, then care over the plus and minus signs must be taken (Rule 1).

Examples

a. $2 \times (a - b) = 2 \times a - 2 \times b = 2a - 2b$
   Thus, each term in the bracket is multiplied by the term outside the bracket, with due regard for the sign convention.

b. $-4(c - 2d) = -4c + 8d$

Note that the multiplication sign, present in Example a, has been omitted, as is usually the case.

c. $-3\left(\dfrac{-2a}{3} + b - \dfrac{1c}{7}\right) = 2a - 3b + \dfrac{3c}{7}$

Multiplying two or more brackets together can become quite involved. However, it is rare for problems in radiography to require even the multiplication of two brackets, but the method is outlined below for the sake of completeness.

Assume we wish to calculate:

$(a + b)(c + d)$
i.e. $(a + b)$ multiplied by $(c + d)$.

To perform this calculation, we take the first term of the first bracket, a, and multiply it by $(c + d)$. Then we add the result to the multiplication of the second term, b, by $(c + d)$:

i.e. $(a + b)(c + d) = a(c + d) + b(c + d)$
$= ac + ad + bc + bd$

Again, we must be careful of the sign convention (Rule 1), as the following two worked examples show.

Examples

a. $(7 + c)(d - 8) = 7(d - 8) + c(d - 8)$
$= 7d - 56 + cd - 8c$

b. $(4 - a)(3 - b + 2c) = 4(3 - b + 2c) - a(3 - b + 2c)$
$= 12 - 4b + 8c - 3a + ab - 2ac$

Exercise A.4

a. $7a - 4(a - 2)$
b. $-6(-x + y - 3)$
c. $2(3a - 4) - 3(-a + 6)$

A.4 SOLVING EQUATIONS

Many of the types of equations encountered in problems associated with radiography are those in which a single 'unknown' (whose numerical value we wish to calculate) is 'mixed up' with several other numbers which may occur on both sides of the equation. (The solution of several equations involving several unknowns, i.e. simultaneous equations, is not normally required, and so will not be discussed here.) Our task, then, in the equations encountered, is to 'unscramble' the unknown so as to leave it on one side of the equation and all the numbers on the other side—the equation is then said to be 'solved'. This process is straightforward, provided that the following simple rule is obeyed.

Rule 3
Always perform the same operation to *both* sides of an equation.

This rule is intuitively obvious if it is imagined that the equals sign of the equation is the pivot of a pair of scales which is in exact balance. Whatever weight we now add to or subtract from one scale-pan must be added to or subtracted from the other or the scales will no longer be in balance. Similarly, if we double (say) the weight on one side we must do the same to the other—thus, provided we multiply by the same factor, balance is preserved and one side is equal to the other side. For example, consider the simple equation:

$$x - 2 = 3$$

If we add 2 to the left-hand side (LHS) of this equation the -2 will be cancelled, leaving x only. However, in accordance with Rule 3 above, we must add 2 to the right-hand side (RHS) in order to preserve equality.

i.e. $\quad x - 2 + 2 = 3 + 2 \quad$ thus $\quad x = 5$

Putting $x = 5$ in the original equation, we have $5 - 2 = 3$, which is correct.
As another example, consider: $15 - y = 7$. Subtracting 15 from both sides so as to eliminate it from the LHS:

$15 - y - 15 = 7 - 15$
i.e. $\quad -y = -8$

Multiplying both sides by -1 in order to make both terms positive (Rule 1), we have:

$-1 \cdot -y = -1 \cdot -8 \quad$ i.e. $\quad y = 8$

(*Note*: The symbol '$\cdot$' is often used, as above, to denote multiplication.)
Substituting our solution into the original equation to serve as a check, as in the previous example, we have:

$15 - 8 = 7$, thus verifying our answer.

It is apparent from these examples that a convenient way of picturing this type of mathematical operation is that of 'transferring a quantity from one side to the other and *changing its sign*'. Obviously, this only applies to the elimination of variables by addition or subtraction, *not* multiplication, which will be discussed in the next example.

Example

$$2 = 7 - \frac{5x}{2}$$

proceeding as before, $\dfrac{5x}{2} = 7 - 2 = 5$

i.e. $\dfrac{5x}{2} = 5$

We cannot now add or subtract anything to leave x on its own—we have to multiply by 2/5:

i.e. $\dfrac{2}{5} \cdot \dfrac{5x}{2} = \dfrac{2}{5} \cdot 5$

i.e. $x = 2$

This last step is known as *cross-multiplication* and may be pictured in the following manner:

 (Cross-multiplication)

The double-ended arrows indicate that movement may be in either direction. Note that there is no change of sign.

One *incorrect* use of cross-multiplication occurs so frequently that it is worth a special mention here. Suppose we have the equation:

$$\frac{7x}{2} = \frac{3}{8} + \frac{x}{3}$$

if we cross-multiply in the following manner:

$$\frac{7x}{2} \diagdown\!\!\!\diagup \frac{3}{8} + \frac{x}{3} \quad \text{(Incorrect)}$$

we obtain:

$$x = \frac{2 \cdot 3}{7 \cdot 8} + \frac{x}{3} \quad \text{(Incorrect)}$$

The fault lies, of course, in the fact that Rule 3 has been disobeyed, i.e. the term $x/3$ remains unaltered although we were intending, by our cross-multiplication, to multiply both sides by $2/7$. Hence, if we wished to cross-multiply at this stage, we should have obtained:

$$x = \frac{2 \cdot 3}{7 \cdot 8} + \frac{2 \cdot x}{7 \cdot 3} \quad \text{(Correct)}$$

which may be further simplified to solve for x.

Exercise A.5

a. $\frac{2}{3}x = 4$

b. $\frac{7}{9}y - 1 = 13$

c. $q + \frac{3}{10} = \frac{5}{12}q$

d. $3\frac{3}{5}z - 12\frac{4}{5} = 1\frac{2}{5}z - \frac{7}{10}$

A.5 POWERS (INDICES)

An *index* is written at the top right of a quantity (the *base*) and refers to the number of times the quantity is multiplied by *itself*. For example, 5^3 means $5 \times 5 \times 5$ (i.e. 125). It is a convenient mathematical 'shorthand' to write powers of a number in this way. In this example, the index is a positive integer (i.e. 3), but this need not be the case for it may be positive, negative, fractional or decimal, as described below.

A.5.1 Combining indices

Let us assume that we have two numbers, 2^3 and 2^2, which we wish to combine by addition, multiplication and division in order to elicit general rules for the handling of indices.

Addition

Using the definition of an index as described above:

$$2^3 + 2^2 = 2 \cdot 2 \cdot 2 + 2 \cdot 2 = 8 + 4 = 12$$

Thus, when adding such numbers, each term is calculated separately prior to addition (or subtraction).

Multiplication

Again, from first principles, we have:

$$2^3 \cdot 2^2 = \underbrace{2 \cdot 2 \cdot 2}_{= 2^3} \cdot \underbrace{2 \cdot 2}_{= 2^2} = 2^5 = 2^{(3+2)}$$

Hence, when multiplying two or more such numbers together, the rule is to *add* the indices.

Division

$$\frac{2^3}{2^2} = \frac{2 \cdot 2 \cdot 2}{2 \cdot 2} = 2 = 2^{(3-2)}$$

Thus, when dividing such numbers, the rule is to *subtract* the indices.

A.5.2 Negative indices

Suppose that we wish to divide 4^2 by 4^4. From first principles (Sect. A.5), we have

$$\frac{4^2}{4^4} = \frac{4 \cdot 4}{4 \cdot 4 \cdot 4 \cdot 4} = \frac{1}{4^2} \qquad \text{Equation A.1}$$

Also, by the rule on division as described above, we may subtract indices:

$$\frac{4^2}{4^4} = 4^{2-4} = 4^{-2} \qquad \text{Equation A.2}$$

Since equations (A.1) and (A.2) are equal:

$$4^{-2} = \frac{1}{4^2}$$

In general, therefore:

$$x^{-n} = \frac{1}{x^n} \qquad \text{Equation A.3}$$

i.e. to change a negative index to a positive index, just take the reciprocal, as shown in Equation A.3.

Examples

a. $10^{-2} = \dfrac{1}{10^2} = \dfrac{1}{100}$

b. $\dfrac{1}{10^{-6}} = \dfrac{1}{\dfrac{1}{10^6}} = 1 \times \dfrac{10^6}{1} = 10^6$

c. $\dfrac{420 \times 10^2}{2 \times 10^4} = 210 \times 10^{-2} = \dfrac{210}{10^2} = \dfrac{210}{100} = 2 \cdot 1$

A.5.3 Fractional indices

What is meant by, say, $x^{1/2}$?

Now, $x^{1/2} \cdot x^{1/2} = x^{1/2+1/2} = x^1 = x$

Also, $\sqrt{x} \cdot \sqrt{x} = x$ from the definition of a square root.

Thus, from inspection of these two equations:

$x^{1/2} = \sqrt{x}$

i.e. $x^{1/2}$ is just the square root of x.

Similarly, $y^{1/3}$ is the cube root of y, $q^{5/8}$ is the eighth root of q raised to the fifth power, etc.

Examples

a. $9^{1/2} = \sqrt{9} = \pm 3$

b. $9^{3/2} = (9^{1/2})^3 = (\pm 3)^3 = \pm 27$

c. $64^{1/3} = \sqrt[3]{64} = 4$

A.5.4 The zero index—x^0

A general number x raised to a power m is x^m. If we divide x^m by itself, the answer will obviously be 1. But $x^m \div x^m$ is x^{m-m} by the rules discussed above. Thus $1 = x^{m-m} = x^0$. Since we took any general number, this result is also general (except for 0^0, which is indeterminate).

Thus any number raised to the power zero is *unity*.

A.5.5 Indices to different bases

A problem on the Inverse Square Law (see Ch. 3) frequently involves calculation of the form:

$$\frac{a \cdot b^2}{c^2}$$

Here a, b and c represent numbers whose values are known, having been specified by the problem. We wish to determine the best way of obtaining the final result, since b and c are frequently large numbers, whose squares are therefore even larger. This means that the probability of making an arithmetical error can be quite high if a laborious method of simplification is undertaken. However, a great simplification is possible if we remember that:

$$\frac{b^2}{c^2} = \left(\frac{b}{c}\right)^2$$
Equation A.4

Example

If $b = 90$ cm and $c = 60$ cm, then $\dfrac{b^2}{c^2}$ the 'hard' way is:

$$\frac{b^2}{c^2} = \frac{90^2}{60^2} = \frac{8100}{3600} = \frac{81}{36}$$

which may be cancelled to give 2.25—this exercise being left to the reader. The 'easy' way is to use Equation A.4:

i.e. $\quad \dfrac{b^2}{c^2} = \left(\dfrac{b}{c}\right)^2 = \left(\dfrac{90}{60}\right)^2 = \left(\dfrac{3}{2}\right)^2 = 1 \cdot 5^2 = 2 \cdot 25$

Note that the answers are the same, as we should expect, but that the second method involves cancelling of smaller numbers so that there is less likelihood of an arithmetical error.

A.6 POWERS OF 10

When 10 is used as a base for indices, all the findings of the previous section apply. In addition, however, powers of 10 are very useful when measuring very large or very small quantities of a given unit, as shown in Table A.1.

Other names not shown in the table exist (see Table A at end of book), but these are all that we shall need. It is advisable for the student to memorise these terms as they are in very common usage in radiography. The following exercise is included for this purpose.

Table A.1 Names for powers of 10

Prefix	Symbol	Power of 10	Example
mega	M	10^6	1 MW = 10^6 watt
kilo	k	10^3	1 kV = 10^3 volt
milli	m	10^{-3}	1 mA = 10^{-3} ampere
micro	μ	10^{-6}	1 μF = 10^{-6} farad
nano	n	10^{-9}	1 nm = 10^{-9} metre
pico	p	10^{-12}	1 pF = 10^{-12} farad

Exercise A.6

a. An X-ray tube has a current of 0·05 amperes passing through it. How many milliamperes (mA) does this correspond to?

b. If the X-ray tube has a peak potential difference of 125 000 volts across it, what is the value in kilovolts (kV_p)?

c. Express a capacitance of 0.000065 farads in microfarads (μF).

d. A photon of light has a wavelength of 550 nanometres (nm). What is this in metres?

A.7 PROPORTIONALITY

A.7.1 Direct proportion

If a car is travelling at constant speed such that the petrol consumption is a steady 40 m.p.g. then:

0·5 gallons have been used after 20 miles
1·0 gallons have been used after 40 miles
1·5 gallons have been used after 60 miles, etc.

Thus, the amount of petrol consumed is in *direct proportion* to the number of miles travelled, and we may write:

gallons $\propto$ mileage

where the sign '$\propto$' means 'is proportional to'. Alternatively, we may write:

$$\text{gallons} = \frac{1}{40} \times \text{mileage}$$

In general, therefore, if two quantities y and x are directly proportional to each other, then:

$y \propto x$ or $y = kx$

where k is called the 'constant of proportionality'. Some examples of direct proportionality which are discussed in the main text include:

- The electric current (I) through a metallic conductor is proportional to the potential difference (V) across it, i.e. $I \propto V$ (Ohm's Law; Ch. 10).
- Intensity of an X-ray beam $\propto$ tube current (mA) (Ch. 29).
- Intensity of an X-ray beam $\propto$ kilovoltage squared, i.e. intensity $\propto kV^2$ (Ch. 29).

A.7.2 Inverse proportion

Suppose that we have many rectangles of equal area, k, but of differing heights (h) and widths (w). However, in each case the area is the same, so that:

$h \times w = \text{constant} (k)$

or, $h = \dfrac{k}{w}$

Then, since k is constant, we may write:

$h \propto \dfrac{1}{w}$

In this case, therefore, h and w are in *inverse* proportion, since w is halved if h is doubled, and vice versa. This is opposite to *direct* proportion, of course, where doubling (say) one quantity also doubles the other.

Examples of inverse proportion discussed in the main text include:

- The capacity (C) of a parallel-plate capacitor is inversely proportional to the separation (d) between its plates, i.e. $C \propto 1/d$ (Ch. 9).
- The intensity (I) from a point source of electromagnetic radiation is inversely proportional to the square of the distance (x) from the course, i.e. $I \propto 1/x^2$ (Ch. 3).
- The electrical resistant (R) of a given length of wire varies inversely as the area of cross-section (A), i.e. $R \propto 1/A$ (Ch. 10).

A.8 GRAPHS

A.8.1 Drawing and interpretation

A good understanding of the construction and interpretation of graphs is of great value in radiography, radiotherapy and nuclear medicine. The following simple, but effective, rules are offered in the drawing of good graphs:

- Each graph should take at least one-third of a page—use as large a scale as practicable so that you can make accurate readings.
- Each graph should have a clear, appropriate title.
- The axes, which should be drawn with a ruler, should be of approximately equal length.
- Both axes must be clearly labelled to show what is being measured and should contain units (cm, sec, kg, etc.) where appropriate.
- The *independent* variable is normally on the X-axis, and the *dependent* variable on the Y-axis, i.e. the variable which is being measured is plotted on the Y-axis while the variable causing the change in Y is plotted on the X-axis. If we consider plotting the radioactivity from a sample over a period of time, then the independent variable is time (plotted on the X-axis) while the dependent variable is the radioactivity (plotted on the Y-axis).

The following examples have been chosen to illustrate both the drawing and the interpretation of graphs.

Example 1—Direct proportion

As described in the last section, two quantities, x and y, are directly proportional to each other if $y = kx$, where k is a constant. Figure A.1 shows $y = kx$ in graphical form. The following points should be noted:

- The graph passes through the origin, since when $x = 0$, y is also equal to zero.
- The slope (or gradient) of the straight line produced is a measure of how steep it is and is defined as *the change in y divided by the corresponding change in x*. Since the graph passes through the origin, this is a convenient place from

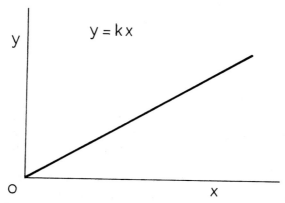

Figure A.1 Graph of $y = kx$, illustrating direct proportion.

which to measure the changes. From this it can be seen that the slope is y/x. But from the equation $y = kx$ it can be seen that $y/x = k$. Thus the slope increases as k increases.

● The general equation for a straight line will be in the form $y = mx + c$ where m is the gradient of the line and c is the intersection of the line with the y axis—the value of x when $y = 0$.

Example 2—Inverse proportion

Figure A.2 shows a graph of the inverse relationship between the capacitance, C, of a parallel-plate capacitor and the distance of separation of its plates, d, where $C \propto 1/d$ or $C = k/d$ for a specific capacitor.

From the graph it can be seen that as the distance between the plates increases, so the capacitance of the capacitor decreases.

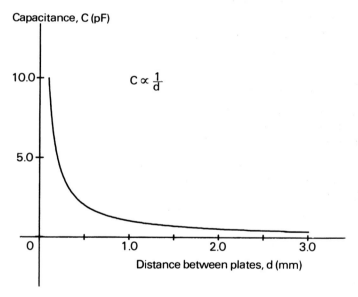

Figure A.2   Graph of $C \propto 1/d$, illustrating inverse proportion.

Example 3—Rating charts

Rating charts are supplied by the manufacturers of X-ray tubes, and contain a lot of information in graphical form which is an essential guide to the radiographer in the selection of 'safe' exposure factors, i.e. the combination of focal-spot size, kV_p, mA, and exposure time which will not cause damage to the X-ray tube. An example of a rating chart is given by Figure A.3, where a family of curves represent the maximum permissible exposure factors for different settings of kV_p. The use of rating charts is discussed in detail in Chapter 23 and we only need to

Figure A.3 Rating chart for an X-ray tube. Note the non-linear (logarithmic) scale on the X-axis.

make the point here that points below a particular curve for one kV$_p$ setting are 'safe', while points above it lead to tube damage by overheating the anode.

Note the non-linear (logarithmic) scale on the X-axis. Logarithmic scales are discussed in Chapter 4.

A.8.2 Interpolation and extrapolation

It is often the case that a graph is drawn using a relatively small number of points, and that these points are joined together with a curve or straight line passing through them. The smooth curve or line makes it possible to 'read off' values from the graph, even when such values lie between the original points used to construct the graph. This procedure is known as *interpolation* and is one of the advantages obtained from the graphical method.

If it is desired to determine the value of one of the plotted variables when it lies outside the range of the points used to plot the graph, the curve may be extended, or *extrapolated*, to reach this region. However, such an extrapolation can lead to large inaccuracies, since several different curves may seem equally suitable and there may be no way of knowing which one is correct!

Exercise A.7

a. Draw a graph of $y = 0.2x$, choosing values of x from 1 to 10 in steps of 1. Hence read from the graph the value of y when x is (i) 1·5, (ii) 9·5, (iii) 12, (iv) 0·5. Verify your answers by substitution into the original equation.

b. Repeat the same procedure for the equation $y = 0.2x^2$. (Note the increased uncertainty in obtaining the extrapolated value of y when $x = 12$.)

A.9 THE GEOMETRY OF TRIANGLES

A.9.1 The right-angled triangle

Consider the right-angled triangle shown in Figure A.4. The trigonometric functions of sine, cosine and tangent are defined as:

$$\sin A = \frac{\text{opposite}}{\text{hypotenuse}} = \frac{a}{b}$$

$$\cos A = \frac{\text{adjacent}}{\text{hypotenuse}} = \frac{c}{b}$$

$$\tan A = \frac{\text{opposite}}{\text{adjacent}} = \frac{a}{c}$$

Note that:

$$\frac{\sin A}{\cos A} = \frac{\frac{a}{b}}{\frac{c}{b}} = \frac{a}{b} \cdot \frac{b}{c} \quad \text{(by Rule 2)}$$

i.e $\quad \dfrac{\sin A}{\cos A} = \dfrac{a}{c} = \tan A$

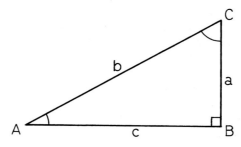

Figure A.4 A right-angled triangle. See text for definition of sine, cosine and tangent of an angle.

Exercise A.8

a. Write down expressions for sin C, cos C, tan C from Figure A.4.

b. What is the value of $\sin^2 A + \cos^2 A$?

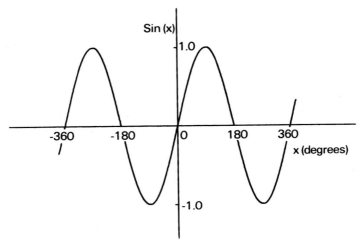

Figure A.5 A sine wave. The curve repeats itself every 360°.

The sine function occurs frequently throughout this book, e.g. in the geometry of triangles and in alternating current theory (Ch. 14). Its graphical form is shown in Figure A.5.

This graph is known as a 'sine wave', and always lies between plus one and minus one. Also, the shape of the curve is *cyclical*, repeating itself every 360°.

A.9.2 Similarity of triangles

The two triangles shown in Figure A.6 are said to be 'similar' because one

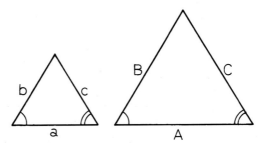

Figure A.6 Two similar triangles.

is just a bigger version of the other, while retaining the same *shape*. Thus, the corresponding angles of the two triangles are equal, but the lengths of the corresponding sides need not necessarily be so. However, if one side has a length which is double (say) that of the corresponding side of the other triangle, than *all* the sides will be doubled compared to the other triangle. Generally, then, we may write:

$$\frac{A}{a} = \frac{B}{b} = \frac{C}{c}$$

Equation A.5

In many practical examples in radiography, however, the similar triangles look more like those shown in Figure A.7.

These two types of similar triangles are discussed further in Chapter 2 (Sects 2.4–2.7). In each case, the ratios of the corresponding sides are equal, in agreement with equation A.5.

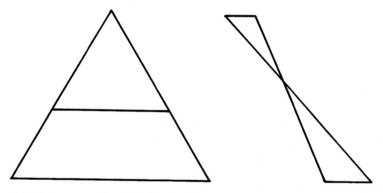

Figure A.7   Further examples of similar triangles.

A.10 POCKET CALCULATORS AND CALCULATIONS IN EXAMINATIONS

Because the price of pocket calculators now puts them within the range of even the most impoverished student, the purchase of such a calculator is strongly recommended. 'Scientific' pocket calculators have the advantage that they can perform calculations which involve trigonometrical and logarithmic functions and so will be found especially useful. Many such calculators are also 'programmable' which means that formulae may be inserted into the calculator memory to allow it to perform certain calculations by simply inserting the appropriate date—a formula for Ohm's Law could be inserted so that when the program is invoked the calculator will automatically calculate the resistance from the value of the potential and the current.

If you are to use a pocket calculator in examinations or if you are about to purchase one, here are some suggestions which you might find helpful:

- Consider the types of calculations which you require from the calculator and do not buy one with lots of unnecessary functions—these simply increase your chance of error.
- Try out a calculator before you buy it (if possible) and, if you are about to use one in an examination, make sure you are familiar with its layout and functions.
- Find out the policy regarding the use of calculators in examinations at your university. Some universities will issue calculators for the purpose of examinations while others have specific regulations regarding programmable calculators.
- Remember that the calculator will only give the correct answer if the correct information is keyed into it. It is important to remember indices and also try to get some 'feel' for the magnitude of the correct answer.

A.11 LOGARITHMS

Although few students would now undertake calculations using logarithms as the chosen method—thanks to the ease of use of the pocket calculator—it is nevertheless helpful to have a basic grasp of the theory of logarithms to explain certain functions in radiography, e.g. it may be easier to understand the exponential equations (see Ch. 4) in their logarithmic form.

Definition

The *logarithm* of a number to a given *base*, is the *power* by which the base must be raised to give the number.

Thus, the logarithm of 100 to the base 10 is 2 as $10^2 = 100$. This would normally be written as $\log_{10}100 = 2$.

The base can be any number but, in practice, logarithms are usually to the base 10 or to the base e where e is the exponential number and is approximately equal to 2.7183.

Consider a situation where we wish to multiply two numbers a and b. If $a = 10^x$ and $b = 10^y$ then:

$$a \times b = 10^x \times 10^y$$
$$= 10^{(x+y)}$$

Thus from our initial definition of logarithms we can say:

$$\log_{10}(a \times b) = \log_{10}a + \log_{10}b$$

By a similar argument it can be shown that:

$$\log_{10}(a/b) = \log_{10}a - \log_{10}b$$

The main use of logarithms in radiography is to allow the simplification of complex formulae—if we consider the intensity of a beam of radiation which has travelled a distance x through a medium, this is given by the equation:

$$I_x = I_0 e^{-\mu x}$$

where I_x is the intensity of the radiation after a thickness x, I_0 is the initial intensity of the radiation, e is the exponential number and μ is the linear attenuation coefficient—these are all explained in Chapter 4. This equation is quite complicated to use in the above form but is much easier to use in its logarithmic form:

$$\log_e I_x = \log_e I_0 - \mu x$$

A.12 VECTOR QUANTITIES

In vector quantities the quantity concerned has direction as well as dimension. Thus in vector addition we need to take both these factors into account. This is probably best illustrated by two simple examples:

a. A man walks 30 metres in an easterly direction and then walks 20 metres in a northerly direction. How far must he walk in a straight line to get back to where he started?

    The situation may be visualised using Figure A.8. By applying Pythagoras' theorem to this we can calculate that the distance from C to A is 36 metres.

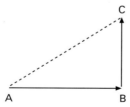

Figure A.8   Distances walked for calculation.

b. Forces $F_1 = 1$ newton, $F_2 = 4$ newtons and $F_3 = 2$ newtons are applied to a point source as shown in Figure A.9. What is the resultant force and what is its direction?

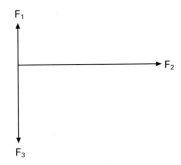

Figure A.9 Forces acting on a point.

As F_1 and F_3 are in opposite directions the resultant force is the difference between F_1 and F_3 and is in the direction of F_3 as this is the larger of the two forces. We can now do vector addition (see Fig. A.10) where AB represents force F_2 and BD represents ($F_3 - F_1$). The resultant force is represented by AD. By application of Pythagoras' theorem the length of this line is 4.12 newtons. Tan A is BD/AB and thus A can be calculated as approximately 14°. Thus we can say that the resultant force measures 4.12 newtons and is in a direction 14° below the horizontal.

Figure A.10 Vector addition of forces.

Appendix summary

- If we multiply or divide two +s or two −s we get a +.
- If we multiply or divide a + and a − sign we get a −.
- When dividing by a fraction we can get the same result if we multiply by the fraction inverted (the fraction turned upside down).
- the following mathematical relationships have been established:

$$x^a \times x^b = x^{(a+b)}$$
$$x^a/x^b = x^{(a-b)}$$
$$x^{-a} = 1/x^a$$
$$x^{1/2} = \sqrt{x}$$
$$x^a/y^a = (x/y)^a$$

- In direct proportion $y \propto x$ or $y = kx$ while in inverse proportion $y \propto 1/x$ or $y = c/x$ where k and c are constants of porportionality.
- $\sin \theta$ = opposite/hypotenuse; $\cos \theta$ = adjacent/hypotenuse and $\tan \theta$ = opposite/adjacent.
- Sine and cosine functions are cyclical, repeating themselves every 360°.
- When drawing graphs, use a manageable scale, use a ruler, label both axes and use a title.

- Similar triangles have the ratio of their corresponding sides equal.
- There are certain factors to consider when purchasing or using a pocket calculator.
- The basic theory of logarithms tells us that if $y = x^n$ then $\log_x y = n$.
- $\log_{10}(x \times y) = \log_{10}x + \log_{10}y$.
- $\log_{10}(x/y) = \log_{10}x - \log_{10}y$.
- In vector addition we can get the resultant vector by joining the vectors end to end. The resultant vector is from the origin to the tip of the last vector.

ANSWERS TO EXERCISES

Exercise A.1

a. $\dfrac{11}{12} - \dfrac{5}{6} = \dfrac{11-10}{12} = \dfrac{1}{12}$

b. $\dfrac{7}{9} + \dfrac{2}{3} = \dfrac{7+6}{9} = \dfrac{13}{9} = 1\dfrac{4}{9}$

c. 20% of $50 = \dfrac{20}{100} \times 50 = 10$

d. $\dfrac{2}{3} - \dfrac{1}{4} + \dfrac{3}{5} = \dfrac{40-15+36}{60} = \dfrac{61}{60} = 1\dfrac{1}{60}$

e. $\dfrac{7}{11} + \dfrac{2}{9} - \dfrac{2}{3} = \dfrac{63+22-66}{99} = \dfrac{19}{99}$

f. Percentage change $= 100 \times \dfrac{(90-80)}{80} = 100 \times \dfrac{10}{80} = 12.5\%$

Exercise A.2

a. $28 \div 7 = 4$

b. $\dfrac{-36}{6} = -6$

c. $\dfrac{144}{-4} = -36$

d. $-13 \times -3 = 39$

e. $-7 \times \dfrac{-8}{-2} = -7 \times 4 = -28$

Exercise A.3

a. $\dfrac{\dfrac{-4}{11}}{\dfrac{7}{22}} = \dfrac{-4}{11} \times \dfrac{22}{7} = \dfrac{-8}{7} = -1\dfrac{1}{7}$

b. $\dfrac{\dfrac{2}{9}}{\dfrac{7}{3} \times \dfrac{-2}{11}} = \dfrac{2}{9} \times \dfrac{3}{7} \times \dfrac{11}{-2} = \dfrac{-11}{21}$

c. $\dfrac{\dfrac{1}{3} \times \dfrac{2}{9}}{\dfrac{9}{1} \times \dfrac{1}{2}} = \dfrac{\dfrac{2}{27}}{\dfrac{9}{2}} = \dfrac{2}{27} \times \dfrac{2}{9} = \dfrac{4}{243}$

Exercise A.4

a. $7a - 4(a - 2) = 7a - 4a + 8 = 3a + 8$

b. $-6(-x + y - 3) = 6x - 6y + 18$

c. $2(3a - 4) - 3(-a + 6) = 6a - 8 + 3a - 18$
$$= 9a - 26$$

Exercise A.5

a. $\dfrac{2}{3}x = 4$
$2x = 12$
$x = 6$

b. $\dfrac{7}{9}y - 1 = 13$
$7y - 9 = 117$
$7y = 126$
$y = 18$

c. $q + \dfrac{3}{10} = \dfrac{5}{12}q$

$12q + \dfrac{36}{10} = 5q$

$12q - 5q = \dfrac{-36}{10}$

$7q = \dfrac{-36}{10}$

$q = \dfrac{-36}{70}$

$= \dfrac{-18}{35}$

d. $3\frac{3}{5}z - 12\frac{4}{5} = 1\frac{2}{5}z - \frac{7}{10}$

$\qquad 3\frac{3}{5}z - 1\frac{2}{5}z = 12\frac{4}{5} - \frac{7}{10}$

$\qquad\qquad 2\frac{1}{5}z = 12\frac{1}{10}$

$\qquad\qquad \frac{11}{5}z = \frac{121}{10}$

$\qquad\qquad 110z = 605$

$\qquad\qquad\quad z = \frac{605}{110}$

$\qquad\qquad\qquad = 5\frac{1}{2}$

Exercise A.6

a. 50 mA
b. 125 kV$_p$
c. 65 µF
d. 0.00000055 m

Exercise A.7

a. From the graph you should obtain the following readings:
   (i)   When $x = 1.5$, $y = 0.3$
   (ii) When $x = 9.5$, $y = 1.9$
   (iii) When $x = 12$, $y = 2.4$
   (iv) When $x = 0.5$, $y = 0.1$.
b. From the graph you should obtain the following readings:
   (i)   When $x = 1.5$, $y = 0.45$
   (ii) When $x = 9.5$, $y = 18.05$
   (iii) When $x = 12$, $y = 28.8$
   (iv) When $x = 0.5$, $y = 0.05$.

Exercise A.8

A. From Figure A.4:
   $\sin C = c/b$
   $\cos C = a/b$
   $\tan C = c/a$
b. From Figure A.4:
   $\sin^2 A + \cos^2 A = (a/b)^2 + (c/b)^2$
   $\qquad\qquad\qquad = \dfrac{a^2 + c^2}{b^2}$
   But $a^2 + c^2 = b^2$—by Pythagoras' theorem.
   Thus, $\sin^2 A + \cos^2 A = 1$.

Appendix B

SCINTILLATION COUNTERS

A scintillation counter may be used to detect minute amounts of X- or γ-radiation. There are two main types of scintillation counter:

- a counter where the detector is in crystalline form usually NaI(Tl)
- a counter where the detector is a liquid scintillation material.

B.1 NaI(Tl) CRYSTALS AND PHOTOMULTIPLIERS

A crystal of sodium iodide with a thallium activator is one of the most efficient scintillators developed. The thallium impurities act as luminescent centres (see Sect. 31.3.1) and about 10–15% of the energy deposited in the crystal is converted to light energy. The maximum light emission is in the blue part of the spectrum with a wavelength of 420 nm. The sodium iodide crystals are mounted in containers called cans to prevent them absorbing moisture from the atmosphere and becoming cloudy. One face of the crystal is attached to a transparent glass window and all other surfaces are in contact with a white reflective powder (magnesium oxide) so that as much light as possible is directed at the back of the crystal.

The back of the crystal is in optical contact with a photomultiplier tube as shown in Figure B.1. If a gamma ray is absorbed by the crystal (at point P on the diagram) this results in the emission of light in all directions. A fairly high percentage of this light reaches the photocathode of the *photomultiplier tube*. The photocathode consists of a thin coating of a mixture of alkaline salts deposited on the inner wall of the face of the photomultiplier tube. About 10–25% of the light photons reaching the photocathode cause it to emit electrons by the photoelectric effect (see Sect. 30.5) and these electrons are accelerated through the tube to a series of positively charged plates called *dynodes*. The surface of these dynodes is coated with a layer of a secondary electron emitter so that each dynode produces approximately six times as many electrons as fall on it. As a result of this process, one electron released at the photocathode may result in one million electrons being collected by the anode of the photomultiplier. The collection of this

Figure B.1 A scintillation detector using sodium iodide. Key: X—NaI(Tl) crystal; R—powdered reflector; C—crystal can; K—photocathode; D1, D2, etc.—dynodes.

charge occurs at a very short time interval after the initial electron is released by the photocathode (normally $<10^{-6}$ s) and so a pulse of electricity is produced, the magnitude of the pulse being proportional to the energy of the absorbed gamma ray photon.

Insight

If the photomultiplier tube contains n dynodes each of which releases 6 electrons for 1 incident electron, then the electron gain in the photomultiplier tube is 6^n. Thus for a 10-dynode tube the gain would be 6^{10} which is just over 60 000 000 electrons and represents a charge at the anode of about 10 picocoulombs.

A spectrum of these pulses will not produce the discrete gamma energies emitted by the radioactive source because of the statistical nature of the light production in the crystal and the electron multiplication in the photomultiplier. This is shown in Figure B.2 where the numbers of pulses of a given height are plotted. The true spectrum would be a line at the centre of the photopeak, as this corresponds to the energy of the gamma rays absorbed by photoelectric absorption. In addition to the gamma rays absorbed by photoelectric absorption, some of the gamma rays undergo Compton scattering (see Sect. 30.6) within the crystal and then escape from the crystal with no further interactions. Such scattering interactions result in energy being deposited in the crystal which is less than the energy of the

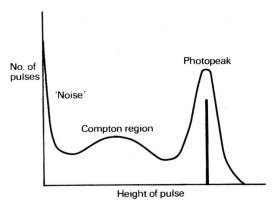

Figure B.2 A typical gamma-ray spectrum using sodium iodide.

gamma rays and so smaller pulses are produced in the photomultiplier. These pulses produce a 'Compton peak' as shown in Figure B.2.

Some very low energy pulses are produced by the release of electrons from the photocathode by thermionic emission (see Sect. 18.2). There are also some positively charged ions produced at the dynodes which may strike the photocathode and cause it to release electrons. The electrons produced by both of the above mechanisms produce no useful signal and are referred to as 'noise pulses' (see Fig. B.2).

B.2 THE USE OF SCINTILLATION COUNTERS IN MEDICINE

It is usual practice to count only the pulses which occur in the photopeak of the spectrum, particularly when investigating the activity and distribution of a radionuclide within a patient's body. This is achieved by the use of a *pulse height analyser* (PHA) which will only produce an electrical output signal if the input pulse lies within a certain range—this range is adjusted to cover the photopeak for the particular radionuclide. Pulses from the PHA are counted on a scalar for a time determined by the timer (see Fig. B.3). The number of counts obtained is related directly to the activity being measured and may be compared to a normal range of values for that structure.

An example of such a study will now be considered. The patient is given iodine-131 in the form of sodium iodide. The iodine component of this is taken up by the thyroid gland. The thyroid uptake may then be counted using equipment similar to that illustrated in Figure B.3. The γ-rays emitted from the thyroid are detected by the lead-shielded sodium iodide crystal and those which lie within the photopeak are counted as described above.

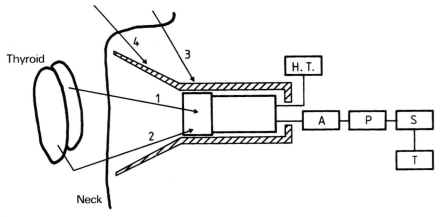

Figure B.3   A scintillation detector used to measure activity within a thyroid gland. Key: A—amplifier; P—pulse height analyser (PHA); S—scalar; T—timer.

The possibility of γ-rays emitted outside the thyroid (see rays 3 and 4) being counted is reduced by the lead collimator—this is the shaded area in Figure B.3. The selection of a specific photopeak by the PHA allows the counter to reject radiations which impinge on the crystals as a result of Compton scattering of the γ-rays (see ray 2). The uptake count is obtained by expressing the thyroid uptake as a percentage of the total radiation ingested by the patient. Typical figures for a '24-hour uptake' lie between 10 and 25%. An overactive thyroid will give a higher figure and an underactive thyroid has a lower figure.

B.3 THE GAMMA CAMERA

The gamma camera was first developed by H. O. Anger in 1958 and the camera and its associated technology have shown considerable progress since then. The gamma camera is a specialised type of scintillation counter where the position as well as the count of the scintillations within a thin NaI(Tl) crystal is obtained by the use of a number of photomultipliers. Such a gamma camera and its associated circuitry is shown in Figure B.4. A multichannel parallel collimator similar to that shown in Figure B.4 ensures that only γ-rays which are at right angles to the crystal face can enter the camera. A geometrical arrangement of photomultiplier tubes—of which there are typically between 61 and 75—allows the position and the intensity of the scintillation produced in the crystal to be measured. This allows us to display a picture of certain physiological processes within the body. This ability to image a dynamic physiological process makes the gamma camera a very powerful tool in the detection of pathologies where the physiology of the structure is disrupted.

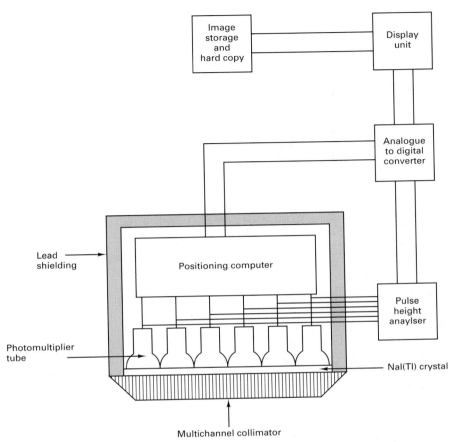

Figure B.4 The main components of a gamma camera and its associated circuitry.

B.4 LIQUID SCINTILLATION COUNTING

Radionuclides which decay solely by beta decay are not suitable for detection by NaI(Tl) crystals because of the low efficiency of detection. This is because many of the β-particles are absorbed by the can around the crystal and others are scattered out of the crystal by interaction with the atoms of the crystal. If we wish to count the activity from samples containing such radionuclides the most efficient way of achieving this is by the use of liquid scintillation counting. A liquid scintillation solution is composed of:

- a solvent (e.g. benzene or toluene)
- a scintillation solute (the *primary* solute)
- a *secondary* solute.

A sample containing the beta-emitting radionuclide is dissolved in a liquid scintillation solution. The β-particles from the radionuclide travel through the liquid and produce ionisation and excitation (see Sect. 26.6) within the molecules of the solvent. This excitation energy is transferred quickly (in less than 10^{-9} s) to the primary solute which fluoresces (see Sect. 31.3.1) when the electrons drop to their original lower-energy state. The secondary solute is introduced into the solution as a *wavelength shifter* and so its function is to absorb photons emitted by the primary solute and re-emit them as photons of a longer wavelength—this increases the efficiency of detection by the photomultiplier tubes. A typical efficiency for a liquid scintillation process is about 3%, i.e. 3% of the energy of the β-particles is converted into photons which can be measured by the photomultiplier tubes.

A typical arrangement for counting the activity in a sample by liquid scintillation is shown in Figure B.5. Two photomultipliers A and B 'view' a plastic or glass bottle into which has been introduced a small quantity (about 10 ml) of the liquid scintillation solution into which has been dissolved the radioactive sample. A scintillation event (for instance at P in the liquid) produces light photons which are detected by both photomultiplier tubes. The output from both photomultiplier tubes is fed to a summing amplifier which is only switched on if the pulses from A and B are received at the same time—the pulses are in coincidence. In this way the random noise pulses from each photomultiplier tube are almost entirely elimi-

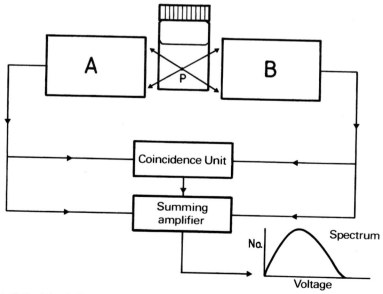

Figure B.5   A basic liquid scintillation counter.

nated. The output pulses from the summing amplifier are then a measure of the continuous beta spectrum (see Fig. 27.8) of the radioactive sample and may be counted using a scalar and timer as described in Section B.3.

Liquid scintillation counting is an extremely sensitive method of measuring the activity of a β-emitting sample because of the intimate contact between the sample and the scintillator. This means that very small quantities of β-emitting radionuclide (as low as 1 part of nuclide in 10^{12} parts of solution) can be detected. Such techniques are used in biochemistry to detect small quantities of substances (e.g. hormones) which it would be difficult to detect by other forms of chemical analysis.

Appendix C

CAT SCANNING

Computer assisted tomographic scanning (CAT scanning) was first described by its inventor Godfrey Hounsfield in the *British Journal of Radiology* in 1973. Since then it has revolutionised the imaging of many body parts, especially soft tissue structures which are difficult to show using 'conventional' radiographic techniques. The physics of CAT scanning is complex and this Appendix merely attempts an overview which will allow the reader to understand the basic principles of the process.

C.1 SCANNING GANTRY

Figure C.1 shows the configuration of the gantry of a typical modern CAT scanner. Note that there is a fixed circular array of detectors (e.g. caesium iodide crystals connected to photomultiplier tubes) and that the X-ray tube moves through a circular field around the patient. Also note that the leading and the trailing edges of the fan of X-rays is wider than the body part being imaged thus enabling calibration of the detectors for the X-ray beam.

If we consider the radiation beam received by detector A on the gantry, it can be seen that this beam passed from the X-ray tube to the detector through a given length of air. As the distance between the X-ray tube and the detector remains constant throughout the rotation of the tube, the attenuation of the radiation (by the air) along this line can be calculated. The radiation arriving at detector B has passed a certain distance through air and a certain distance through the patient. The difference between the readings on detectors A and B must be caused by attenuation of the radiation along the line through the patient to detector B. A similar situation exists for other detectors which are struck by the fan of X-rays. The information from the detectors is sent to a computer via an analogue–digital converter. This changes the analogue information from the detectors to digitised information which the computer is able to store and manipulate. As the tube rotates around the patient, a matrix of readings is taken—this is the scanning phase.

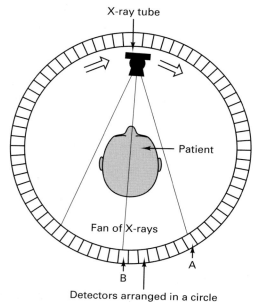

Figure C.1   Line diagram to show the main features of the scanning gantry of a CAT scanner. The thick arrows show the direction of tube rotation. For further explanation of the actions of the gantry, see the text.

C.2 IMAGE RECONSTRUCTION

The computer now processes the information and can produce an image of the 'slice' through the patient by a process called *back projection*. The image is divided into a series of small boxes called *pixels* and each pixel is given a certain value of brightness on the display monitor depending on the absorption within that particular box—usually the higher the absorption the brighter the pixel. The greater the number of pixels that are used to form the image, the higher the resolution but the greater the demands made on the detectors and the computer for processing of larger amounts of information. On a modern system the minimum display would be a 512×512 matrix and in this, each image consists of a total of 262 144 pixels.

C.3 IMAGE MANIPULATION

Because of the very wide range of X-ray absorptions which can be displayed on such a system, it is often convenient to use a technique called *windowing*. If we know the attenuation figures for certain tissue types, it is possible to instruct the computer to display only absorptions which lie within (or close to) this band. This allows us—with our limited grey scale vision—to see subtle changes in structure within these tissues. Both the window centre and the window width may be altered but further discussion of this is beyond the scope of this brief overview.

The images from such a CAT scanner may be stored on floppy disks or magnetic tape and 'hard copies' may be made using either a laser imager of a multiformat camera.

The information from CAT images may be used to aid the diagnosis of the patient's condition; it is also very useful in planning radiotherapy treatment.

C.4 SPIRAL CAT

Many modern scanners use spiral scanning; here the tube rotates around the patient at the same time as the patient moves longitudinally with respect to the gantry. One of the advantages of this technique is the ease with which it facilitates high-quality three-dimensional reconstructions of images of body parts.

C.5 RADIATION DOSES AND CAT

The main disadvantage of CAT scanning is the large dose delivered to the area under investigation—the typical dose for a chest scan may be up to 400 times the dose for a postero-anterior (PA) chest radiograph.

Appendix D

MAGNETIC RESONANCE IMAGING

D.1 NUCLEAR MAGNETIC RESONANCE

The phenomenon of nuclear magnetic resonance (NMR) has been used in chemistry since the 1940s but it was not used for magnetic resonance imaging (MRI) until the mid 1970s.

In the nucleus of the hydrogen atom is a single proton which carries a positive charge. This proton spins on an axis and so has a magnetic field which is coincident with its axis of rotation. Under normal circumstances there are many million such protons in body tissues (mainly as part of water molecules) and the magnetic axes are randomly aligned so that there is no significant net magnetic effect produced.

If we place a bar magnet in an external magnetic field, it will align itself with the magnetic field as described in Chapter 11. Similarly, if protons are subjected to a strong external magnetic field—most magnets in magnetic resonance imaging are around 1 tesla—a small percentage of the protons will attempt to align with the magnetic field. This situation is shown in Figure D.1. Because of the proton's spin there is an extra force in existence which will cause the proton's axis to describe a circle in the direction in which it is pointing. This movement is called *precession*. The frequency of this precession for all hydrogen nuclei is the same if all the nuclei are exposed to the same strength of magnetic field—in a field of 1 tesla the nuclei will precess with a frequency of 42.6 MHz; doubling the field strength will double the precession frequency. The frequency of precession is known as the *Larmor frequency*.

D.2 MAGNETIC RESONANCE IMAGING

In magnetic resonance imaging, the patient is placed in the centre of a magnet similar to that shown in Figure D.2. The main magnet coils produce the external magnetic field with which the hydrogen protons align themselves. The gradient coils superimpose a magnetic field on top of this so that hydrogen protons along the long axis of the patient will resonate

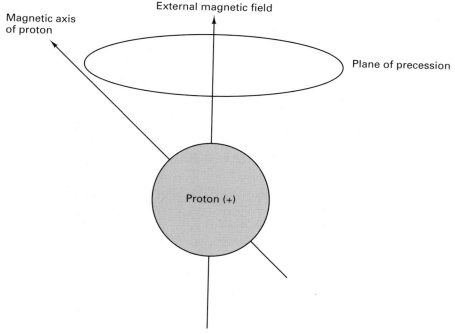

Magnetic axis
of proton

External magnetic field

Plane of precession

Proton (+)

Figure D.1 A spinning proton has a distinct magnetic axis. If this proton is placed in an external magnetic field, the proton will align with the field so that its axis of rotation sweeps out a cone, rather like a spinning top as it is about to fall over. This movement is called precession.

at different values of Larmor frequency. The protons aligned with the external magnetic field are in their lowest energy state. If we wish to get a signal to produce a magnetic resonance image, the protons must be excited by giving them energy. This can be done by energising the protons with a radio-frequency (RF) pulse. To allow maximum absorption of this energy, the pulse must have the same frequency as the Larmor frequency of the proton. This situation is illustrated in Figure D.3 where some of the protons are precessing at too low or too high a frequency to resonate with the RF pulse but others—the central section—are precessing in frequency with the pulse and so will produce maximum absorption of energy. This section will therefore form the 'slice' through the structure which will be imaged. Exposure of these protons to the RF pulse will cause their magnetisation vector to swing through either 90° or 180°. After the RF pulse the protons will again turn to precess in alignment with the external magnetic field. This turning of the spinning proton on its axis produces an RF signal which can be detected on suitable equipment (e.g. on the RF coils) and so the density of the protons and the time it takes them to turn can be established.

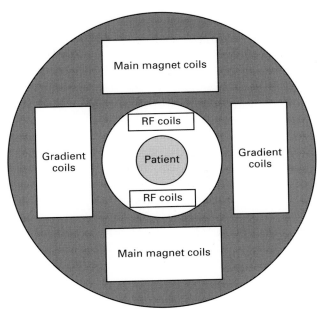

Figure D.2   Diagrammatic representation of the coils in a magnetic resonance imager; RF—radio-frequency.

The main magnets of such a device are very powerful and could generate a large amount of heat because of the resistance of the coils. This is prevented by cooling the coils until they are superconductive (see Ch. 10).

The relaxation time is different for water molecules bound into different tissue or chemical types. Analysis of the relaxation time allows MR spectroscopy to be performed.

D.3 CONTRAST AGENTS FOR MAGNETIC RESONANCE IMAGING

The contrast of certain structures in the MR signal may be enhanced by the addition of a contrast agent. Such contrast agents are usually paramagnetic—the most common, currently used agents are compounds of gadolinium.

D.4 SAFETY OF MAGNETIC RESONANCE IMAGING

The presence of a large magnetic field may pose problems to patients with certain metallic prostheses, and great care must be taken to prevent the introduction of ferromagnetic material into the bore of the magnet, but, generally speaking, magnetic resonance imaging has none of the hazards associated with imaging using ionising radiations.

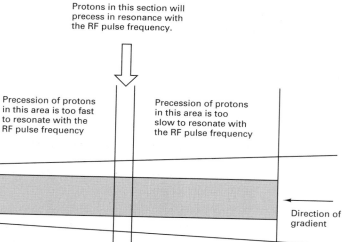

Protons in this section will
precess in resonance with
the RF pulse frequency.

Precession of protons
in this area is too fast
to resonate with the
RF pulse frequency

Precession of protons
in this area is too
slow to resonate with
the RF pulse frequency

Structure

Direction of
gradient

RF pulse direction

Figure D.3 The position of a transverse plane may be set by altering the gradient along the structure. The protons which resonate in frequency with the radio-frequency (RF) pulse are imaged and so this sets the position of the plane.

Appendix E

DIGITAL IMAGING

E.1 DIGITAL IMAGE CONSTRUCTION

A 'conventional' radiograph produced using film and intensifying screens is an example of an *analogue image*. If such an image is scanned as a series of horizontal lines and the contents of each line is divided into a series of small boxes we have set up the basic mechanism which will allow us to produce digital images. Such an *image matrix* is shown in Figure E.1 and each of the small boxes is called a *pixel*. The contents of each box is now given a numerical whole number value to produce our *digitised image*—if we consider our initial radiograph we could call the blackest area –1000 and the lightest area +1000 and so we have a digital scale of 2000. This process of measuring the contents of each box and giving it a number is known as *sampling*. The rate of sampling (number of pixels per line) is important as this controls the resolution of the image. A high rate of sampling gives a high-resolution image but is more demanding on the computing facilities. Many modern digital imaging systems will have sampling rates of over 1000 pixels per line and 1000 lines per image—thus the image is made up of 1 000 000 pixels. In such a situation, if the image is displayed on a 20 cm × 20 cm section of a monitor, each pixel will be a square of side 0.2 mm and so will be below the resolving power of the eye—thus we are aware of the overall image and do not see the individual pixels. We can see this by viewing Figure E.2. If you look at this from a distance of about 1 metre you will simply see the image but if you examine it from close range, using a magnifying glass if necessary, you will see that the image is composed of a series of black and white blocks—the pixels can be resolved by the eye at the closer distance.

E.2 DIGITAL RADIOGRAPHY SYSTEMS

The production of radiographic images in this way—by first using a film and then digitising the image—imposes a number of restrictions because of the limitations of film as an imaging medium. For this reason it is more

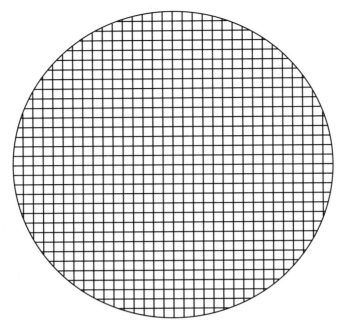

Figure E.1 This shows an example of the matrix used for a digitised image. Each box of this matrix is a pixel.

Figure E.2 An example of a digitised image where the pixels are so large that they can be seen at close range.

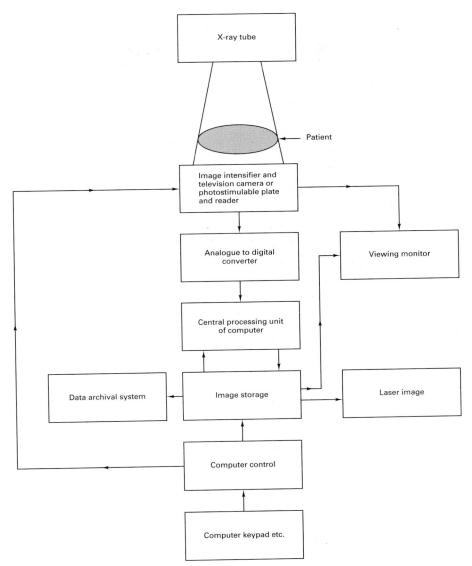

Figure E.3 Block diagram of the major components of a digital imaging system.

likely that digitised images will be produced using the type of equipment shown in the box diagram in Figure E.3.

The initial image is either produced as a signal from a television camera attached to an image intensifier (in digital fluoroscopy) or from the reader of a photostimulable plate (in digital radiography). This image is simultaneously sent to a viewing monitor and to the central processing unit in a computer, via an analogue–digital converter. Having been processed this image can now be displayed on the viewing monitor. The image may be altered or manipulated using the computer keyboard and computer controls. These facilities allow us to alter the contrast and brightness of the image, to window on specific absorption levels within the image so that only structures of interest are displayed, to enhance the edges of structures and to subtract one image from another. This facility is especially useful in studies using a contrast agent. Having manipulated the image as required, hard copies may be produced on a laser imager and the data stored in a data archival system.

E.3 DISPLAY, STORAGE AND TRANSMISSION OF DIGITISED IMAGES

The digitised images from such a system may be stored on suitable optical disks and can be recalled by hospital staff in other parts of the hospital by insertion of the appropriate codes into the computer. Digitised images may also be sent from one part of the country to another using suitable linking systems thus allowing the possibility of *tele-radiology*.

Such systems may, in the not too distant future, replace the film and intensifying screens as the principal method of production of radiographic images.

Appendix F

ULTRASOUND IMAGING

Sound is a series of compressions and rarefactions of a medium. Thus sound travelling through air will cause the tympanic membrane in our ears to vibrate and so we appreciate the existence of sound. The higher the frequency of vibration the higher the pitch of the sound. The human ear is able to detect sound with a frequency range from 20 Hz to 20 kHz. Frequencies above 20 kHz are inaudible to us—but may be heard by bats, dogs and dolphins—and are described as *ultrasound*. For the purposes of medical imaging, the ultrasound is normally in the range 1–10 MHz.

F.1 PRODUCTION OF ULTRASOUND

Ultrasound used in medical imaging is produced using the piezoelectric effect. This effect is illustrated in Figure F.1. If a potential difference is applied to the faces of a suitable crystal, then the crystal will distort as

Figure F.1 When a potential difference is applied across the faces of a crystal ABCD it will distort to form the shape EFGH. When the potential is removed it returns to its original shape. If mechanical stress is applied to ABCD until it adopts the shape EFGH, then a potential difference will be established between surface AB and surface CD. This is known as the piezoelectric effect.

shown. If the potential difference is removed, then the crystal will return to its original shape in a series of oscillations. Such oscillations are in the ultrasound frequency range. Similarly, if a suitable crystal is compressed by mechanical stress then a potential difference is established between the opposing faces of the crystal. Thus the crystal can not only produce ultrasound but can also detect the presence of ultrasound because of the mechanical stress which this imposes on the crystal.

If a pulse of high potential is applied across the opposing faces of a crystal and then removed, the crystal will oscillate with reducing amplitude until it returns to its original shape—this is rather like the effect produced by striking a cymbal with a drumstick. To prevent this happening, the ultrasound production from the crystal is *damped* either using mechanical damping or electronic damping. This means that only a short pulse of ultrasound is produced—if we return to the cymbal analogy this is similar to striking the cymbal with a drumstick and then pinching the cymbal between our fingers.

F.2 PULSE-ECHO IMAGING

In pulse-echo imaging, the device responsible for the production and the detection of ultrasound is called a *transducer*. This produces a pulse of ultrasound every millisecond. The pulse of ultrasound lasts for a time of 1 μs and so for the next 999 μs the transducer is capable of detecting the returning echoes. Such a set-up for ultrasound imaging is shown in Figure F.2.

The transducer produces pulses of ultrasound as described and also detects the returning echoes. Any air between the transducer and the patient is excluded by the use of a coupling gel. The ultrasound energy travels through the patient and will produce echoes at the interfaces of structures which have different values of *acoustic impedance*. The acoustic impedance of a substance is given by the equation:

$Z = \rho c$

where Z is the acoustic impedance, ρ is the density of the medium and c is the velocity of ultrasound travelling through that medium. Thus we can get detectable echoes at the interfaces between most tissue types within the body.

In Figure F.2, a pulse of ultrasound is transmitted from the transducer under the influence of the pulse transmission control. This pulse travels through body tissues and encounters faces A and B of a structure within the patient. Each of the faces will send an echo back to the transducer and this information is detected by the echo receiving and timing unit. If we know the velocity of the ultrasound in tissue and the time taken from

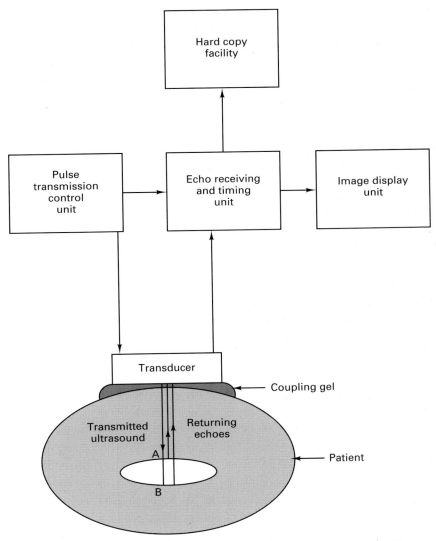

Figure F.2   Block diagram showing the basic functions of a pulse-echo ultrasound imager. For clarity the returning echoes have been displaced to the right.

the transmission of the pulse until the receipt of the return echoes, then we can calculate the distance from the transducer to the interface using the formula:

$$d = \tfrac{1}{2}ct$$

where d is the distance between the transducer and the interface, c is the velocity of ultrasound in that particular tissue and t is the time taken from the transmission of the ultrasound pulse until the detection of the returning echo. By suitable sweeping of the ultrasound beam the echoes from all the structures can be collected, the positions of the interfaces calculated and the image displayed on an image display unit—usually a television monitor. Hard copies of the image may be made on a suitable hard copy facility—e.g. a thermal imager.

F.3 DOPPLER ULTRASOUND IMAGING

If ultrasound echoes return from a moving structure, then there is a frequency shift in the returning echo. The amount and direction of this frequency shift depends on the velocity and the direction of the moving interface relative to the transducer. This effect is known as the *Doppler effect*. Using this effect and a suitably designed transducer—this time the transducer face is in two halves, one continuously transmitting ultrasound and the other continuously receiving it—it is possible to detect the position and the velocity of structures in the body. Such techniques are now used for studies of blood flow.

Appendix G

MODULATION TRANSFER FUNCTION (MTF)

The MTF is a mathematical method of assessing the performance of an imaging system, whether it be optical, radiographic or radioactive (e.g. gamma camera—App. B.3). The use of the MTF for this purpose was pioneered in the field of optics when it was discovered that a lens which was excellent at imaging the structure of very fine objects was not necessarily as good as another lens of lower resolving power when imaging coarser (i.e. larger) objects.

G.1 SPATIAL FREQUENCIES AND MODULATION

The concept of spatial frequencies is inherent in any description of the MTF and will therefore be considered first before the MTF is defined in Section G.2.

An object with a spatial frequency of ν cycles per cm (say) is shown in Figure G.1. The object has an amplitude which is sinusoidal with a wavelength of λ. The spatial frequency is the number of cycles per unit length, and is therefore given by $1/\lambda$. The *modulation* of the object, m_0, is defined as:

$$m_0 = \frac{a-b}{a+b} \qquad\qquad \text{Equation G.1}$$

where a and b are the height of the peaks and the troughs of the waveform respectively.

The amplitude of the sine wave is the intensity of light for lenses, the activity for gamma cameras and the X-ray intensity in radiography. If it is supposed that an absorber is placed in the path of an X-ray beam such that it would produce a sinusoidal variation of intensity of the transmitted beam, then a perfect imaging system would produce a sine wave of photographic exposure on the film of the *same* modulation. The *image modulation* would then be the same as the *object modulation*. However, in practice, the relative amplitude of the image modulation is reduced by the finite size

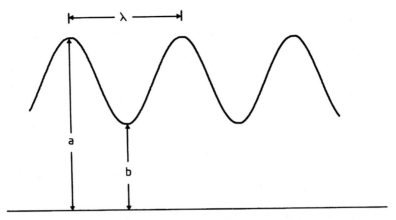

Figure G.1   The definition of modulation (see text).

of the focal spot and the characteristics of the film/screen combination, which tend to spread the image on to a larger area than theoretically desirable. Thus, the 'peaks' of the sinusoidal exposure tend to contribute to the 'troughs', so that an overall reduction in amplitude (and therefore modulation) is experienced.

This effect of a reduction in image modulation is small when the sinusoidal object has a long wavelength (low spatial frequency), but is of increasing importance as the wavelength is reduced to about 1 mm or less (spatial frequencies of 10 per cm or more). The image modulation therefore depends upon the spatial frequency of the object, and this forms the basis of the MTF described below.

G.2 MTF AND SPATIAL FREQUENCY

The modulation transfer function is defined as:

$$\text{MTF} = \frac{\text{image modulation}}{\text{object modulation}} \qquad \text{Equation G.2}$$

In a perfect imaging system, the image is an exact copy of the object and so has the same modulation at all spatial frequencies. The MTF is therefore always unity for such a system. However, we have seen that the image modulation is reduced as the spatial frequency increases (Sect. G.1) and so a graph of the MTF plotted against spatial frequency has a general appearance as shown in Figure G.2. Three cases are considered: an 'ideal' imaging system, where the MTF is 1·0 and is independent of the spatial frequency, a curve where the MTF is reduced at the higher frequencies due to geometric unsharpness only, and a curve obtained when using screens.

It is to be expected that the imaging of fine detail (high spatial frequencies) would be worse when using screens because of the spreading of the light from the fluorescent screens over the film. The MTF is particularly useful in separating the individual causes of image degradation. MTFs due to each cause may be measured separately (MTF$_1$, MTF$_2$, . . . etc.) and may be combined to produce the overall MTF of the system:

$$MTF = MTF_1 \times MTF_2 \ldots$$

Equation G.3

It thus becomes possible to predict the response of the overall system with various combinations of focal spot size, film/screen combinations, etc. if the MTF of each is known.

G.3 OBJECTS AS SPATIAL FREQUENCIES

A 'sinusoidal' object does not bear much similarity to the objects which are normally radiographed. However, it may be shown that the shape of any object may be obtained from the summation of sine and cosine waves of different amplitudes and frequencies (Fourier's theorem). Thus, if the MTF of the X-ray unit is known at each frequency, the overall response to the object may be determined.

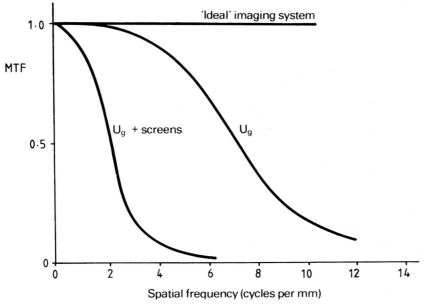

Figure G.2 The variation of the modulation transfer function (MTF) with spatial frequency for an ideal system, that due to geometric unsharpness (U_g), and that due to geometric unsharpness and screens (U_g + screens).

As an example of the summation of amplitudes of different frequencies forming a shape, consider the flat-topped object shown by the dotted lines in Figure G.3(a). The height of the object may be considered to represent the degree of absorption of the X-rays by the object, and the width is the physical size of the object. It may be shown that such a shape may be obtained by adding an infinite series of cosine waves (which are just sine

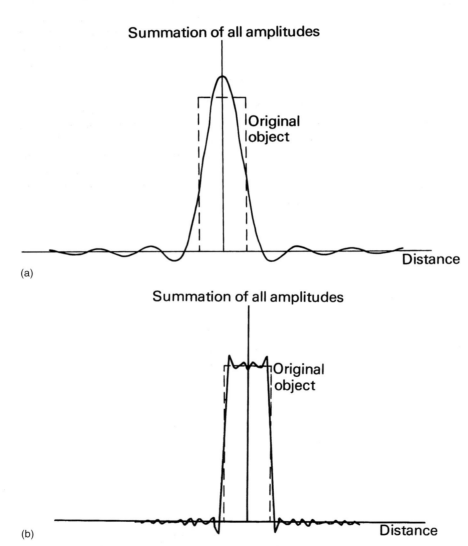

(a)

(b)

Figure G.3 The representation of a 'square' object (dotted lines) by the summation of frequencies of different amplitudes: (a) 500 terms; (b) 2500 terms. An infinite number of terms reproduces the object exactly.

waves displaced by 90°) of increasing frequency (f), where the amplitudes (g) are given by:

$$g = \frac{\sin(\pi f d)}{2\pi f}$$

Equation G.4

   The sum of the first 500 terms of such amplitudes is shown in Figure G.3(a). The effect of including 2500 terms (i.e. containing higher frequencies) is shown in Figure G.3(b), where a closer approximation to the square shape is obtained. The agreement is exact when an infinite number of terms is included. However, the higher spatial frequencies present in the object are poorly reproduced in the image, because the MTF is low at high frequencies. Since the high frequencies are responsible for the 'squareness' of the corners for objects such as shown in Figure G.3, sharp objects will be shown as being slightly blurred or 'out of focus'. This is in accordance with the concept of *unsharpness* as discussed earlier, and the two approaches are just two ways of looking at the same thing. The MTF is more mathematically rigorous as a complete description of the imaging properties of the X-ray unit, but even this does not consider other problems such as statistical 'noise' within the image, known as 'quantum mottle'.

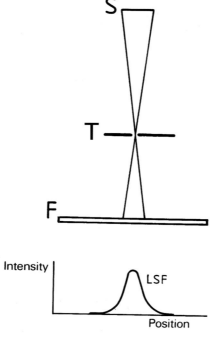

Figure G.4   The line spread function. Key: S—source of X-rays; T—test object with narrow slit; F—film.

G.4 MEASUREMENT OF MTF

It would be difficult in practice to manufacture sinusoidal objects in the numbers and the small wavelengths required. It would also be time-consuming to measure the object and image modulation for each conceivable combination of frequency, position of absorber and screen/film combination. Fortunately, there is no need to do this, since the MTF may be calculated from the line spread function (LSF). This calculation is best accomplished using a computer program and is beyond the scope of this book. The LSF is the profile of the intensity curve obtained by shining the X-ray beam through a very narrow slit (Fig. G.4).

Appendix H

SI BASE UNITS

SI base units were discussed in Chapter 6. Below are the precise definitions of these units.

Mass

The unit of mass is the *kilogram*. The mass of one kilogram is equal to the mass of the international platinum-iridium prototype of the kilogram.

Length

The unit of length is the *metre*. The metre is the length equal to 1 650 763.73 wavelengths in a vacuum of the radiation corresponding to the transition between the levels $2p_{10}$ and $5d_5$ of the krypton-86 atom.

Time

The unit of time is the *second*. The second is the duration of 9 192 631 770 periods of the radiation corresponding to the transition between the two hyperfine levels of the ground state of the caesium-133 atom.

Electric current

The unit of electric current is the *ampere*. The ampere is the constant current which, if maintained in two straight parallel conductors of infinite length, of negligible circular cross-section and placed 1 metre apart in a vacuum, would produce between these conductors a force equal to 2×10^{-7} newton per metre of length.

Temperature

The unit of temperature is the *kelvin*. The kelvin is the fraction $1/273.16$ of the thermodynamic temperature of the triple point of water.

Luminous intensity

The unit of luminous intensity is the *candela*. The candela is the luminous intensity, in the perpendicular direction, of the surface of 1/600 000 square metre of a black body at the temperature of freezing platinum under a pressure of 101 325 newtons per square metre.

Amount of substance

The unit of amount of substance is the *mole*. The mole is the amount of substance of a system which contains as many elementary entities as there are atoms in 0.012 kilogram of carbon-12.

Tables

Table A Powers of 10

Prefix	Symbol	Factor
exa	E	10^{18}
peta	P	10^{15}
tera	T	10^{12}
giga	G	10^{9}
mega	M	10^{6}
kilo	k	10^{3}
milli	m	10^{-3}
micro	μ	10^{-6}
nano	n	10^{-9}
pico	p	10^{-12}
femto	f	10^{-15}
atto	a	10^{-18}

Table B Physical constants

Quantity	Value
Avogadro's number, N_A	*6.02×10^{23} mole^{-1}
Velocity of light in a vacuum, c	3.00×10^{8} m$\cdot$s^{-1}
Permittivity of vacuum, ε_0	8.8×10^{-12} F$\cdot$m^{-1}
Permeability of vacuum, μ_0	1.26×10^{-6} H$\cdot$m^{-1}
Electron rest mass, m_e	9.11×10^{-31} kg
Proton rest mass, m_p	1.672×10^{-27} kg
Neutron rest mass, m_n	1.675×10^{-27} kg
Planck's constant, h	6.63×10^{-34} J$\cdot$s
Electronic charge, e	-1.60×10^{-19} C

* Or 6.02×10^{26} (kg-mole)$^{-1}$

Table C Important conversion factors

1 atomic mass unit (amu)	$= 1.66 \times 10^{-27}$ kg
1 electron volt (eV)	$= 1.60 \times 10^{-19}$ J
1 joule (J)	$= 6.24 \times 10^{18}$ eV
Electron mass	$= 0.511$ MeV
Proton mass	$= 938$ MeV
Neutron mass	$= 940$ MeV
1 angstrom (Å)	$= 0.1$ nm

Table D Greek symbols and their common usage

Name	Symbol		Usage
	Capital	Lower case	
Alpha	A	α	α-particle (He nucleus)
Beta	B	β	β-particle (electron or positron)
Gamma	Γ	γ	γ-ray; slope of photographic density curve
Delta	Δ	δ	Δx or δx used to indicate change in x
Epsilon	E	ε	
Zeta	Z	ζ	
Eta	H	η	
Theta	Θ	θ	Used to represent an angle
Iota	I	ι	
Kappa	K	κ	
Lambda	Λ	λ	Wavelength; decay constant
Mu	M	μ	Attenuation coefficient
Nu	N	ν	Frequency of electromagnetic radiation
Xi	Ξ	ξ	
Omicron	O	o	
Pi	Π	π	Circumference/diameter of circle; pair production
Rho	P	ρ	Density of matter
Sigma	Σ	σ	Standard deviation (σ); summation of terms (Σ)
Tau	T	τ	Photoelectric absorption
Upsilon	Y	υ	
Phi	Φ	ϕ	Used to represent an angle
Chi	X	χ	
Psi	Ψ	ψ	
Omega	Ω	ω	Symbol for resistance in ohm (Ω)

Answers to self-tests

CHAPTER 2

a. Fine 3.46 × 0.6 mm; broad 6.91 × 1.2 mm
If your answer differs substantially from the outline answer, refer to Section 2.3.

b. 2.5 × 3.0 cm
If your answer differs substantially from the outline answer, refer to Section 2.4.

c. 1.02 cm
If your answer differs substantially from the outline answer, refer to Section 2.5.

d. (i) 0.043 mm
   (ii) 0.021 mm
If your answer differs substantially from the outline answer, refer to Section 2.6.

e. 71.2 cm
If your answer differs substantially from the outline answer, refer to Section 2.7.

f. (i) The images of points on the plane of the fulcrum move at the same velocity as the film and are thus sharp. The images of points above the plane of the fulcrum move with a higher velocity than the film, whereas those of points below the plane of the fulcrum move with a lower velocity than the film. Because their velocity differs from that of the film they will show movement unsharpness.
   (ii) The tomographic angle and the tomographic layer thickness are inversely related, i.e. as the tomographic angle is increased so the layer thickness decreases.
If your answer differs substantially from the outline answer, refer to Section 2.8.

CHAPTER 3

a. The intensity of a beam of electromagnetic radiation at a point is the total energy per second flowing past that point when normalised to a unit area.
If your answer differs substantially from the outline answer, refer to Section 3.2.

b. The intensity of the radiation emitted from a small isotropic source is inversely proportional to the square of the distance from the source, provided there is negligible absorption or scattering of the radiation by the medium through which it passes.
If your answer differs substantially from the outline answer, refer to Section 3.3.

c. (i) $0.8\,mGy{\cdot}s^{-1}$
 (ii) 300 cm
If your answer differs substantially from the outline answer, refer to Section 3.5.

d. 6 mAs
If your answer differs substantially from the outline answer, refer to Section 3.6.

CHAPTER 4

a. 17:00 on 17 February
If your answer differs substantially from the outline answer, refer to Section 4.5.

b. 121.58 days
If your answer differs substantially from the outline answer, refer to Section 4.5.

c. 67.2 MBq
If your answer differs substantially from the outline answer, refer to Section 4.5.

d. $1/t_{\frac{1}{2}\,(eff)} = 1/t_{\frac{1}{2}\,(phys)} + 1/t_{\frac{1}{2}\,(biol)}$
If your answer differs substantially from the outline answer, refer to Section 4.6.

e. 19.8 mm
If your answer differs substantially from the outline answer, refer to Section 4.8.

f. (ii) 6 hours
 (iii) $0.1155\,h^{-1}$
 (iv) 0.24 MBq
If your answer differs substantially from the outline answer, refer to Section 4.10.

CHAPTER 5

a. Matter is neither created nor destroyed, but it may change its chemical form as the result of a chemical reaction.
If your answer differs substantially from the outline answer, refer to Section 5.2.

b. Energy can neither be created nor destroyed but can be changed from one form to another. The amount of energy in a system is thus constant.
If your answer differs substantially from the outline answer, refer to Section 5.3.

c. The total linear or rotational momentum in a given system is constant.
If your answer differs substantially from the outline answer, refer to Section 5.4.

d. *Law 1:* A body will remain at rest or will travel with a constant velocity unless acted upon by a net external force.
Law 2: The rate of change of momentum of a body is proportional to the applied force.
Law 3: The action of one body on a second body is always accompanied by an equal and opposite action of the second body on the first.
If your answer differs substantially from the outline answer, refer to Section 5.5.

e. 187.4×10^6 m·s^{-1}
If your answer differs substantially from the outline answer, refer to Section 5.5.

f. 0.262 kg
If your answer differs substantially from the outline answer, refer to Section 5.6.

CHAPTER 6

a. Velocity = *metre per second;* acceleration = *metre per second per second;* force = *newton;* pressure = *pascal;* weight = *newton;* energy = *joule;* power = *watt.*
If your answer differs substantially from the outline answer, refer to Table 6.2.

b. Exposure generates 7500 HU. As the maximum heat storage capacity of the anode disk is 10 000 HU a second exposure would generate a total heat of 15 000 HU which is outwith the capacity of the disk.
If your answer differs substantially from the outline answer, refer to Section 6.4.

CHAPTER 7

a. 0.1; 10%
If your answer differs substantially from the outline answer, refer to Section 7.3.3.

b. 6%
If your answer differs substantially from the outline answer, refer to Section 7.3.4.

c. (i) 100%
   (ii) 50%
   (iii) 10%
   (iv) 2%
   (v) 1%
If your answer differs substantially from the outline answer, refer to Section 7.3.3.

d. (i) = 10%
   (ii) = approx. 21%
If your answer differs substantially from the outline answer, refer to Section 7.3.4.

e. (i) Mean = 36; median = 36
   (ii) Mean = 9; median = 10
   (iii) Mean = 47.7; median = 47
If your answer differs substantially from the outline answer, refer to Section 7.4.1.

f. Mean = 70.07; standard deviation = 1.111; standard error = 0.035; 2 standard deviation limits = 69.85–70.29
If your answer differs substantially from the outline answer, refer to Section 7.4.1.

CHAPTER 8

a. When thermal energy is applied, this causes increased vibrational energy in the atoms of the bar. Because of this they occupy more room causing an expansion of the bar.
If your answer differs substantially from the outline answer, refer to Section 8.3.

b. 373 K
If your answer differs substantially from the outline answer, refer to Section 8.3.1.

c. 840 W
If your answer differs substantially from the outline answer, refer to Section 8.3.2.

d. The temperature rise in the molybdenum disk will be half of the temperature rise produced in the tungsten disk.
If your answer differs substantially from the outline answer, refer to Section 8.3.2.

e. Kinetic energy is given to the atoms at the point of heating. These atoms transfer some of their vibrational energy to neighbouring atoms. Heat is transmitted along the structure by these interatomic collisions.
If your answer differs substantially from the outline answer, refer to Section 8.4.1.

f. Heat is transferred to atoms at its point of application by conduction. These atoms have increased vibrational energy and so occupy more space. This causes a decrease in the density of the fluid and so it will rise because of hydrostatic pressure. The rising molecules will dissipate heat to the surrounding molecules. In this way convection currents are established and the whole of the fluid is heated.
If your answer differs substantially from the outline answer, refer to Section 8.4.2.

g. When atoms are heated they increase their vibrational energy. Atoms may get rid of this energy in the form of photons of electromagnetic radiation in the infra-red part of the spectrum. These photons are absorbed by other bodies and so the energy is transferred.

If your answer differs substantially from the outline answer, refer to Section 8.4.3.

h. *Stationary anode:* heat is dissipated from the target by conduction to the copper anode and along the copper anode to the oil by conduction. *Rotating anode:* heat is dissipated from the anode disk by radiation to the oil. In both types heat is dissipated through the oil by convection, through the housing by conduction and to the air in the X-ray room by convection.

If your answer differs substantially from the outline answer, refer to Sections 8.7.1 and 8.7.2.

CHAPTER 9

a. The general properties of electrical charges are as follows:

- Charges can be considered as being of two types: positive and negative.
- The smallest unit of negative charge which can exist in isolation is that possessed by an electron and the smallest unit of positive charge which can exist in isolation is that possessed by the proton.
- Electrical charges exert forces on each other even when they are separated by a vacuum. The forces are mutual, equal and opposite.
- Like charges (i.e. charges of the same sign) *repel* each other while unlike charges (of opposite signs) *attract* each other.
- The magnitude of the mutual forces between the charges is influenced by:
  —the magnitude of the individual charges
  —the medium in which they are embedded, being greatest when the medium is a vacuum
  —the inverse square of the distance between the charged bodies.
- Electrical charges may be *induced* in a body by the proximity of a charged body, leading to a force of attraction between the two bodies.
- Electrical charges may flow easily in some materials (called *electrical conductors*) and with difficulty in other materials (called *electrical insulators*). Both types of material are capable of having charges induced in them.
- When electrical charges move they produce a magnetic field.

If your answer differs substantially from the outline answer, refer to Section 9.3.

b. The force is proportional to the magnitude of each of the charges and inversely proportional to the square of the distance between them.

If your answer differs substantially from the outline answer, refer to Section 9.4.

c. (i) *Conductor.* Proximity of a positively charged body will attract electrons on to the surface of the conductor next to the charged body. This leaves positive charges on the opposite surface. A state of equilibrium is set up where the force of attraction on the electrons from the positively charged body is equal to the attraction from the positive charges on the opposite surface of the conductor. At this point there is no further flow of charge.

(ii) *Insulator.* This involves a description of the action of a positively charged body on the molecules of an insulator either to produce molecular distortion or to cause rotation of polar molecules so that they align with the electrical field.

If your answer differs substantially from the outline answer, refer to Sections 9.7.1 and 9.7.2.

d. Earth is assumed to be electrically neutral in that it contains equal numbers of positive and negative charges. Thus there is no force between neutral earth and a unit positive charge and so no work is needed to move the latter towards earth. As no work is done the electrical potential of earth is zero.

If your answer differs substantially from the outline answer, refer to Section 9.8.1.

e. (i) On a conducting sphere the charges experience mutual repulsion so that we get a regular distribution of charge on the external surface of the sphere.

(ii) On an irregularly shaped body the charges repel each other so that the distribution of charge varies with the radius of curvature of the body surface. The highest concentration of charge is on the parts of the body with the smallest radius of curvature.

If your answer differs substantially from the outline answer, refer to Sections 9.8.5 and 9.9.

CHAPTER 10

a. An electrical conductor will readily allow the flow of electric charge whereas an insulator will have a very large resistance to the flow of charge. This is explained by the fact that conductors have an ample supply of electrons in the conduction band whereas, in insulators, the conduction band is empty of electrons.

If your answer differs substantially from the outline answer, refer to Section 10.3.

b. Length of the conductor ($R \propto l$); cross-sectional area ($R \propto 1/A$); resistivity ($R \propto \rho$) and temperature ($R \propto T$).

If your answer differs substantially from the outline answer, refer to Section 10.7.1.

c. 2 metres

If your answer differs substantially from the outline answer, refer to Section 10.7.1.

d. *Ohm's Law* states that the current flowing through a metallic conductor is proportional to the potential difference which exists across it provided that all physical conditions remain constant.

A body is said to have an electrical resistance of 1 *ohm* if a potential difference of 1 volt across it produces an electrical current through it of 1 ampere.
If your answer differs substantially from the outline answer, refer to Section 10.8.

e. $R = 24\ \Omega$; $I = 0.25$ A; $I_1 = 0.2$ A; $I_2 = 0.05$ A; $V_1 = 2$ V; $V_2 = 4$ V.
If your answer differs substantially from the outline answer, refer to Section 10.8.

f. Energy $= 30$ kJ; power $= 250$ W.
If your answer differs substantially from the outline answer, refer to Section 10.9.

g. Volt drop in the cables is 20 V and the potential difference across the set is 380 V.
If your answer differs substantially from the outline answer, refer to Section 10.10.

CHAPTER 11

a. $F = m_1 m_2 / 4 \pi \mu_0 d^2$
If your answer differs substantially from the outline answer, refer to Section 11.2.1.

b. This requires a diagram similar to Figure 11.3.
If your answer differs substantially from the outline answer, refer to Section 11.3.

c. The three terms refer to the magnetism induced in a material as a result of an external magnetic field.

In *diamagnetism*, the electrons orbiting a nucleus have their orbits changed as a result of the external magnetic field. They remain in this condition until the field is removed and then revert to their original orbitals. Thus all materials are diamagnetic. The magnetic induction produced within the sample opposes the applied magnetic field and so the relative permeability is less than unity.

In *paramagnetism* the atoms of the material can be considered as elementary bar magnets since the magnetic effect of the electrons complement each other. Such materials are rapidly demagnetised at room temperature when the external magnetic field is removed. Materials have a temperature above which the paramagnetic effect is lost and only the diamagnetic effect remains. Paramagnetic materials have a relative permeability of just over unity.

Ferromagnetic materials are easily magnetised. The atoms within the material rotate as domains when influenced by an external magnetic field. Such materials have relative permeabilities measured in hundreds or thousands.
If your answer differs substantially from the outline answer, refer to Section 11.6.

d. In ferromagnetic materials, the induced magnetism always lags behind the magnetising force because of the frictional forces between magnetic domains. This phenomenon is known as hysteresis.
If your answer differs substantially from the outline answer, refer to Section 11.7.

CHAPTER 12

a. In a bar magnet the atomic magnets predominantly face in one direction and so produce a magnetic field as shown in Figure 11.3. When electrons flow through a wire, they produce a magnetic field as shown in Figure 12.3(a). By comparing the two diagrams the similarities between the two fields can be seen.
If your answer differs substantially from the outline answer, refer to Sections 11.3 and 12.6.

b. Iron has higher magnetic permeability than air and so there is an increase in the lines of magnetic force in the vicinity of the iron core. As the current through the solenoid is increased, so the magnetising force is also increased. This is initially accompanied by an increase in the magnetic intensity as the molecular magnets align with the magnetic field. Eventually the point is reached where there is no further increase in the magnetic intensity as all the molecular magnets have now aligned with the field from the solenoid—magnetic saturation has been produced.
If your answer differs substantially from the outline answer, refer to Sections 12.6 and 11.6.3.

c. This requires a diagram similar to Figure 12.5. When switch S is open, no current flows through the solenoid and so the soft iron piece M is held in the position shown by the spring P. Contacts C_1 and C_3 are in contact, while C_1 and C_2 are 'open'. When S is closed, the current passing through the solenoid magnetises the soft iron core which attracts M by induced magnetism. M pivots about O so that the arm L lifts C_1 away from C_3 and into contact with C_2. Thus, if the external circuit is joined, current will flow between C_1 and C_2 but no current will flow between C_1 and C_3. Opening S reduces the current in the solenoid to zero and hence restores the system to its original condition, since M loses its magnetism and is pulled quickly away under the action of the spring P (C_1 and C_3 are closed and C_1 and C_2 are open).
If your answer differs substantially from the outline answer, refer to Section 12.7.

CHAPTER 13

a. Electromagnetic induction is where electricity is produced by the interlinking of a conductor with a changing magnetic field. Electromagnetism is the production of a magnetic field by the passage of an electric current.
If your answer differs substantially from the outline answer, refer to Section 13.2.

b. Faraday's First Law states: a change in the magnetic flux linked with a conductor induces an EMF in the conductor. This means that the conductor must be in close proximity to the magnetic field (to produce linkage) and that the magnitude or position of the magnetic field relative to the conductor must be changing in order to produce an EMF.

Faraday's Second Law states: the magnitude of the induced EMF is proportional to the rate of change of the magnetic flux linkage. This means that the EMF will alter if the strength of the magnet alters, if the rate of change of the magnetic field alters and if the linkage between the magnetic field and the conductor alters.

Lenz's Law states: the direction of the induced current in a conductor caused by a changing magnetic flux is such that its own magnetic field opposes the changing magnetic flux. This means that when an EMF is induced in a conductor this will be in such a way as to cause a current to flow which will have an associated magnetic field in opposition to the changing magnetic flux which created it.

The magnitude of the induced EMF depends on:

- the magnitude of the magnetic flux
- the efficiency by which this flux is interlinked with the conductor (e.g. how many turns in the coil)
- the rate of change of the magnetic flux.

If your answer differs substantially from the outline answer, refer to Sections 13.4 and 13.5.

c. If a conductor is moved through a magnetic field but no external circuit is connected to the ends of the conductor, an EMF will be generated in the conductor but no current will flow through it.
If your answer differs substantially from the outline answer, refer to Section 13.4.

d. If the conductor is moved in the direction indicated, the EMF will be such as to cause a flow of electrons into the page. The maximum EMF is produced when the conductor is moved at right angles to the magnetic field. Zero EMF is produced if the conductor is moved parallel to the magnetic field.
If your answer differs substantially from the outline answer, refer to Section 13.6.

e. (i)   When the magnet moves downwards above the wire the current induced in the wire will be in a clockwise direction.
(ii) When the magnet moves downwards below the wire the current in the wire will be in an anticlockwise direction.
If your answer differs substantially from the outline answer, refer to Section 13.6.

f. If a changing current is passed through one conductor, then this will produce a changing magnetic field around this conductor. If a second conductor is placed within this changing magnetic field, then (by Faraday's Laws) an EMF will be generated in the conductor and a current will flow in it if the conducting loop is complete. By Lenz's Law this current will be in the opposite direction to the original current. The size of this secondary current will vary with the magnetic field—it will be a current of changing magnitude as there is a changing magnetic field. This changing secondary current will produce its own changing magnetic field which will induce an EMF and current in the first conductor. Thus *each conductor induces electricity in the other* and the effect is known as *mutual induction.*

If a solenoid is connected across a source of EMF, current flow starts to build up in the solenoid. As this current increases, *each turn* of the solenoid produces a changing magnetic flux which is linked to the *other turns* of the solenoid. Thus from Faraday's and Lenz's Laws, an EMF in the opposite direction to the EMF from the source will be induced in the solenoid—this is known as a *back EMF.* This effect is known as *self-induction.*

A mutual inductance of 1 *henry* exists between two conductors if 1 volt is induced in one conductor where there is a current change of 1 ampere per second in the other.

A conductor has a self-inductance of 1 *henry* if a back EMF of 1 volt is induced when the current flowing through it changes at 1 ampere per second. *If your answer differs substantially from the outline answer, refer to Sections 13.7 and 13.8.*

g. This would require a simple diagram similar to Figure 13.6 and an explanation as follows. Consider the situation where the coil shown is rotated in a clockwise direction. Thus, from the initial position, side X of the coil will move upwards through the magnetic field and side Y will move downwards. At this point in its movement the coil is cutting the maximum number of lines of flux as it is moving at right angles to the flux lines, and so the maximum EMF will be generated. We can see that electrons will travel towards us on side X and away from us on side Y. Thus an excess of electrons will exist at brush A and a shortage of electrons will exist at brush B—brush A is negative and brush B is positive. This situation is shown as position 1 on the graph. Now consider the situation when the coil had turned in a clockwise direction from its initial position through 90°— this is the second position of the coil shown. In this position both side X and side Y of the coil are moving parallel with the lines of magnetic flux and so no current is generated—this is again shown as 2 on the graph. In position 3 the coil has rotated through 180° from its original position. Side X of the coil is now moving downwards through the magnetic field and side Y is moving upwards. As in position 1, a maximum number of lines of flux are being cut as the conductor is moving at right angles to the flux, and so, again, the maximum EMF will be generated. The polarity of A and B is now the reverse of position 1. In position 4 the conductor is again moving parallel to the lines of flux so no EMF is generated. The conductor then returns to position 1 and so one cycle is complete. The process is then repeated. The type of current shown in the graph is known as an *alternating current.*

In cases where there is no external circuit connected, then no current is able to flow and only sufficient work to overcome the frictional resistance is necessary to keep the rotational movement at the same speed. As soon as an external circuit is connected, then a current is able to flow in the circuit and in the winding. This current will flow in such a direction as to oppose the motion of the coil. This means that mechanical work must be performed to overcome this resisting force, i.e. mechanical energy is converted into electrical energy.

The effect of suddenly increasing the electrical load demanded from the generator is to suddenly increase the opposition to its rotation. Hence the generator slows down momentarily and the induced EMF (which depends on the speed of rotation) is reduced. Thus we find that, in times of increased demand on the generators, there is a drop in the voltage they supply.

If your answer differs substantially from the outline answer, refer to Section 13.9.

CHAPTER 14

a. A sinusoidal alternating current is one where the current can be illustrated in graphical form to describe a sine wave. A graph similar to the one in Figure 14.2 should be included.

If your answer differs substantially from the outline answer, refer to Section 14.4.

b. The *peak* value of the current is the same as the amplitude and represents the maximum positive or negative value of the current. The *average* value of the current is the mean current which flows during a complete cycle. The *RMS* value of the current is that value of constant current which, flowing for the same time, would produce the same expenditure of electrical energy in a circuit.

For an alternating current: $I_{AV} = 0$; $I_{RMS} = 0.707 I_P$
For a full-wave rectified current: $I_{AV} = 0.636 I_P$; $I_{RMS} = 0.707 I_P$.

If your answer differs substantially from the outline answer, refer to Sections 14.4.1, 14.4.2 and 14.4.3.

c. (i) RMS current = 0.1 A
   (ii) Peak current = 0.1414 A
   (iii) Average current = 0
   (iv) Average power = 1 W

If your answer differs substantially from the outline answer, refer to Sections 14.4.1, 14.4.2 and 14.4.3.

d. Impedance = 46 1 Ω; phase angle = 29.9°; peak current = 6.5 A.

If your answer differs substantially from the outline answer, refer to Section 14.7.4

e. The resonance frequency for a circuit is that frequency of the supply to the circuit which results in the highest current flow through the circuit for a given potential across its ends. The resonance frequency for the circuit given is 39.8 Hz.

If your answer differs substantially from the outline answer, refer to Section 14.7.4.

f. Phase voltages = 230 V; line voltages = 398 V.
If your answer differs substantially from the outline answer, refer to Section 14.8.1.

CHAPTER 15

a. A current-carrying conductor will experience a force when placed in a magnetic field.
If your answer differs substantially from the outline answer, refer to Section 15.2.

b. The magnitude of the force is proportional to:

- the magnetic flux density (B)
- the magnitude of the electric current (I)
- the length of the wire (l)
- the sine of the angle between the magnetic field and the wire ($\sin \theta$).

The equation is $F = BIl \sin \theta$
If your answer differs substantially from the outline answer, refer to Section 15.3.

c. A diagram similar to Fig 15.4 is required. A simplified DC electric motor is shown in the diagram where a battery is connected to a coil of wire KLMN via brushes B at a commutator C. The coil of wire is in the magnetic field of a permanent magnet, the direction of whose field is from left to right in the figure. When the current is switched on, the electron flow is in the direction indicated in the diagram, and the coil is affected by a clockwise force due to the motor principle (i.e. an *upward* force on KL and a *downward* force on MN). The commutator C turns with the coil KLMN so that the current always flows in the same direction relative to the permanent magnet. Hence the coil always experiences a clockwise force and keeps turning. Without the commutator, KLMN would eventually stop at right angles to the permanent magnetic field.
If your answer differs substantially from the outline answer, refer to Section 15.6.

d. Three uses might include:

- drive motors for mobile X-ray machines
- production of the rotation of the rotating anode X-ray tube
- electron beam scanning in the television monitor

or other reasonable examples.
If your answer differs substantially from the outline answer, refer to Section 15.9.

CHAPTER 16

a. Capacitance is the ratio of the charge on the body to its potential. The unit of capacitance is the *farad*. The capacitance of a body is 1 *farad* if a charge of 1 coulomb held by the body results in a potential of 1 volt.
If your answer differs substantially from the outline answer, refer to Section 16.3.

b. 80×10^{-3} C, 70 kV
If your answer differs substantially from the outline answer, refer to Section 16.3.

c. The capacitance depends on the area of the plates, A, the separation of the plates, d, and the dielectric constant, K, of the material between the plates. The equation is $C = \varepsilon_0 KA/d$.
If your answer differs substantially from the outline answer, refer to Section 16.4.

d. (i) Connect the three capacitors in parallel
   (ii) Connect the three capacitors in series.
If your answer differs substantially from the outline answer, refer to Sections 16.6 and 16.7.

e. 20 µF
If your answer differs substantially from the outline answer, refer to Sections 16.6 and 16.7.

f. 27.38 V; 273.8 µC
If your answer differs substantially from the outline answer, refer to Section 16.9.

g. Examples are: capacitor discharge mobile units; electronic timers; voltage smoothing; phase splitting for AC induction motors.
If your answer differs substantially from the outline answer, refer to Section 16.11.

h. The voltage rating of the capacitor; the leakage of the capacitor; whether the capacitor is to be used for AC or DC; the physical size of the capacitor; the price of the capacitor.
If your answer differs substantially from the outline answer, refer to Section 16.12.

CHAPTER 17

a. 55 kV$_{RMS}$; 77.8 kV$_P$
If your answer differs substantially from the outline answer, refer to Section 17.3 or Section 14.4.3 to convert RMS value to peak value.

b. The efficiency of a transformer is the ratio of the output power to the input power.
    The primary current is 0.2 A$_{RMS}$.
If your answer differs substantially from the outline answer, refer to Section 17.5

c. When a current flows through the secondary of the high-tension transformer there is a volt drop because of the resistance of the secondary winding given by $V = IR$ where R is the resistance of the secondary winding and I is the current through it. The potential difference across the secondary is $V_0 - IR$ where V_0 is

the off-load voltage. Thus an increase in current produces an increase in IR and thus a reduction in the output voltage.
If your answer differs substantially from the outline answer, refer to Section 17.6.3

d. 98 kV
If your answer differs substantially from the outline answer, refer to Section 17.6.3

e. (i) 600 turns
    (ii) 120 V
    (iii) 640 turns
If your answer differs substantially from the outline answer, refer to Section 17.7

f. Transformer rating is the maximum combination of voltage and current which a transformer can withstand for a specific time without damage to the transformer. If the voltage is exceeded, then the insulation in the transformer may be insufficient for the electrical potential involved thus leading to insulation breakdown. If too large a current flows for too long a time, then there may be overheating of either the transformer core or the transformer windings. Some transformers as part of their normal function generate significant amounts of heat. Such transformers are cooled by immersing the transformer in an oil bath.
If your answer differs substantially from the outline answer, refer to Section 17.9

CHAPTER 18

a. In the atoms which make up a body, the outer shell electrons are more loosely bound than the inner electrons because they are further away from the nucleus. The application of heat to a body increases the kinetic energy of its atoms and so increases the violence of their collisions. As a result of these collisions the outer electrons may be dislodged from the atom. Electrons so released near the centre of a body travel only a relatively short distance, but if they are released near the surface of the material they may have sufficient kinetic energy to leave the body. In thermionic emission this is the mechanism by which the electrons are emitted. The higher the temperature of a body, the greater the kinetic energy of the atoms and so a greater number of electrons will have sufficient energy to break free from the influence of the surface atoms of the body.
If your answer differs substantially from the outline answer, refer to Section 18.2.

b. If we assume that a body is electrically neutral before the application of heat, then each electron which leaves the body by thermionic emission will cause the body to have a net positive charge. After a very short period of time a state of equilibrium is set up where electrons leave the body and enter a 'cloud' of electrons near its surface and are then attracted back to the body, i.e. electrons are attracted back to the body as fast as they are emitted. The number of electrons in this cloud remains fairly constant since electrons are entering and

leaving the cloud at equal rates. This cloud of electrons is known as the *space charge*. If the temperature of the body is increased, then the number of electrons in the space charge will also increase due to the increased electron emission from the body. If the body is left to cool, it will reduce the space charge to zero by attracting electrons from it back to the body.
If your answer differs substantially from the outline answer, refer to Section 18.2.1.

c. Devices are the vacuum diode, the X-ray tube and the vacuum triode.
If your answer differs substantially from the outline answer, refer to Section 18.3.

d. When the filament is heated, electrons will be produced by thermionic emission and will gather close to the filament to form the space charge. If a source of potential is connected across the diode so that the anode has a positive potential with respect to the cathode, the effect is to move the position of the space charge from the immediate vicinity of the cathode to a position somewhere between the cathode and the anode. Under these circumstances some of the electrons produced at the filament will gain sufficient kinetic energy to pass through the space charge and reach the anode. Other electrons will be repelled by the space charge and return to the filament. Thus, the space charge has a limiting effect on the flow of current across the diode, and the diode is said to be *space-charge limited*. If we make the anode more positive, then the space charge will move further away from the cathode and more electrons will flow across the diode—there is an increase in the diode current. At a particular value of anode potential, all the space charge is collected by the anode as soon as it is produced by the filament. This represents the maximum flow of electrons through the diode at that filament temperature, as electrons will travel across the diode as soon as they are produced by the filament. The diode is then said to be *saturated* or *temperature limited*.
If your answer differs substantially from the outline answer, refer to Section 18.4.

e. In the triode valve, electrons flow from the cathode (or filament) to the anode by passing through the grid. The current through the triode is controlled by the negative bias on the grid. If the grid is very negative, then it will repel electrons from the cathode so that none pass through it. Thus there is no current through the triode. If the grid is made less negative, then current will flow through the triode, the amount of current being controlled by the bias on the grid. Like the diode, the triode will eventually saturate.
If your answer differs substantially from the outline answer, refer to Section 18.5.

CHAPTER 19

a. An intrinsic semiconductor is a chemically pure semiconductor which is also assumed to have perfect regularity of atoms within its crystal lattice. In such materials there is a narrow gap between the valence band and the conduction band so that, at normal room temperatures, many electrons have sufficient energy to jump up to the conduction band and so take part in electrical conductivity.

If your answer differs substantially from the outline answer, refer to Section 19.3.

b. If small amounts of trivalent or pentavalent impurities are added to an intrinsic semiconductor, its conductivity is greatly increased. It is now classed as an extrinsic semiconductor. If the impurity added is a trivalent impurity, then the substance is a *P*-type semiconductor, whereas a pentavalent impurity produces an *N*-type semiconductor.

If your answer differs substantially from the outline answer, refer to Sections 19.4 to 19.4.2.

c. In the *P*-type semiconductor the majority carriers are positive holes in the valence band and the minority carriers are thermally generated free electrons in the conduction band. In the *N*-type semiconductor the majority carriers are free electrons in the conduction band and the minority carriers are free holes in the valence band.

If your answer differs substantially from the outline answer, refer to Sections 19.4.1 and 19.4.2.

d. A *PN* junction is produced when a *P*-type semiconductor and an *N*-type semiconductor are heat fused together. When *P*- and *N*-types are brought together and heat fused in intimate contact, then free electrons from the *N*-type and free positive holes from the *P*-type are able to penetrate across the boundary between them. This diffusion of charge across the barrier results in recombination of the positive holes and the free electrons (the free electrons drop into the positive holes so that their charges are cancelled). Thus for a short distance on either side of the *PN* junction (about 0.5×10^{-6} m) no free carriers exist—this is therefore known as a *depletion layer*. However, a net charge exists on either side of the junction because the *N*-type has lost electrons and the *P*-type has lost positive holes. Thus there is a negatively charged area just within the *P*-type region and a positively charged area just within the *N*-type region. The two peaks of charge increase in size until no further net flow of majority carriers takes place. For example, a free electron from the *N*-type will only be able to pass over to the *P*-type if it has sufficient energy to overcome the repulsion of the negative peak at the *PN* junction. The charge distribution produces its own potential difference known as the *potential barrier* since it acts in opposition to the flow of majority carriers from either side of the barrier. When the *PN* junction is forward biased, the potential barrier is lowered, so free charges readily cross the junction. If the *PN* junction is reverse biased, the height of the potential barrier is increased, thus preventing any charge flow across the barrier.

If your answer differs substantially from the outline answer, refer to Section 19.5.

e. The solid-state rectifier has the following advantages over the thermionic diode valve:

- it contains no filament and thus has a longer life, consumes less power and produces less heat
- it is smaller in size than the thermionic diode thus enabling the production of a more compact X-ray unit
- it has a smaller forward voltage drop thus enabling a higher kV_p to be applied to the X-ray tube
- the reverse current is less than a vacuum diode and so it is a more efficient rectifier.

If your answer differs substantially from the outline answer, refer to Section 19.5.4.

f. When electrons are injected into the base from the emitter across the *NP* junction, they become *minority carriers* within the base and so readily cross the collector-to-base *PN* junction. This process is so efficient that approximately 98% of the electrons injected into the base from the emitter are able to diffuse across the base and form the collector current. The remaining 2% form the base current. This ratio of approximately 50 : 1 for the collector current and the base current remains constant for a particular transistor. Thus the base current may be used to control the collector current, as an increase in the base current will allow a subsequent increase in the collector current.

If your answer differs substantially from the outline answer, refer to Section 19.6.1.

g. This requires a diagram similar to Figure 18.13 together with the following explanation.

Junctions *J1* and *J3* are forward biased but junction *J2* is reverse biased. Consequently, if the thyristor is connected into a circuit, only a small leakage current flows through it—it behaves as an open switch. If a positive pulse is applied to the *P*-type layer (the gate) at junction *J1*, then positive holes are injected into the *P*-type material and flow across the junction *J1* so that the potential barrier at that junction is greatly reduced. The reduced potential difference across *J1* means that a higher reverse potential difference than before exists across *J2* and, if high enough, will cause electrical breakdown to occur at this junction due to the avalanche effect. Once this breakdown occurs, a large current may flow through the thyristor—it behaves as a closed switch. It is not possible to switch the thyristor off by applying a negative pulse to the gate but it will switch off when the potential difference across it is zero—the avalanching effect can no longer be maintained under such conditions.

If your answer differs substantially from the outline answer, refer to Section 19.7.

CHAPTER 20

a. In the X-ray unit it is necessary to step-up voltage before it is applied across the

X-ray tube and it is also necessary to step-down voltage before it is applied across the tube filament. The most convenient method of achieving this is to use transformers which require an AC supply. The X-ray tube will only produce useful X-rays when the anode is positive and the cathode is negative, and so it is desirable to have a unidirectional supply to the tube. This is achieved by the use of rectification.

If your answer differs substantially from the outline answer, refer to Section 20.2.

b. The self-rectified unit has the following advantages:

- the circuit is simple and thus little can go wrong
- the unit is relatively inexpensive
- because of the absence of rectifiers it is possible to incorporate the circuit in a single tank and thus eliminate the need for external high-tension cables.

In the modern X-ray unit solid-state rectifiers are employed. These are reliable, relatively cheap and small enough to allow single-tank construction if this is desirable.

If your answer differs substantially from the outline answer, refer to Section 20.3.1.

c. A diagram similar to Figure 20.3 is required with an explanation to indicate that during one half-cycle the electron flow is through one pair of diodes and through the other pair in the other half-cycle. For both half-cycles, electrons can flow through the X-ray tube from cathode to anode.

If your answer differs substantially from the outline answer, refer to Section 20.4.

d. This requires a diagram similar to Figure 20.6 with an explanation that the pulsating output from the high-tension transformer is first capacitor smoothed to reduce the voltage ripple. This ripple is then removed by the use of triode valves where the grid bias is most negative at the peak of the voltage and least negative at the trough. Thus a constant potential is applied to the X-ray tube.

If your answer differs substantially from the outline answer, refer to Section 20.5.2.

e. A box diagram similar to Figure 20.9 would help the explanation. The mains supply is rectified and capacitor smoothed to produce an almost constant potential. This is then passed through a frequency invertor to produce an alternating voltage of frequency 5000 Hz. This high-frequency AC is now passed through the high-tension transformer and the resultant voltage is again rectified and capacitor smoothed before being applied to the X-ray tube. The voltage thus applied to the tube is almost a constant potential.

If your answer differs substantially from the outline answer, refer to Section 20.7.

CHAPTER 21

a. During the 'prep' stage of the exposure sequence two major things happen:

- The appropriate filament of the X-ray tube is raised to its working temperature so that it emits the required number of electrons by thermionic emission, thus allowing the tube current (mA) to flow during the exposure.
- The anode is made to rotate at the required speed prior to the exposure being made.

If your answer differs substantially from the outline answer, refer to Section 21.2.

b. This requires a simple diagram similar to Figure 21.1 followed by a description similar to the one below.

This type of switching has no moving parts and utilises two thyristors connected as a flip-flop circuit to perform the switching sequence. Two thyristors are required to switch an alternating current as each conducts the half-cycle when that thyristor is forward biased. At the end of each half-cycle, each thyristor will cease to conduct as the potential difference across it drops to zero, and so a voltage pulse must be applied to its gate if it is required to conduct during the next half-cycle. Thus, during the exposure, the timer is simply required to apply a train of synchronised pulses to the gates of the thyristors at a time slightly later than the mains zero to ensure their continued conduction. At the end of the exposure these pulses stop and the thyristors cease to conduct at the end of the next half-cycle. This system is inertia free and allows an accuracy of one voltage pulse (i.e. an exposure time of 0.01 second in the case of a two-pulse unit).

If your answer differs substantially from the outline answer, refer to Section 21.3.1.

c. X-rays are produced when electrons flow from the cathode to the anode of the X-ray tube. These electrons are normally focused on to the target of the tube by a focusing cup which is at a negative potential equal to that of the filament. If a separate bias is applied to the focusing cup, then it is possible to make it more negative than the filament. Tubes which offer this facility are known as grid-controlled tubes. If the focusing cup is made about 3 kV more negative than the filament, it will produce a sufficiently large electrostatic field to prevent any electrons from crossing the X-ray tube and therefore no exposure is made. When the bias is reduced to make it equal that of the filament, electrons will flow across the tube and X-rays will be produced. At the end of the exposure the high negative bias is re-established on the focusing cup, thus stopping electron flow. The grid-controlled tube is therefore acting as an electronic exposure switch as well as a producer of X-rays. This arrangement is used in cine-radiography and in capacitor discharge units.

If your answer differs substantially from the outline answer, refer to Section 21.3.2.

d. This requires a diagram similar to Figure 21.3 and an explanation of the operation of the circuit as follows.

The time taken to charge a capacitor so that there is a predetermined potential across its plates is determined by the resistance in the line. When this trigger voltage is achieved, then a signal is sent to the switching system which terminates the X-ray exposure by stopping current flow through the X-ray tube. For thyristor switching, the exposure can be terminated by simply removing the triggering voltage pulses from the gates of the thyristors. Thus at the end of the next half-cycle, the thyristors will cease to conduct and the exposure will terminate.

If your answer differs substantially from the outline answer, refer to Section 21.4.

e. This requires a diagram similar to Figure 21.4 and an explanation of the operation of the circuit as follows.

The capacitor is charged from two sources V_1 and V_2. V_1 is a stable source of voltage (e.g. a rectified supply from the autotransformer). The amount of charge which the capacitor receives from V_1 is controlled by the variable resistor R. V_2 is a rectified supply from the mid-point of the high-tension transformer so that the amount of charge from this source is directly related to the amount of charge passing through the X-ray tube (the mAs). The radiographer will position the variable resistor, R, to determine the charge from V_2 and hence the charge passing through the X-ray tube during the exposure—the radiographer selects the required mAs.

If your answer differs substantially from the outline answer, refer to Section 21.4.2.

f. This requires a diagram similar to Figure 21.6 and an explanation of the operation of the circuit as follows.

The capacitor is charged from two sources V_1 and V_2. V_1 is a stable source of voltage (e.g. a rectified supply from the autotransformer). The amount of charge which the capacitor receives from V_1 is controlled by the variable resistor R. V_2 is an amplified supply from an ionisation chamber or a photocell either of which can measure the amount of radiation which has passed through the patient. If we assume that the amount of charge from V_1 is determined by the position of the variable resistor, R, then the remainder of the charge required to raise the potential of the capacitor to the trigger voltage of the switching device must be from the source V_2. As this is directly related to the amount of radiation passing through the patient on to the imaging device, this will be constant irrespective of the amount of radiation absorbed by the patient. The timer, in this case, terminates the exposure when the correct amount of radiation has passed through the ionisation chamber or photocell. Thus, if the ionisation chamber or photocell is positioned over the correct part of the patient, the radiograph should always receive the correct exposure. If we vary the position of the variable resistor, R, we can vary the amount of charge required from V_2 thus allowing imaging devices of differing sensitivities (speeds) to be used.

If your answer differs substantially from the outline answer, refer to Section 21.4.3.

CHAPTER 22

a. A diagram similar to Figure 22.1 without the light beam diaphragm is required. The functions of the major components are as follows:

- *Filament*—production of a given number of electrons by thermionic emission.
- *Focusing cup*—this prevents the spread of the electron beam by the electrostatic repulsion of the electrons and focuses the electron beam on to the target at the anode.
- *Target*—this is responsible for converting some of the kinetic energy of the electrons which cross the tube into X-rays.
- *Anode*—the anode mass is responsible for removing heat from the target by conduction and dissipating this heat to the oil.
- *Oil*—the oil has the functions of a coolant and an insulator.
- *Expansion bellows*—these allow for the expansion of the oil when heated.
- *Microswitch*—this prevents further X-ray exposures being made if the oil is overheated.
- *Tube port*—this allows the useful X-ray beam to leave the tube.
- *Lead lining*—this reduces the radiation leakage from the tube to the required limits.
- *Tube shield*—this protects the components and holds them in place. It also restricts access to the 'live' components.

If your answer differs substantially from the outline answer, refer to Sections 22.4.1–22.4.3.

b. A diagram similar to Figure 22.6 is required. The functions of the major components are as follows:

- *Filament*—production of a given number of electrons by thermionic emission.
- *Focusing cup*—this prevents the spread of the electron beam by the electrostatic repulsion of the electrons and focuses the electron beam on to the target at the anode.
- *Focal track*—this is responsible for converting some of the kinetic energy of the electrons which cross the tube into X-rays.
- *Anode disk*—the anode disk is responsible for removing heat from the focal track by conduction and dissipating this heat to the oil by radiation.
- *Anode stem*—this connects the anode disk to the rotor. It is designed to allow minimal heat dissipation through it by conduction.
- *Rotor assembly*—this is responsive to the induced currents from the stator coils to produce a torque which rotates the disk.
- *Ball bearings*—these allow rotation of the rotor which is free from vibration and only has limited frictional forces.
- *Stator coils*—these produce the 'rotating field' which induces currents in the rotor to produce rotation of the anode of the tube.
- *Oil*—the oil has the functions of a coolant and an insulator.
- *Expansion bellows*—these allow for the expansion of the oil when heated.
- *Tube port*—this allows the useful X-ray beam to leave the tube.
- *Lead lining*—this reduces the radiation leakage from the tube to the required limits.

- *Tube shield*—this protects the components and holds them in place. It also restricts access to the 'live' components.

If your answer differs substantially from the outline answer, refer to Sections 22.5.1–22.5.2.

c. Tungsten is used in the construction of the filament because:

- Tungsten has a low thermionic work function and so will readily emit electrons by thermionic emission.
- Tungsten has a low vapour pressure and so does not easily evaporate. This helps prolong the life of the filament as evaporation would cause the wire to become thin. It also prolongs the life of the tube as it prevents the formation of a tungsten film on the inner wall of the glass envelope.
- Tungsten is a rugged metal which can be drawn into a thin wire which will not easily distort. This helps to maintain the shape of the filament helix over a period of time.

Tungsten is used in the construction of the target because:

- Tungsten has a high atomic number ($Z = 74$) and so is an efficient producer of X-rays.
- Tungsten has a high melting point (3387°C) so it can withstand the heat generated during the X-ray exposure without melting.
- Tungsten has a low vapour pressure so it does not readily vaporise at its normal working temperature.
- Tungsten can be readily machined to give the smooth surface required for X-ray production.

If your answer differs substantially from the outline answer, refer to Sections 22.4.2 and 22.4.3.

d. Your table should be similar to Table 22.1 on page 319.
If your answer differs substantially from the outline answer, refer to Section 22.5.2.

e. If the filament heating current is increased, there will be an increase in the amount of heat released within the filament. This will produce an increase in the temperature of the filament. An increase in the temperature of the filament will produce an increase in the number of electrons released by thermionic emission. Assuming that the X-ray tube is operating under saturation conditions, then the release of more electrons by thermionic emission will result in an increase in the current through the X-ray tube. A reduction in the filament heating current will have the opposite effect.
If your answer differs substantially from the outline answer, refer to Section 22.7.1.

f. If a normal filament heating current flows through the filament, electrons will be released by thermionic emission but will only flow across the X-ray tube as a tube current if the correct potential difference is applied—this happens during the exposure. Thus during the 'prep' stage of the exposure, there is a filament heating current but no tube current.

If there is no filament heating current, no electrons are produced by thermionic emission at the filament and so, under normal circumstances, no current will flow through the X-ray tube. This situation might occur in the case of a break in the electrical supply to the filament when an exposure is attempted.
If your answer differs substantially from the outline answer, refer to Section 22.7.1.

CHAPTER 23

a. The rating of an X-ray unit is the combination of exposure settings which the unit can withstand without incurring unacceptable damage.
If your answer differs substantially from the outline answer, refer to Section 23.2.

b. (i) If the focal spot size is increased, the electrons will dissipate their energy over a larger area. This will produce a smaller temperature rise and so will increase the rating.
If your answer differs substantially from the outline answer, refer to Section 23.3.

   (ii) The heat produced at the target of the X-ray tube is related to the number of electrons striking the target per unit time (mA) and the energy of the electrons (related to the kV_p). Thus, for a given exposure time, the mA and the kV_p are reciprocal factors in that if the mA is halved the kV_p can be doubled.
If your answer differs substantially from the outline answer, refer to Section 23.3 'Insight'.

   (iii) For a given value of kV_p and mA the amount of heat produced in the target is related to the exposure time. If the exposure time is very short, then insignificant cooling takes place at the target and the rating is principally affected by the target area. If the exposure time is long, then significant dissipation of heat from the target takes place and the rating is more affected by the thermal characteristics of the anode disk.
If your answer differs substantially from the outline answer, refer to Section 23.3.

   (iv) The self-rectified circuit has the poorest rating while the constant potential circuit has the best rating. The differences in rating are most marked at short exposure times. This is because the heating effect of individual pulses is most apparent in this situation. The more constant the heat production the less likelihood of thermal damage to the target—hence the best rating for constant potential. For longer exposure times, the thermal capacity of the anode disk is the dominating factor. This is independent of the type of rectification and so the curves all tend to come closer together as the exposure time increases.
If your answer differs substantially from the outline answer, refer to Section 23.3.

   (v) If we increase the anode diameter, we will also increase its circumference.

This means that the heat energy is now deposited over a larger area and so leads to more efficient cooling, thus improving the rating. Doubling the diameter of the disk will increase its rating by 40–50% but this has practical limitations because of the extra mechanical stress this imposes on the bearings.

If your answer differs substantially from the outline answer, refer to Section 23.5.

(vi) Doubling the speed of rotation will again increase the rating by about 40–50%. It should also be noticed that the difference in rating diminishes with longer exposure times since it is the overall thermal capacity of the anode that is the dominant factor.

If your answer differs substantially from the outline answer, refer to Section 23.5.

c. For short exposure times the rating is determined by the temperature rise at the target surface. This is affected by rectification, focal spot size, etc. and so all of the above will cause a separation of the curves at short exposure times. For longer exposure times, the rating is more affected by the thermal properties of the anode disk. As these are constant for any one tube irrespective of the choice of focus etc., the curves therefore become closer together.

If your answer differs substantially from the outline answer, refer to Section 23.3.

d. The single exposure rating chart assumes that there is no significant heat stored in the anode before the exposure is made. If this is not the case, then the heat stored in the anode plus the heat produced by the exposure may cause thermal damage to the anode. This can be avoided by reference to the heating and cooling charts for multiple exposures.

If your answer differs substantially from the outline answer, refer to Section 23.6.

e. (i) Referring to rating chart A it can be seen that the coordinates for 200 mA and 0.5 s meet at a point which indicates that kV_ps in excess of 125 kV_p are available and so the exposure is within the rating of the tube.

If your answer differs substantially from the outline answer, refer to Section 23.3.

(ii) Referring to rating chart B it can be seen that the coordinates for 1250 mA and 0.5 s meet at a point above the 80 kV_p line indicating that the exposure is not within the rating of the tube.

If your answer differs substantially from the outline answer, refer to Sections 23.3 and 23.6.1.

(iii) Referring to chart D it can be seen that the line required for checking the rating is 500 HU per second and that after a time of 4 minutes the heat generated is less than 900 000 HU. The anode storage capacity is 220 000 HU and so the proposed cinefluoroscopy is within the rating.

If your answer differs substantially from the outline answer, refer to Section 23.6.2.

(iv) Referring to rating chart B, it can be seen that the coordinates for 500 mA and 0.8 s allow kV_ps of greater than 110 kV_p to be used and so the single exposure is within the tube rating. If we now refer to the angiographic rating chart (C)—the load is $80 \times 10^3 \times 500 \times 10^{-3} = 40$ kW—we can see that for an exposure time of 80 msec and 4 exposures per second the maximum number of exposures is 18. The proposed series was 4 exposures per second for 6 seconds, which is 24 exposures and so is not within the rating of the tube.

If your answer differs substantially from the outline answer, refer to Section 23.6.3.

CHAPTER 24

a. The mass of a body, m, and its energy, E (excluding potential energy), are related by the formula $E = mc^2$, where c is the velocity of electromagnetic radiation. Thus the energy of a body is proportional to its mass (and vice versa) since c is a constant. If we consider a stationary body with a rest mass m_0, then the rest energy of this body is given by $E_0 = m_0c^2$. If we now consider this body travelling with a velocity, V, then its energy is now E_v and Einstein's equation is $E_v = m_vc^2$. Since the energy of the body when moving, E_v, is greater than the energy of the body when at rest, E_0, and since c is a constant then m_v must be greater than m_0—a body increases in mass as its velocity increases. For this reason it is usual to define the mass of the body when it has zero velocity as its *rest mass* and the mass of the body when it is travelling with a known velocity, V, as its *relativistic mass*.

If your answer differs substantially from the outline answer, refer to Section 24.4.1.

b. Sometimes electromagnetic radiation behaves as 'packets' of energy which have an associated momentum. Such a packet of energy is called a photon or a quantum and the quantum theory predicts that the quantum will have an energy, E, given by $E = h\nu$ where h is a constant known as Planck's constant and ν is the frequency of vibration of the associated wave. Thus, the electromagnetic wave may also behave like a particle, possessing energy and momentum. An electromagnetic wave may behave like a particle in the case of photoelectric absorption and an electron (a particle) behaves like a wave in part of the electron microscope.

If your answer differs substantially from the outline answer, refer to Section 24.6.

c. The central point of the principle is that measuring one quantity affects another quantity so that it is never possible to measure both quantities simultaneously with complete accuracy.

If your answer differs substantially from the outline answer, refer to Section 24.7.

CHAPTER 25

a. The general properties of all electromagnetic radiations are:

- The waves of the radiations are composed of transverse vibrations of electric and magnetic fields.
- The vibrations have a wide range of wavelengths and frequencies.
- All electromagnetic radiations travel through a vacuum with the same velocity—3×10^8 m·s^{-1}.
- All electromagnetic radiations travel in straight lines.
- The radiations are unaffected by electric or magnetic fields.
- The radiations may be polarised so that they vibrate in one plane only.
- The radiations are able to produce constructive or destructive interference.
- All the radiations obey the duality principle and so can either be considered as waves or as quanta with energy and momentum.

If your answer differs substantially from the outline answer, refer to Section 25.3.

b. (i) *Cycle*—one complete waveform (this can start from any point on the wave and end at the corresponding point on another wave).
   (ii) *Wavelength*—the distance travelled in completing one cycle.
   (iii) *Frequency*—the number of cycles per second.
   (iv) *Amplitude*—the magnitude of the peak of the wave above the X axis.

If your answer differs substantially from the outline answer, refer to Section 25.3.1.

c. $E = hc/\lambda$ or $E = 0.124/\lambda$

Using the equation: $E = 0.124/\lambda$
$$\lambda = 1.24/E$$
$$= 1.24/50 \text{ nm}$$
$$= 0.0248 \text{ nm}$$

Using the equation: $E = 0.124/\lambda$
$$\lambda = 1.24/0.0124 \text{ keV}$$
$$= 100 \text{ keV}$$

If your answer differs substantially from the outline answer, refer to Section 25.3.2.

d. Radio waves, microwaves, infra-red radiation, visible, ultra-violet radiation, X-rays and gamma-rays.

If your answer differs substantially from the outline answer, refer to Section 25.4.

e. When the anode of the X-ray tube is bombarded by electrons it emits both heat and light as well as X-rays. The X-ray spectrum is composed of a continuous or Bremsstrahlung spectrum upon which is superimposed a characteristic or line spectrum from the tungsten target. The absorption processes within the aluminium filter and the lead collimators also produce characteristic radiation from these elements, although these are of fairly low intensity. When the radiation beam passes through the patient, some of the photons are absorbed and some are scattered. The above processes produce a minute amount of heat and other characteristic radiations from the elements which make up the body tissues. When the transmitted X-ray beam strikes the intensifying screens in the cassette, these produce fluorescent radiation in the ultra-violet and visible parts of the spectrum. This is principally responsible for the production of the radiographic image on the film.

If your answer differs substantially from the outline answer, refer to Section 25.5.

f. A wide range of answers are possible. Some of these might include:

- The emission of light from image intensifiers when bombarded with X-rays.
- The emission of light from cathode ray tubes and television monitors when the phosphors are bombarded by electrons.
- The emission of light from fluorescent tubes to allow us to view radiographs.
- The emission of X-rays and γ-rays from certain radioisotopes which allow imaging or treatment of organs.
- The emission of light from sodium iodide crystals (in gamma cameras and CAT scanners) when bombarded with γ-rays or X-rays.
- The emission of light from photostimulable plates when scanned using a laser beam.
- The use of a laser beam to 'write' information on to the film in a laser imager.

If your answer differs substantially from the outline answer, refer to Section 25.5.

CHAPTER 26

a. This requires a simple planetary model diagram of the nitrogen atom to demonstrate that the nucleus contains 7 protons and 7 neutrons. The *K*-shell contains 2 electrons and the *L*-shell contains 5 electrons.

If your answer differs substantially from the outline answer, refer to Section 26.2.

b. (i) A *nuclide* is a nucleus with a particular value of atomic mass number and atomic number.

 (ii) A *radionuclide* is a nuclide where the atomic nucleus is unstable and therefore likely to undergo radioactive decay.

 (iii) An *isotope* is a nucleus which has the same atomic number but a different mass number compared to another nucleus, e.g. $^{14}_{6}C$ and $^{12}_{6}C$ are both isotopes of carbon.

 (iv) An *isobar* is a nucleus which has the same atomic mass number as another nucleus, e.g. ^{14}C and ^{14}N are isobars.

 (v) The *atomic number* of an element is the number of protons in the atomic nucleus.

 (vi) The *atomic mass number* is the total number of nucleons (protons and neutrons) in the nucleus.

If your answer differs substantially from the outline answer, refer to Section 26.3.

c. (i) The *discrete electron orbital* is the pathway followed by a particular electron around the atomic nucleus.

(ii) These orbitals are grouped together to give *electron shells*, e.g. the two electrons in the *K*-shell each have discrete electron orbitals.

(iii) Electrons in a particular shell have an *electron binding energy* which is the amount of work which must be done to remove the electron from that shell and create a free electron. The electron binding energy varies with electron shell (*K* being highest) and also increases, for a shell, with the atomic number of the element.

If your answer differs substantially from the outline answer, refer to Sections 26.4 and 26.7.

d. There are two Bury–Bohr Rules:

- An electron shell, *n*, cannot contain more than $2n^2$ electrons.
- The outer shell cannot contain more than 8 electrons.

Using these rules we can say that potassium will have the following electron configuration:

K-shell	2
L-shell	8
M-shell	8
N-shell	1

If your answer differs substantially from the outline answer, refer to Section 26.5.

e. (i) *Ionic bonds.* This type of bond is caused when one or more electrons are transferred from one atom to another, forming charged atoms (*ions*) which are attracted to one another by electrostatic attraction, thus forming the bond. After the electron exchange, the shells of each ion appear to be closed.

(ii) *Covalent bonds.* These bonds are formed by the apparent sharing of electrons such that each atom appears to increase its number of electrons thus forming an apparently closed shell.

If your answer differs substantially from the outline answer, refer to Section 26.5.

f. If the electron within an orbital is given sufficient energy to cause it to move to a higher energy level but not overcome its binding energy, then the process is called *excitation*. The excited electron will return to its original orbital with the emission of a photon of electromagnetic radiation. In *ionisation* the electron is given sufficient energy to overcome its binding energy and leave the atom. The atom has now lost one of its electrons and so becomes a positive ion.

If your answer differs substantially from the outline answer, refer to Section 26.6.

CHAPTER 27

a. For the spontaneous emission of an alpha (α) particle from a nucleus, the nuclide must have an atomic mass number greater than 150. The nucleus must also have too few neutrons for the number of protons—a higher neutron : proton ratio would be required to produce nuclear stability. The alpha particle consists of two protons and two neutrons tightly bound together (a helium nucleus). It may be considered as a free particle having high kinetic energy, which is trapped in the nucleus. Thus the daughter nucleus has two protons and two neutrons fewer than the parent nucleus.

The mechanism of production of the α-particle is quite complex. The nucleus depends on a balance of disruptive electrostatic (Coulomb) forces and attractive forces between the nucleons caused by the short-range nuclear forces. In very large nuclei there is a large amount of electrostatic repulsion between the protons which extends across the whole nucleus. This is balanced by the short-range nuclear force which exists between adjacent nucleons. Thus, if the nucleus becomes elongated, the electrostatic forces dominate and the nucleus becomes even more elongated. This process continues until the nucleus divides into two fragments, the daughter nuclide and the α-particle.

An example of α-decay is the decay of bismuth-212 to thallium-208 with the emission of an α-particle as shown in the equation below:

$$^{212}_{83}\text{Bi} \rightarrow \ ^{208}_{81}\text{Tl} + \ ^{4}_{2}\alpha$$

If your answer differs substantially from the outline answer, refer to Section 27.4.

b. *Negatron (β^-) emission.* β^--particles are emitted from nuclei which have too many neutrons for nuclear stability. Nucleons are being constantly changed from proton to neutron and back within the atomic nucleus. A neutron may be thought of as consisting of a proton and a negatron:

$$n \rightarrow p^+ + \beta^-$$

It appears that in nuclei which have too many neutrons, there is a finite possibility that a neutron becomes isolated within the nucleus and then decays to form a proton and a negatron. The proton rejoins the nucleus and the negatron is ejected. This transformation results in the atomic mass number remaining unchanged (the combined number of protons and neutrons is still the same) but the atomic number will increase by 1 as one extra proton has been added to the nucleus (this results in the formation of a different element with the consequent rearrangement of electron orbitals to suit the new element).

An example of β^--particle decay is where carbon-14 decays to form nitrogen with the emission of a β^--particle.

$$^{14}_{6}\text{C} \rightarrow \ ^{14}_{7}\text{N} + \beta^-$$

Positron (β^+) emission.   Protons are continuously changing into neutrons and back. In these reactions we can consider a proton as consisting of a neutron and a positron.

$p^+ \rightarrow n + \beta^+$

Positron emission takes place from nuclei which have too many protons to achieve stability. In such cases, protons appear to become isolated within the nucleus and then to decay to form a neutron which rejoins the nucleus and a positron which is ejected from the nucleus. In this reaction the atomic mass number will remain the same but the atomic number will decrease by 1 (the total number of protons and neutrons is unchanged but one proton has been converted into a neutron).

An example of such a reaction is the decay of carbon-11 to boron as shown below:

$$^{11}_{6}C \rightarrow ^{11}_{5}B + \beta^+$$

If your answer differs substantially from the outline answer, refer to Sections 27.5.1 and 27.5.2.

c. When cobalt-60 decays with the emission of a β^--particle the daughter nucleus is left in an excited state. The $^{60}_{28}Ni$ nucleus is left at an energy 2.5 MeV above its ground state. It immediately decays to its ground state in two jumps:

- it decays to 1.33 MeV above its ground state by the emission of a 1.17 MeV γ-ray
- it then drops to its ground state by the emission of a second γ-ray of energy 1.33 MeV.

In the case of $^{60}_{27}Co$ decaying to $^{60}_{28}Ni$, the nucleus remains in an excited state before the emission of the γ-rays for a time so short that it is incapable of accurate measurement. However, this is not always the case, and those excited states which last sufficiently long for their durations to be measured are known as *metastable states*. The transition from a metastable state to a more stable state is known as an *isomeric transition*.

If your answer differs substantially from the outline answer, refer to Sections 27.6 and 27.6.1.

d. If a nucleus of low mass number has too few neutrons for stability but has insufficient excess energy (<1.02 MeV) to eject a positron, then an alternative way by which the nucleus may undergo an isobaric transformation and lose energy is by electron capture. In this process the nucleus captures one of the orbiting electrons, the most likely being a capture of a *K*-shell electron.

The capture of an electron by the nucleus results in one of the protons in the nucleus changing into a neutron. During the process of electron capture a neutrino is emitted by the nucleus. The processes involved in electron capture may be shown thus:

$$p^+ + e^- \rightarrow n + \nu$$

If your answer differs substantially from the outline answer, refer to Section 27.7.

e. The short-range forces holding the nucleus together exist between adjacent nucleons, whereas the Coulomb forces act across the whole of the nucleus. This fact becomes increasingly important as the size of the nucleus increases. A very large nucleus may be pictured rather like a liquid drop in which the nucleons are moving about with very high energy and continuously deforming the shape of the nucleus.

During this process, it is possible for the nucleus to become very elongated and then to break into two fragments—usually of fairly similar sizes. Such a phenomenon is known as *spontaneous fission* and can occur for very large nuclei, e.g. Thorium-232 is capable of spontaneous fission. As well as the *fission fragments* from such a reaction, one or more neutrons are usually liberated and the whole fission process is accompanied by the release of large amounts of energy.

Neutron activated fission is a more controllable process than spontaneous fission. This occurs as a result of a heavy nucleus capturing an incoming neutron and then breaking into large fragments in a similar way to spontaneous fission. An example of such a reaction is the disintegration of $^{238}_{92}U$ into two fission fragments of $^{145}_{56}Ba$ and $^{94}_{36}Kr$ if the uranium-238 nucleus is made to absorb a neutron. The fission of the nucleus is normally accompanied by the release of gamma rays and neutrons. Both of the fissile fragments are extremely rich in neutrons and so each will usually release a neutron. The neutrons from both of the above processes can now react with two $^{238}_{92}U$ nuclei resulting in the release of four fissile fragments and four neutrons and so a *chain reaction* can be set up. Such a process is accompanied by the release of large amounts of energy.

If your answer differs substantially from the outline answer, refer to Section 27.9.

f. This requires a diagram similar to Figure 27.15 followed by the following description. If molybdenum-98 is placed in a neutron stream, the nuclei of the molybdenum atoms can be made to absorb the neutrons to produce molybdenum-99. The capture of a neutron raises the energy of the resulting molybdenum-99 nuclei and each loses this energy by the prompt emission of a γ-ray. The reaction may be shown using the equation below:

$$^{98}_{42}Mo + n \rightarrow {}^{99}_{42}Mo + \gamma$$

A molybdenum-99/alumina column is in the centre of the generator. The molybdenum-99 has a half-life of 67 hours and decays to form technetium-99m by β⁻-particle emission as shown below:

$$^{99}_{42}Mo \rightarrow {}^{99}_{43}Tc^m + \beta^- + \bar{\nu}$$

The $^{99}_{43}Tc^m$ is eluted from the generator at regular intervals as sodium pertechnetate. This isotope, which is in liquid form, may then be used for a number of radionuclide imaging situations. The $^{99}_{43}Tc^m$ decays to $^{99}_{43}Tc$ by the emission of a γ-ray of energy 140 keV. The metastable isotope has a half-life of 6 hours.

If your answer differs substantially from the outline answer, refer to Section 27.11.1.

g. The ideal radionuclide for imaging should:

- have a short half-life—approximately twice the length of time from injection into the patient to completion of the scan—the half-life of $^{99}_{43}\text{Tc}^m$ is 6 hours
- emit γ-rays of relatively low energy, so that these are easily detected and do not pose a major hazard to others because of their penetrating power—the γ-rays emitted from $^{99}_{43}\text{Tc}^m$ have an energy of 140 keV
- emit no particles as part of its decay pattern as these add significantly to the patient dose—90% of the radiation from $^{99}_{43}\text{Tc}^m$ is in the form of γ-radiation; the remaining 10% consists of energy emitted as a result of internal conversion, X-rays and Auger electrons
- be readily labelled to allow its uptake by specific organs—$^{99}_{43}\text{Tc}^m$ is readily labelled
- be readily excreted by the patient—$^{99}_{43}\text{Tc}^m$ is readily excreted by the patient, normally through the urinary system although other routes are possible depending on the labelling
- be easily generated in the radio-pharmacy—$^{99}_{43}\text{Tc}^m$ is readily generated in the radio-pharmacy using a technetium generator.

If your answer differs substantially from the outline answer, refer to Section 27.12.

CHAPTER 28

a. This requires a diagram similar to Figure 28.1 followed by the following text. There are a number of ways in which high-energy electrons from the filament of the X-ray tube may lose their energy when they collide with the atoms of the target. These are:

- the loss of energy by the electrons from the filament because of interactions between them and the outer electrons surrounding the atoms of the target material
- the loss of energy by electrons from the filament because of interactions between them and the nuclei of the atoms of the target material
- the loss of energy by electrons from the filament because of interactions between them and individual electrons of the target atoms.

If your answer differs substantially from the outline answer, refer to Section 28.2.

b. To produce Bremsstrahlung radiation, electrons which are accelerated from the filament of the X-ray tube must interact with the positive nucleus of the atoms of the tube target. When such a quantum is emitted, the kinetic energy of the electron is suddenly reduced by an amount equal to the energy of the quantum, and so the electron is suddenly slowed down or *braked*. This is an example of an inelastic interaction since the total kinetic energy of the electron and of the nucleus are not conserved because some energy is removed by the emission of the quantum of radiation. The energy of the quantum may be in the X-ray part of the electromagnetic spectrum and the radiation is known as *braking* or *Bremsstrahlung radiation*. The exact energy of this quantum will vary and may be very small if the electron does not lose much energy in its interaction with the nucleus, or it may be up to the total kinetic energy of the electron if it is involved in a direct collision with the nucleus. This means that the Bremsstrahlung radiation will form a continuous spectrum.

If your answer differs substantially from the outline answer, refer to Section 28.4.2.

c. If the energy of the electrons accelerated across the tube from the filament is greater than the binding energy of a particular orbital electron, it is possible for a filament electron to be involved in an inelastic collision with one of the orbital electrons of the target atoms. The orbital electron will be given sufficient energy to overcome its binding energy and thus be liberated from the atom. This causes a vacancy in the electron shell involved, e.g. the *K*-shell. This vacancy is quickly filled by one of the outer electrons undergoing a quantum jump downwards to fill the vacancy and emitting a quantum of electromagnetic radiation in the process. The energy of the quantum emitted is given by:

$$E = E_1 - E_2$$

where E_1 is the energy of the electron before the jump and E_2 is the energy of the electron after the jump. As this energy varies for the same transition in different materials it is known as *characteristic radiation* as it is characteristic of the material emitting the radiation.

If your answer differs substantially from the outline answer, refer to Section 28.5.

d. This requires a diagram similar to Figure 28.6 followed by the following description. The energy of the Bremsstrahlung radiation is expressed in keV and lies somewhere between zero and a maximum value. This maximum photon energy is achieved if an electron which has the maximum kinetic energy gives up all its energy to form a single photon. The value of this photon in the case of the beam will be 100 keV as the maximum potential across the X-ray tube will be 100 kV$_p$. The Bremsstrahlung radiation is a continuous spectrum. The intensity of the low-energy photons within this spectrum is decreased because of absorption of these photons by the target material. The average energy of the X-ray beam is about one-third to one-half of its maximum energy. The total intensity of the beam—the quantity of the radiation—is given by the area under the curve. The energies of the *K*, *L*, *M*, etc. lines are always in the same position although the energy of lines from *M* onwards is so small that it is likely to be totally absorbed in the X-ray tube. These discrete energies form a line spectrum—the exact energy of the line is determined by the difference between the initial energy of the electron and its final energy. The line spectra will not be produced in this case for all lines from K outwards as the energy of the electrons from the filament is sufficiently large to displace any electron from its orbital within the tungsten target atom.

The relationship between the kV_p across the tube and the minimum wavelength is given by the equation:

$$\lambda_{min} = 1.24/kV_p$$

If your answer differs substantially from the outline answer, refer to Section 28.6.

CHAPTER 29

a. The quality of the radiation is a measure of the penetrating power of the X-ray beam. The more penetrating the X-ray beam the higher the beam quality. The quantity of the radiation is a measure of the number of X-ray photons present in a beam of radiation. The larger the number of photons present the greater the quantity of radiation.

If your answer differs substantially from the outline answer, refer to Section 29.2.

b. This should have a graph similar to Figure 29.1. The tube current is a measure of the number of electrons crossing the X-ray tube in unit time. An increase in the number of electrons per unit time (with all other factors remaining unchanged) produces an increase in the chance of producing X-ray photons and thus will produce an increase in the intensity or quantity of the radiation. A reduction in the tube current has the opposite effect. As the energy of the electrons is unaffected by the tube current, then the quality of the X-ray beam is not affected by the mA.

If your answer differs substantially from the outline answer, refer to Section 29.3.

c. This should be accompanied by a graph similar to Figure 29.2. An increase in the potential difference across the X-ray tube will produce an increase in the kinetic energy of the electrons at the point of contact with the target. This has two effects on the Bremsstrahlung spectrum:

- As the electrons have more energy, they are more likely to have some of this energy converted into X-ray photons—thus there will be an increase in the quantity of radiation from the tube.
- As the electrons have an increase in their energy, there will be an increase in the average energy of the photons in the X-ray beam—thus there will be an increase in the quality of the X-ray beam.

The use of a lower kV_p has the opposite effect. The use of a lower kV_p may also mean that the kinetic energy of the filament electrons is less than the binding energy of the K-shell electrons of the target atoms and so no characteristic radiation will be produced as a result of quantum leaps by electrons to fill the vacancy in the K-shell (see graph for lower kV_p in Figure 29.2).

If your answer differs substantially from the outline answer, refer to Section 29.4.

d. This should be accompanied by a graph similar to Figure 29.3. The higher the atomic number of the target material, the more positive the nucleus of each target atom. This means that the material is more efficient at producing radiation by the Bremsstrahlung process. Thus, the quantity of the Bremsstrahlung radiation is affected but not the quality. A material with a higher atomic number will also produce characteristic radiation at a higher photon energy than is produced by a target of a lower atomic number. This has a marginal effect on the quality of the overall spectrum from the X-ray tube.

If your answer differs substantially from the outline answer, refer to Section 29.5.

e. This should be accompanied by a graph similar to Figure 29.4(b). The closer the waveform across the X-ray tube is to a constant potential, the higher the average kinetic energy of the electrons at the point of contact with the target. This will produce an increase in the quality and in the quantity of the radiation from the tube.

If your answer differs substantially from the outline answer, refer to Section 29.6.

f. This should be accompanied by a diagram similar to Figure 29.5. Filtration absorbs X-ray photons by the photoelectric effect. Thus, there is a selective absorption of low-energy photons compared with high-energy photons. As a result, the average photon energy of a beam is increased—filtration increases the quality of the radiation beam. However, as some of the photons have been absorbed by the filter, there are fewer photons in the beam after filtration than there were before filtration—filtration produces a reduction in the quantity of a beam of radiation.

If your answer differs substantially from the outline answer, refer to Section 29.7.

CHAPTER 30

a. (i) If we measure the intensity of the radiation before it enters an attenuator and measure the intensity again when it leaves the attenuator, we find that there is less intensity at the point of exit than there was at the point of entrance. This reduction in intensity is known as attenuation.

(ii) When the beam of radiation passes through matter, some of the energy of the photons may be transferred to the atoms of the material. This process is known as absorption.

(iii) When a beam of radiation passes through matter, some of the photons may interact with atoms of the material and, as a consequence of this interaction, the photons may be deflected from their original paths. This may or may not be accompanied by a loss of energy. This process is known as scattering.

If your answer differs substantially from the outline answer, refer to Section 30.2.

b. The total linear attenuation coefficient, μ, is the fraction of the radiation removed from a beam per unit thickness of an attenuating medium. This would be used as a measure of attenuation when it is important to establish the amount of radiation absorbed along a straight line.

The total mass attenuation coefficient, μ/ρ, is the fraction of the radiation removed from a beam of unit cross-sectional area as it passes through unit mass of a medium. This measure of attenuation would be used if we wish to see how the photon energy influences the amount of attenuation, as it is independent of the state of the medium.

If your answer differs substantially from the outline answer, refer to Sections 30.2.2 and 30.2.3.

c. In photoelectric absorption the photon interacts with a bound electron. The maximum chance of the process occurring is when the energy of the photon is equal to or just greater than the binding energy of the particular electron shell. The photon displaces the electron from its orbital, some of the photon energy being used to overcome the binding energy of the electron and the rest being given to the electron as kinetic energy. The vacancy is filled by electrons further from the nucleus undergoing quantum jumps and giving off characteristic radiation. The mass attenuation coefficient due to the photoelectric effect (τ/ρ) is influenced by the atomic number of the absorber and by the energy of the incident photon as shown in the following equation:

$$\tau/\rho \propto Z^3/E^3$$

If your answer differs substantially from the outline answer, refer to Section 30.5.

d. In Compton scattering the photon interacts with a free electron. As a result of this interaction, the photon is deflected from its path and loses some of its energy which the electron gets as kinetic energy. As the photon is deflected from its path, it is said to be scattered. The likelihood of the process occurring depends on the electron density of the attenuator and the energy of the incident photon as shown in the equation below:

$$\sigma/\rho \propto \text{electron density}/E$$

As the electron density of all materials (with the exception of hydrogen) is approximately the same, the amount of Compton scattering is largely unaffected by the material.

If your answer differs substantially from the outline answer, refer to Section 30.6.

e. Pair production involves an interaction between a high-energy photon (≥ 1.02 MeV) and the field around an atomic nucleus. This interaction results in the energy of the photon being converted to matter in the form of an electron and positron pair. Any excess energy is given to the pair as kinetic energy. The positron will eventually interact with an electron and both will be annihilated producing two photons, each of energy 0.51 MeV. These photons are known as annihilation radiation. The likelihood of the process occurring is linked to the photon energy and the atomic number of the attenuator by the equation shown below:

$$\pi/\rho \propto (E - 1.02)Z$$

If your answer differs substantially from the outline answer, refer to Section 30.7.

CHAPTER 31

a. If a substance is bombarded with high-energy radiation and the atoms of the substance absorb the radiation, this will cause an increase in the energy of some of the electrons within the atoms of the absorber. If this energy is re-emitted in the form of light, then the whole process is called luminescence. If the light emission stops within 10^{-8} s of the end of the radiation bombardment, then the process can be termed fluorescence; if it continues beyond this point then it is known as phosphorescence or afterglow.
If your answer differs substantially from the outline answer, refer to Section 31.3.

b. When an X-ray photon is involved in a photoelectric interaction with an atom of a phosphor crystal then this liberates an electron and gives it kinetic energy. This electron will now move within the conduction band, leaving a hole in the valence band. As the electron passes close to other atoms it liberates further electrons and so a large number of electrons will enter the conduction band. Some of the electrons in this band will collide with one another and so will lose small amounts of energy and will thus adjust their energy to the upper energy level of the luminescent centre. At the same time, some holes in the valence band will raise their energy to the lower level of the luminescent centre. Some of the electrons at the upper level of the centre will perform quantum jumps to neutralise the holes at the lower level of the centre and in so doing will give up energy in the visible part of the spectrum. As a result of one photoelectric interaction, a large number of electrons can perform this transition; thus the number of light photons liberated is much greater than the number of X-ray photons absorbed.
If your answer differs substantially from the outline answer, refer to Section 31.3.1.

c. When an X-ray photon is involved in a photoelectric interaction with an atom of a phosphor crystal, this liberates an electron and gives it kinetic energy. This electron will now move within the conduction band, leaving a hole in the valence band. As the electron passes close to other atoms it liberates further electrons and so a large number of electrons will enter the conduction band. Some of the electrons in this band will collide with one another and so will lose small amounts of energy and will thus drop into the deep traps in the forbidden energy gap. Thus, the number of electrons in the traps is proportional to the amount of radiation. If the substance is heated, these electrons can have their energy raised to allow them to re-enter the conduction band and some will adjust to the energy level of the luminescent centre. At the same time, some holes in the valence band will raise their energy to the lower level of the luminescent centre. Some of the electrons at the upper level of the centre will perform quantum jumps to neutralise the holes at the lower level of the centre and in so doing will give up energy in the visible part of the spectrum. The number of light photons liberated is proportional to the number of X-ray photons absorbed.

If your answer differs substantially from the outline answer, refer to Section 31.4.

d. A diagram similar to Figure 31.4 would help the description. The intensifying screen consists of a base material—normally a flexible plastic—which provides support for the rest of the system. On one side of this is coated a substratum layer which may be reflective or absorptive depending on the function of the screen. The phosphor layer is coated on top of the substratum layer and consists of phosphor crystals in a binder material. The binder may be clear or tinted and may also contain carbon microgranules. On the outer surface of the screen is a clear supercoat which protects the phosphor from abrasion and from chemical contamination.

If your answer differs substantially from the outline answer, refer to Section 31.5.1.

e. When an X-ray photon is involved in a photoelectric interaction with an atom of a barium fluorohalide crystal, this liberates an electron and gives it kinetic energy. This electron will now move to the conduction band, leaving a hole in the valence band. As the electron passes close to other atoms it liberates further electrons and so a large number of electrons will enter the conduction band. Some of the electrons in this band will collide with one another and so will lose small amounts of energy and will thus drop into the deep traps in the forbidden energy gap. Thus, the number of electrons in the traps is proportional to the amount of radiation. If the substance is scanned with a laser beam, then these electrons can have their energy raised to allow them to re-enter the conduction band and some will adjust to the energy level of the luminescent centre. At the same time, some holes in the valence band will raise their energy to the lower level of the luminescent centre. Some of the electrons at the upper level of the centre will perform quantum jumps to neutralise the holes at the lower level of the centre and in so doing will give up energy in the visible part of the spectrum. The number of light photons liberated is proportional to the number of X-ray photons absorbed. This light may be measured and used to produce a digitised image.

If your answer differs substantially from the outline answer, refer to Section 31.7.

CHAPTER 32

a. The density of bone is approximately twice that of soft tissue and so (if all the other factors are equal) bone will attenuate twice as much radiation as soft tissue. Bone and soft tissue also differ in atomic number. This is important for photoelectric absorption as shown by the equation $\tau \propto \rho \times Z^3/E^3$. Since the atomic number of bone is approximately twice that of soft tissue, the combination of this with its higher density results in it attenuating about 16 times as much radiation as the same thickness of soft tissue. Because of this the intensity of the X-ray beam transmitted through bone will be less than that transmitted through soft tissue.

If your answer differs substantially from the outline answer, refer to Section 32.3.1.

b. The kV_p selected affects the quality and the quantity of the radiation from the X-ray tube. Increasing the kV_p will increase the average photon energy and so will cause an appreciable reduction in the amount of photoelectric absorption. This will cause a reduction in the contrast on the radiograph. An increase in the kV_p also increases the amount of scattered radiation reaching the radiograph, again reducing the contrast. However, if the kV_p selected is too low, then more dense structures such as bone will be underpenetrated. The kV_p also affects the quantity of radiation which in turn affects the average density on the radiograph.

If your answer differs substantially from the outline answer, refer to Sections 32.3.5 and 32.6.

c. Scatter to the radiograph can be limited by:

- the use of collimation, thus limiting the amount of scatter formed
- the use of low kV_p techniques so that the scatter is largely absorbed by the patient—this does produce an increase in patient dose
- the use of a secondary radiation grid to absorb the scatter formed.

If your answer differs substantially from the outline answer, refer to Sections 32.3.3 and 32.3.4.

d. Characteristic curves may be used to compare the speed, contrast and film latitude of the two emulsions.

If your answer differs substantially from the outline answer, refer to Sections 32.5.2, 32.5.3 and 32.5.4.

CHAPTER 33

a. The exposure at a particular point in a beam of radiation is a measure of the amount of ionisation which will occur as the beam passes through unit mass of air. The absorbed dose is a measure of the energy imparted to a unit mass of the medium as a result of the radiation beam being directed at the medium. The dose equivalent is the absorbed dose multiplied by the quality factor for the radiation. For the same exposure, different media will absorb different absorbed doses of radiation. The amount of biological damage to tissue is dependent on the dose equivalent and so it is necessary to convert the absorbed dose in gray to the dose equivalent in sievert.

If your answer differs substantially from the outline answer, refer to Sections 33.3, 33.3.3 and 33.4.

b. The methods which can be used include calorimetry, the free air ionisation chamber or chemical methods of radiation dose measurement. One of these methods should then be described in detail.

If your answer differs substantially from the outline answer, refer to Sections 33.5.1, 33.5.2 and 33.5.3.

c. This requires a diagram similar to Figure 33.6. The chamber wall is made of graphite, bakelite or plastic and as it has an atomic number similar to air it is said to be air equivalent, i.e. it absorbs the same amount of radiation as the same mass of air. When the wall absorbs radiation it emits electrons which will enter the air of the chamber and cause a loss of charge from the positive central electrode. The amount of charge lost is proportional to the radiation exposure to the chamber. This can then be corrected for the calibration factor against the standard chamber. When we know the exposure we can calculate the absorbed dose in air as we know the energy required to produce an ion pair in air.

If your answer differs substantially from the outline answer, refer to Section 33.6.1.

d. Methods used include the thimble ionisation chamber, the Geiger–Müller counter, scintillation detectors, thermoluminescent dosemeters, photographic film and semiconductor detectors. One of these methods should then be described in detail.

If your answer differs substantially from the outline answer, refer to Sections 33.6.1–33.6.6.

CHAPTER 34

a. When a photon of ionising radiation interacts with an atom of a tissue cell, the photon can have sufficient energy to cause ionisation of the atom. The secondary electrons emitted by this process may also have sufficient energy to ionise other atoms. The free radicals produced by such ionisations can produce new chemicals within the cell. If the original chemical was important to the cell function, this new chemical can cause a change in the cell's function—a biological effect of radiation.

If your answer differs substantially from the outline answer, refer to Section 34.4.

b. Both stochastic and deterministic effects are possible biological effects of ionising radiation. The effects are contrasted in the table below:

Stochastic effects	Deterministic effects
No safe lower limit below which the effect will not occur	Threshold limit exists below which the effect will not occur
The greater the dose received the greater the risk of the effect occurring	The effect always occurs once the threshold has been exceeded
The severity of the effect when it occurs is not related to the dose received	The greater the dose received above the threshold, the more severe the effect

If your answer differs substantially from the outline answer, refer to Sections 34.4.1 and 34.4.2.

c. As the sum of the weighting factors of all the organs is unity, the effective whole-body dose is 2×1 mSv = 2 mSv.
If your answer differs substantially from the outline answer, refer to Section 34.8.

d. The factors to be considered include:

- the effective half-life of the material
- the level of the radioactivity in the body organs
- whether the level is uniform or if there is increased uptake by certain organs
- the decay system of the radionuclide
- the quality factor(s) of the radiation(s) emitted during the decay
- the size of the organs involved
- the weighting factor of the organs involved.

If your answer differs substantially from the outline answer, refer to Section 34.9.

e. (i) 5 mSv
   (ii) 15 mSv
   (iii) 5 mSv
   (iv) 13 mSv in 3 months
   (v) 10 mSv during the declared period of a pregnancy.
If your answer differs substantially from the outline answer, refer to Table 34.4.

f. A classified radiation worker is someone who is likely to receive a dose of radiation which exceeds more than three-tenths of any relevant dose limit. The person concerned must be over 18 years of age, must be medically fit to be a classified person and must be informed of his/her classification.
If your answer differs substantially from the outline answer, refer to Section 34.10.

g. The three general principles are:

- Every practice resulting in an exposure to ionising radiation should be justified by the advantages it produces.
- All exposures should be kept as low as reasonably achievable (ALARA).
- The sum of the doses and committed doses should not exceed specified limits.

If your answer differs substantially from the outline answer, refer to Section 34.11.

h. The radiation protection advisor is usually responsible for ensuring that the employer complies with the current radiation protection legislation. Duties would include giving advice on:

- dosimetry and monitoring
- the designation and control of restricted areas
- drawing up systems of work and Local Rules
- investigation of radiation incidents
- ensuring adequate training and update of radiation workers
- commenting on the design of new, or modification of old, premises from a radiation protection aspect
- preparation of contingency plans
- selection and training of radiation protection supervisors.

Radiation protection supervisors (RPSs) are persons directly involved in working with ionising radiation on a day-to-day basis. It is normal to have an RPS in each department to ensure safe working practice within that department. All RPSs must have sufficient knowledge and experience to allow them to carry out their duties in their department.

If your answer differs substantially from the outline answer, refer to Section 34.11.1.

i. The three common methods of personnel monitoring are:

- the film badge method
- thermoluminescent dosimetry
- the use of pocket dosemeters.

The advantages and disadvantages depend on the method selected. The main advantage of the film badge method is that there is a permanent record of the dose received, as the film is kept after processing. The disadvantages include the fact that the reading is obtained some time after the exposure to radiation, the film is expensive and it will deteriorate if not stored in proper conditions prior to processing. A similar list of advantages and disadvantages for TLD or pocket dosemeters is acceptable.

If your answer differs substantially from the outline answer, refer to Section 34.11.3.

j. A controlled area is one where the instantaneous dose rate exceeds $7.5\ \mu Sv\cdot h^{-1}$ or where an adult employee is likely to receive more than three-tenths of any relevant dose limit. The following have access to such an area:

- classified radiation workers
- other workers for whom there is a written scheme of work
- patients undergoing diagnostic or therapeutic procedures.

If your answer differs substantially from the outline answer, refer to Section 34.11.4.

k. The radiation field size may be limited by the use of collimation. The fastest film/intensifying screen combination consistent with good image quality should be used. The number of repeat examinations should be eliminated/reduced by the use of good radiographic technique (positioning, exposure, patient preparation, etc.). There should be consistent optimum film processing. The highest practicable kV_p for the particular examination should be used. Autotimers should (if possible) be used to control exposure time. Gonad shields should be used where appropriate. An appropriate secondary radiation grid should be selected. It may be possible to use compression or tissue displacement for obese patients. Digital techniques should be used where appropriate.

If your answer differs substantially from the outline answer, refer to Section 34.11.5.

Index